HLA AND ASSOCIATED IMPORTANT DISEASES

Edited by **Yongzhi Xi**

HLA and Associated Important Diseases
http://dx.doi.org/10.5772/57022
Edited by Yongzhi Xi

Contributors

Yongzhi Xi, Christina Bade-Doeding, Ranji Rani, Amanda Vansan Marangon, Daniela Cardozo, Ana Maria Sell, Jeane Visentainer, Mª Isabel Torres, Masahito Katahira, Attapon Cheepsattayakorn, Jacome Bruges-Armas, Ana Rita Couto Rendeiro, Iris Foroni, Bruno Filipe Bettencourt, Manuela Lima, Margarida Santos, Jerzy Kazimierz Kulski, Shingo Suzuki, Yuki Ozaki, Shigeki Mitsunaga, Hidetoshi Inoko, Takashi Shiina

Published by InTech

Janeza Trdine 9, 51000 Rijeka, Croatia

Publishing Process Manager Iva Lipovic

Technical Editor InTech DTP team

Cover InTech Design team

First published May, 2014

Printed in Croatia

Additional hard copies can be obtained from orders@intechopen.com

HLA and Associated Important Diseases, Edited by Yongzhi Xi

p. cm.

ISBN 978-953-51-1230-3

For EU product safety concerns:
IN TECH d.o.o., Prolaz Marije Krucifikse Kozulić 3, 51000 Rijeka, Croatia, info@intechopen.com or visit our website at intechopen.com.

Meet the editor

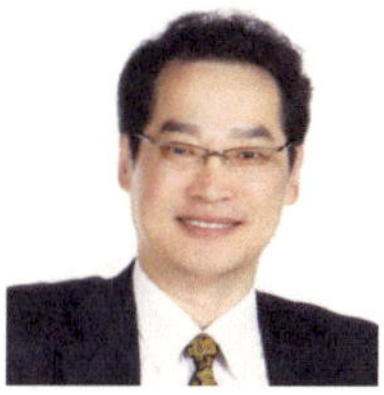

Dr. Yongzhi Xi graduated from BINZHOU Medical College and Academy of Military Medical Sciences, P.R. China, in 1982 and 1988 respectively, and trained at the Institute of Applied Radiobiology Immunology/TNO, The Netherlands, during 1991-1992. Since 1996 he has been Professor of Medicine and Hematology/Immunology, Chief of Immunology Laboratory, Beijing 307 Hospital Affiliated to Academy of Medical Sciences, Beijing. He has been engaged in studies on hematology/immunology, especially for HLA structure, function and clinical typing for HSC and organ transplantation. He has published over 180 articles in the scientific literature, covering various aspects of hematology/immunology research and has authored 6 books. Also, he has been the recipient of many science/technology awards and the member of many Science Societies/Associations.

Contents

Preface

This year marks the 60th anniversary (1954) of the discovery of the human major histocompatibility complex (MHC), or the human leukocyte antigen (HLA) system, by the French Nobel laureate physician Jean Dausset, as well as the 55th anniversary (1958) of the identification and naming of the first human leukocyte antigen, MAC (equivalent to the HLA-A2 antigen). Sixty years ago, Dausset first discovered that sera from patients with leukopenia or from patients who had received multiple blood transfusions were capable of agglutinating 56–100% of leukocytes from normal donors. The discovery preluded a massive international collaboration for investigation of the HLA system. Furthermore, also in 1958, independent studies by Rose Payne and Jon van Rood found that the sera from some parous women contained leukocyte antibodies. A subsequent study by van Rood used a computer-assisted statistical method to establish an HLA antisera cluster analysis method and identified the HLA-Bw4/6 antigen. In addition, in the early- and mid-1960s, a series of major breakthroughs by scientists from many international collaborative laboratories, combined with the discoveries outlined above, confirmed that humans and mice have the same major histocompatibility complex system, called HLA and H-2, respectively, thus providing a perfect ending to the journey of HLA discovery. The entire history of HLA research involves great international and inter-disciplinary collaborations. World experts in HLA research collaborated closely; shared experience, discoveries, and valuable antisera; and unified experimental techniques and nomenclatures. Through frequent conferences, laboratories in different countries formed massive international collaborations and thereby greatly accelerated the discovery of the HLA system and progress in the field.

It should be emphasized that although human HLA and mouse H-2 belong to the MHC system, the discoveries of these two systems did not have a consequential or causal relationship. This is because the study of the mouse H-2 system relied mainly on serological analysis of mouse red blood cells, whereas the discovery of the human HLA system was based on the finding that sera from leukopenia patients contained leukoagglutinin. Just as Dausset described in *"The HLA Adventure"* in 1990, "It would not, however, be altogether accurate to claim that the HLA pioneers were stimulated by the H-2 model to seek a counterpart in man. In actually, the effort to study men and mice progressed quite independently of each other for many years."

HLA is by far the most complex and polymorphic human gene system ever discovered. Since the first official naming by HLA Nomenclature Committee of the World Health Organization in 1968 and with the rapid advances in molecular biology techniques, many new HLA and HLA-related alleles have been discovered each year. As of January 2014, more than 10,000 HLA and HLA-related alleles had been identified. The currently recognized and confirmed numerous biomedical functions of HLA contrast sharply with the original view that HLA serve only as major transplantation antigens involved in the transplant rejection response and are relevant only to immunogenetics. It has been proved that the characteristics of MHC systems in various species are similar to those of the human HLA system, including the following: (1) the antigens are widely distributed on the surfaces of lymphocytes and other nucleated cells, are closely related to allogeneic and xenogeneic transplantation rejections, and are the major transplantation antigens stimulating the mixed lymphocyte reaction and graft-versus-host reactions; (2) the system is directly involved in the processing of endogenous and exogenous antigens by antigen-presenting cells (APCs), a key factor determining whether specific immune responses can be induced; (3) in the specific recognition by T-cell receptors (TCRs) of peptide antigens presented by APCs, TCRs need to recognize the MHC/HLA molecules associated with the peptide antigen simultaneously in order to generate a signal that triggers T-cell activation and consequently controls the immune response of an organism to an antigen, as well as the interactions between immunocompetent cells; (4) the system encodes some components of the complement system; and (5) the frequency of certain antigens/alleles is related to many human diseases involving all systems in the body, manifested as either susceptibility or antagonism.

Ever since the discovery of HLA, scientists have been studying the role of HLA in the relationship between organ matching and organ transplant survival. Today, HLA is considered the most important factor affecting organ transplant survival rates. At the same time, scientists are also very interested in the relationship between HLA and disease. In 1973, Paul Terasaki and colleagues first reported that the HLA-B27 antigen is strongly associated with ankylosing spondylitis, a finding subsequently confirmed by many scientists in several countries. This discovery sparked extensive research on HLA antigen-associated diseases worldwide, which peaked in the 1970s and 1980s. Thus far, research papers on HLA-related diseases number over 10,000 and pertain to over 500 diseases, of which autoimmune diseases, infectious diseases, and cancer are the most prominent.

Compared with the discovery of the human ABO red-blood cell group system by Austrian genetic pathologist Karl Landsteiner, the history of MHC research in various species is short, and the history of human HLA exploration is even shorter. However, the achievements within such a short period are remarkable. We can say that the discovery of HLA is not only an adventure in the history of scientific discovery but also a tale of the unremitting persistence of scientists and an epic of great scientific discoveries. Other scientific discoveries generally result from a scientific hypothesis derived from a scientific theory, which, with scientific innovation and investigation, often change a specific discipline, but rarely revolutionize multiple disciplines, much less science as a whole; however, the discovery and confirmation of HLA were entirely different. In addition to elucidating the gene structure, protein structure, and various biological functions of the HLA system, HLA research has shaped research in modern basic medicine, clinical medicine, and human sociology. It not only brought revolutionary changes to basic sciences, such as biology, immunology, genetics, genomics, and human sociology, but also brought unprecedented breakthroughs to many disciplines in clinical medicine, such as organ transplantation, oncology, transfusion science, forensic science, laboratory science, reproductive science, vaccinology, and internal medicine. It is no exaggeration to say that HLA has become one of the hottest and most active fields in modern basic medicine, clinical medicine, and other scientific disciplines.

Under such circumstances, both basic HLA research and its clinical application need a new monograph that comprehensively reflects the latest achievements in the field (although monographs covering achievements at different stages of HLA research have been published earlier). Therefore, in early 2013, InTech Publisher, with great vision and a sense of responsibility, started work on publishing a book about new achievements in HLA research. Upon kind invitation from the former Publishing Process Manager Ana Pantar, Professor Xi gladly agreed to serve as Editor of the book. Thus, Professor Xi was fortunate to contribute both as an author and as Editor, to organize international experts in the areas of HLA-related basic research and clinical application, to unite their knowledge in chapters covering various related topics, and finally to finish the book "HLA and Associated Important Diseases" which is dedicated to its readers.

The book consists of three sections: The first section comprises Chapters 1–5, which mainly cover basic theoretical and technological developments and independently describe HLA data and statistical analysis, HLA class I polymorphism and Tapasin dependency, HLA-E, -F and -G the non-classical side of the MHC cluster and HLA matching strategy. The second section, Chapters 6–9, introduces research progress pertaining to several important HLA-associated autoimmune diseases. The third section, Chapters 10–13, outlines progress on several important HLA-associated infectious diseases. The contents of this book are relatively comprehensive and novel, covering HLA-related basic theory, advanced matching techniques, and important HLA-associated autoimmune and infectious diseases. Thus, this book is ideal for experts, clinicians, technicians, and graduate students working in HLA-related research and clinical areas. I hope this book will become a valuable reference for basic and clinical research.

Of note, the progress of HLA research could be described as “dazzling,” that is, information and knowledge in this field have accumulated rapidly. The moment you put pen to paper, new studies and data emerge. Thus, it is always difficult to present an up-to-date and accurate account of the latest developments in this field. Therefore, this book can only describe the current state of the field and introduce developments in several main areas of HLA research. Some omissions are inevitable. Fortunately, since the beginning, this book has received strong support and positive responses from many experts in the field, which has helped establish this book as an authoritative resource. In addition, the authors of this book were scrupulous in their writing, which guarantees that the content is of good scientific quality and is novel, up-to-date, and practical. Necessarily, the chapters have some overlap in content, different writing styles, and different scientific points of view. However, in order to ensure the integrity and continuity of each chapter, as Editor of the book, with full respect for the authors, decided not to delete or modify content.

This book was written with tireless dedication by many experts in the HLA field, despite their busy work schedules. Their efforts contributed to the book’s smooth publication. Thus, we need to take this opportunity to first express a heartfelt thanks and deep respect to them. We also want to thank former researchers for their significant contributions to the HLA field, as well as colleagues who are still on the front lines of HLA research. Without their contributions, HLA research would not be so brilliantly significant today. Lastly, we also want to thank the former Publishing Process Manager, Ana Pantar, the current Publishing Process Manager, Iva Lipovic, and the staff at InTech Publisher for their valuable contributions to the editing and publication of this book.

Xi Yongzhi, M.D
Department of Immunology and National Center for Biomedicine Analysis,
Beijing 307 Hospital Affiliated to Academy of Medical Sciences,
Beijing, P.R.China

He Fuchu, Ph.D
Academician & Professor of Genetics and Cell Biology
Academy of Military Medical Sciences, P.R.China

Section 1

Basic Aspects of Human Leukocyte Antigens

Chapter 1

Statistic and Analytical Strategies for HLA Data

Fang Yuan and Yongzhi Xi

Additional information is available at the end of the chapter

http://dx.doi.org/10.5772/57493

1. Introduction

To date, the HLA system is the most complex and polymorphic human gene system identified. Although the research history of HLA is not very long, we have made rapid advancements in our understanding of the HLA system during this short time. Research in the HLA field involves elucidating the structure and various biological functions of genes and proteins associated with the HLA system; in addition, it can be directly applied in the study of basic medicine, clinical medicine, anthroposociology, and other fields. HLA research has led to not only revolutionary reforms in basic medical disciplines, such as biology, immunology, heredity, genetics, and anthroposociology, but also unprecedented breakthroughs in many clinical medicine specialties, including organ transplants, oncology, transfusion science, forensic medicine, ecsomatics, genesiology, and vaccination, as well as in disease-related fields of internal medicine. Therefore, it is critical to organize and process HLA study data using appropriate statistical analysis.

Undoubtedly, the proper use of statistics can directly affect the scientific nature, truth, and objectivity of HLA-related studies. Moreover, in addition to the principles and methods of biomedical statistics commonly used in other life sciences, the statistical analysis of HLA study data has its own specific requirements, which integrate the theories and methods of modern bioinformatics. Bioinformatics is a significant research frontier in biomedical statistics and an important field of biomedical research, expanding from macrocosm to microcosm. It integrates numerous methods of biotechnology, computer technology, mathematics, and statistics and is gradually becoming a major discipline yielding discoveries of the secrets of biology, thereby playing an irreplaceable role in organizing and processing relative HLA study data. However, these methods are not within the scope of basic statistical and analytical strategies used for evaluating HLA study data. Thus, due to the limited space and contents of this book, this Chapter will not discuss them. If appropriate, we will describe these methods in a specific chapter of a new monograph about the progress of HLA basic research in the future.

2. Basic concepts of HLA genetic statistics

2.1. Genetics basis for statistical analysis of HLA data

Hardy-Weinberg law: The Hardy-Weinberg law is also referred to as the hereditary equilibrium law or genetic equilibrium law. The basis of the Hardy-Weinberg law is as follows: in an infinite, randomly mating group, when there is no migration, mutation, selection, or genetic drift, the genotype frequency and gene frequency at a locus in the group will remain unchanged generation by generation, achieving a genetic equilibrium state, known as the Hardy-Weinberg equilibrium. This law was proposed by G.H. Hardy, a British mathematician, and W. Weinberg, a German medical scientist, in 1908.

The factors that influence the Hardy-Weinberg equilibrium are as follows:

1. Mutation: Under natural conditions, the rate of gene mutation caused by the reparation effects of DNA replicase is 1×10^{-6}–10^{-8}/gamete/locus/generation in higher animals, demonstrating that the frequency of natural mutation is very low.
2. Selection: a) Reproductive fitness: This is a measure of the ability of providing genes for progeny, i.e., the relative capability of a certain genotype to survive and produce progeny in comparison with other genotypes; in HLA studies, the normal fitness 1 is often used as a reference. b) Heterozygote dominance: In some recessive hereditary diseases and under certain conditions, the heterozygote may be more favorable to survival and progeny reproduction in comparison to homozygous normal individuals.
3. Random genetic drift: The random fluctuation of gene frequency in a small or separated group is referred to as genetic drift.
4. Migration: Gene frequencies may vary among individuals of different races and nationalities. Migration makes different populations intermate, and foreign genes are mutually introduced, which leads to gene flow and thus alters the gene frequency of the original group.
5. Genetic heterogeneity: Individuals with consistent phenotypes or identical clinical symptoms of a specific type of disease may have different genotypes. If they are not strictly distinguished, the Hardy-Weinberg equilibrium will likely become complex.
6. Founder effect: This is a form of genetic drift and refers to a new group established by minor individuals with some alleles of the parent group. The population size of this new group may increase later; however, its gene variance is very small because there is no mating or proliferation between this group and other biological groups. This situation generally occurs in an isolated island or a self-enclosed, newly established village.

Generally, the circumstances meeting the criteria of ideal populations do not exist in practical applications. However, the Hardy-Weinberg equilibrium is still the basis for studies of gene distribution because it is impossible to model all of the factors influencing the investigated group, and various factors can counteract each other (e.g., mutation and selection).

Now we will explain this concept with an example.

Assume that there is an autosomal locus, in brief, alleles A and A′. If the frequencies of genes A and A′ are p_m and q_m in males and p_f and q_f in females, then sperm frequencies with genes A and A′ are p_m and q_m, respectively, and ovum frequencies with genes A and A′ are p_f and q_f, respectively. Obviously, $p_m+q_m=1$ and $p_f+q_f=1$. If mating is completely random, the genotype frequency of the next generation will be as shown in Table 1.

		Sperm	
		A(p_m)	A′(q_m)
Ovum	A(p_f)	AA(p_m*p_f)	AA′(q_m*p_f)
	A′(q_m)	AA′(p_m*q_f)	A′A′(q_m*q_f)

Table 1. Genotype frequencies of progeny generated by random combinations of sperm and ovum

The investigated genes are in autosomes and are unrelated to genotypes; therefore, the frequencies of the three genotypes are identical in male and female progeny. Assume that the frequencies of the three genotypes AA, AA′, and A′A′ are *P*, *Q*, and *R*, respectively. From the table above, we can obtain:

$$P = p_m \times p_f$$

$$Q = q_m \times p_f + p_m \times q_f$$

$$R = q_m \times q_f$$

If we assume that the frequencies of genes A and A′ in progeny are p and q, respectively, then $p+q=1$, $p=P+1/2Q=p_m{}^{*}\, p_f+1/2(q_m{}^{*}\, p_f+ p_m{}^{*}\, q_f)=1/2p_m+1/2p_f$; similarly, $q=1/2q_m+1/2q_f$.

That is to say, when gene frequencies are different between males and females, they will be averaged in the next generation and thus become equal in both sexes. Therefore, when mating is completely random, and selection, mutation, and migration are absent, the gene frequencies and the frequencies of the three genotypes will maintain unchanged generation by generation. If the frequency series of genes A and A′ in gamete is expressed as:

$$(p_A + q_{A'})$$

then the genotype frequency series in progeny is:

$$\left(p^2{}_{AA} + 2pq_{AA'} + q^2{}_{A'A'}\right)$$

By generalizing the results above, if we assume that the frequencies of n alleles "A_1, A_2…A_n" in a group are p_1, p_2 …p_n, then ($\sum_{i=1}^{n} p_i = 1$), and it may be proved that the genotype frequency series in progeny can be expressed as

$$(p_{1A1} + p_{1A1} + \dots \dots + p_{nAn})^2$$

This is the presentation formula of the Hardy-Weinberg equilibrium. From this formula, we can see that the frequency of homozygotes AA or A′A′ is equal to the square of the gene frequency, while the heterozygote frequency is twice the product of the corresponding two gene frequencies. We will explain this concept using ABO blood groups as an example. ABO blood groups are known to be controlled by three alleles A, B, and O, found at the same locus. We can assume that the gene frequencies are p, q, and r, respectively. According to the presentation formula of the Hardy-Weinberg equilibrium, various genotype frequencies of ABO blood groups are expressed with the expansion equation of $(pA+pB+pO)^2$. See the following table.

Phenotype	Genotype	Genotype frequency
A	AA	p^2
	AO	$2pr$
B	BB	q^2
	BO	$2qr$
O	OO	r^2
AB	AB	$2pq$

Table 2. Genotype frequency of ABO blood groups

2.2. Statistical basis of HLA data analysis

2.2.1. Population and sample

The study subjects of HLA statistical data analysis are mostly specific groups, such as individuals with a disease, of the same race, or from the same region, etc. However, due to the limitations of the study method, it is usually impossible to investigate every individual in the group, and the features of the whole group can only be presumed by analyzing some individuals of the group. Thus, two concepts should be defined, i.e., population and sample. The core issue of statistical data analysis is how to deduce the population from a sample.

Population refers to all subjects in a study. The population can also be divided into the infinite population and the limited population. For example, we want to investigate the distribution of a certain HLA phenotype in Asian individuals; because it is difficult to estimate the total number of Asian individuals, we can assume that this population is infinite. Alternatively, if we want to study the recombination characteristics of the HLA system in a specific family, this population is limited. In HLA data analysis, most populations are infinite. Every member constituting the population is referred to as an individual.

A sample is a part of the population, and the number of individuals contained in a sample is the sample size. The core issue of statistical data analysis is that we presume the characteristics of a population from a sample. In order to accurately estimate the population parameters, an appropriate sample size is the foundation of data analysis.

Many factors need to be considered when determining the sample size, such as study objectives, precision, degree of confidence, reliability of statistical testing, sampling method, basic information of the population, study protocol, and study funds. Determination of the appropriate sample size fully reflects the repeatability rule in statistical analysis. Now, we will discuss how to determine the sample size in several common cases of HLA statistical analysis.

1. Determination of sample size when estimating population parameters

For example, if we want to understand the distribution of HLA-B*27 in healthy residents of a certain region and the frequency of the HLA-B*27 gene in patients with ankylosing arthritis, how many individuals should be included in the sample? According to the principle of the hypothesis test, if the sample size is too small, then the pre-existing differences cannot be shown; thus, it is hard to obtain correct study results, and the conclusion lacks sufficient basis. Conversely, an oversized sample can increase the practical difficulties of such analyses and unnecessarily waste labor, materials, financial resources, and time; in addition, sample excess may cause inadequate investment and decrease quality control during the scientific research process, thereby introducing potential interference with the study results.

When determining the sample size, the first thing to do is to define the test level or significance level "α", i.e., specifying in advance the allowable probability (α) of false-positive errors in this test (generally, α=0.05); additionally, you should decide whether a one-sided test or two-sided test will be used. The smaller α is, the larger the sample size must be.

The test power should also be defined. The higher the test power is, the larger the sample size must be. The test power is determined by the probability of type-II errors (β). In the design of scientific studies, the test power should be not lower than 0.75; otherwise, it is possible that the test results will not reflect true differences in the population, thereby yielding false-negative results.

In this example, the population represents healthy residents in a certain region, and the individuals investigated in the study constitute the sample. The frequency of gene HLA-B*27 in the population is presumed from the distribution proportion of HLA-B*27 in the sample. If we assume that the distribution frequency of gene HLA-B*27 is P, then the minimal sample (n) meeting the statistical conditions is calculated with the following formula:

When P is close to 0.5:

$$n=\left(\frac{u_{1-\alpha/2}}{\delta}\right)^2 P(1-P)$$

When P is close to 0 or 1:

$$n=\left[\frac{57.3u_{1-\alpha/2}}{\sin^{-1}\left(\delta/\sqrt{P(1-P)}\right)}\right]^2$$

When P is unknown:

$$n=0.25\left(\frac{u_{1-\alpha/2}}{\delta}\right)^2$$

In the formulas above, u indicates "u distribution", and δ indicates permissible error.

In this example, we want to investigate the frequency of HLA-B*27 in healthy residents of a certain region. We assume that P in the previous investigation is 10%, the permissible error of this investigation is 1%, and α=0.05 (two-sided), and we can attempt to estimate the number of individuals required for the study. From the critical value form of the u distribution or the u distribution function, we know that $u_{(1-0.05/2)}$=1.96, and the calculated n is about 3457 cases.

2. Estimation of the sample size when comparing the ratio of two populations

When comparing a certain ratio between two populations, for example assessing the differences in the morbidities of cardiovascular diseases between blue collar and white collar workers in a city, HLA analysis often involves determining the distribution differences of a certain gene in diseased and control groups. We can assume that at least two samples with samples sizes of n_1 and n_2, respectively, will be sampled from each population, and the estimated values of the population ratio obtained from the two samples are p_1 and p_2, respectively.

If n_1 is equal to n_2, then:

$$n_1 = n_2 = \frac{[u_{1-\alpha/2}\sqrt{2p(1-p)} + u_{1-\beta}\sqrt{p_1(1-p_1) + p_2(1-p_2)}]^2}{(p_1 - p_2)^2}$$

If n_1 is not equal to n_2, then $n_2=k\times n_1$:

$$n_1 = \frac{[u_{1-\alpha/2}\sqrt{2p(1-p)(1+k)/k} + u_{1-\beta}\sqrt{p_1(1-p_1) + p_2(1-p_2)/k}]^2}{(p_1 - p_2)^2},$$

where u = u distribution, β = test power, and p = integrated rate of both groups.

2.2.2. Sampling: The process of obtaining a sample from the population

The purpose of sampling is to determine the characteristics of a population by studying a sample (subset) of the population. For example, we want to determine the distribution of genotype HLA-B*07 in a marrow bank from the gene frequencies of 1000 individuals in the bank. This requires that the sample can maximally represent the population features. Therefore, every individual in the population should have the same chance to be sampled, and the sample should be free from bias. For example, in a study investigating a certain HLA phenotype and disease, we generally hope to determine the relationship between the disease and the specific HLA phenotype. In order to do this, researchers must be careful not to deliberately exclude cases without the specific HLA phenotype during sampling. The resulting sample would then not be representative of the total population; this is a bias sample and would not represent the total population profile. The sample we use should be a miniature, accurate representation of the population. In order to achieve this goal, we should use the method of random sampling to obtain samples.

Many randomization methods are commonly used. Initially, drawing lots, casting coins, and casting lots were used; later, researchers adopted random number form, random arrangement form, and the computer-based methods to generate random numbers. For sampling studies in medical science and the grouping of trial subjects, random number form and random arrangement form are relatively convenient. They both perform random sampling and work out a tool table according to the equal probability principle of mathematical statistics, and the sampling results are better than those obtained by drawing lots or casting coins. Study subjects should be randomly and uniformly assigned into each treatment group (all control and trial groups), thereby preventing various objective factors from intervening with the study results. The greater the number of study subjects, the higher the randomization level. However, it is unnecessary to maximize the amount of study subjects; we should select an appropriate randomization method depending on the trial features. Some common randomization methods are detailed below.

1. Drawing lots: This method is easy to perform. For example, if we want to divide 12 animals into two groups, we should number the animals with 1, 2, 3, …, 12 and prepare the 12 lots, each having a number from 1 to 12. The lots are then mixed, and 6 lots are drawn as per prior specifications; the animals with these 6 lots are assigned into Group 1, and the remaining animals are assigned into Group 2.

2. Random number form: The random number form is carried out according to the principle of random sampling. It can be used for both random assignment and random sampling. All of the numbers in the form are mutually independent. Regardless of horizontal, longitudinal, or slant order, the numbers can randomly occur; therefore, random numbers can be obtained in order by starting from any direction and any location. Some examples are given below.

a. Dividing into two groups: We planned to observe 20 patients with gastric ulcers (patient No. 1–20); one group uses an effective drug ranitidine as a control, and the other group uses a lily decoction. Twenty2-digit random numbers are generated by looking up the random number form, and the random numbers are arranged from small to large, allowing us to obtain the grouping order number "R". If R is between 1 and 10, then the patient is assigned into Group A; if R is between 11 and 20, then the patient is assigned into Group B. The grouping results are presented in Table 3 (reference: TianheXu, Jiu Wang. Design of Medical Experiments: Lecture 2 – Rules of randomization and blinding method. *Chinese Medical Journal*, 2005, 40(8): p.54).

Patient No.	1	2	3	4	5	6	7	8	9	10	11	12	13	14	15	16	17	18	19	20
Random number	93	22	53	64	39	7	10	63	76	35	87	3	4	79	88	8	13	85	51	34
Grouping order number (R)	20	7	12	14	10	3	5	13	15	9	18	1	2	16	19	4	6	17	11	8
Group	B	A	B	B	A	A	A	B	B	A	B	A	A	B	B	A	A	B	B	A

Table 3. Randomized grouping results of 20 patients

b. Randomized division of three or more groups: If we want to randomly divide 15 animals into 3 groups, we should number the animals from 1 to 15.Then, fifteen 2-digit random numbers are generated by looking up the random number form, and the random numbers should be arranged from small to large. The order number "R" can then be obtained. If R is between 1 and 5, then the animal is assigned into Group A. If R is between 6 and 10, then the animal is assigned to Group B. If R is between 11 and 15, then the animal is assigned to Group C. The grouping results are presented in Table 4 (TianheXu, Jiu Wang. Design of Medical Experiments: Lecture 2 – Rules of randomization and blinding method. *Chinese Medical Journal*, 2005, 40(8): p.54).

Animal No.	1	2	3	4	5	6	7	8	9	10	11	12	13	14	15
Random number	33	35	72	67	47	77	34	55	45	70	8	18	27	38	90
Grouping order number (R)	4	6	13	11	9	14	5	10	8	12	1	2	3	7	15
Group	A	B	C	C	B	C	A	B	B	C	A	A	A	B	C

Table 4. Randomized grouping of 15 animals

2.3. Definitions of relative terms in HLA statistical data analysis

2.3.1. Definitions of HLA phenotype, haplotype, and genotype

HLA antigens have their own allele code on the chromosome; generally, the HLA antibody-antigen specificity of an individual can be detected using available typing reagents and committed cells. The antigen-specific type obtained by this method is referred to as the phenotype. However, the antigen phenotype does not reflect the individual's allele combination pattern on the chromosome. The combination of HLA alleles on the chromosome is referred to as the haplotype. If this combination expands from type-I and type-II alleles to type-III genes or adjacent loci, it is often referred to as an extended haplotype. Two haplotypes form the HLA genotype of an individual, i.e., the pattern of the HLA allele combination on two chromosomes in the individual (Table 5). Generally, the haplotype and genotype can only be determined by performing phenotype analysis of all the members of a family or by using special experimental methods, such as monospermal analysis. The phenotype of every individual has many potential combinations that depend on different genotypes. It is therefore important to understand an individual's haplotype and genotype in allogeneic organ transplant, transplantation of hematopoietic stem cells, and forensic identification.

Individual	Individual 1	Individual 2	Individual 3
Typing results	A*11:01 A*24:01 B*07:02 B*27:04	A*11:01 B*07:02 B*27:04	A*11:01 B*27:04
Phenotype	HLA-A11, A24, B7, B27	HLA-A11, B7, 27	HLA-A11, B27
Genotype	HLA-A*11:01,A*24:01 HLA-B*07:02, B*27:04	HLA-A*11:01, A*11:01 HLA-B*07:02, B*27:04	HLA-A*11:01, A*11:01 HLA-B*27:04, B*27:04
Haplotype	HLA-A*11:01, B*07:02 & HLA-A*24:01, B*27:04 or HLA- A*11:01, B*27:04 & HLA-A*24:01, B*07:02	HLA- A*11:01, B*07:02 & HLA- A*11:01, B*27:04	HLA- A*11:01, B*27:04 & HLA- A*11:01, B*27:04

Table 5. Differences in HLA phenotypes, haplotypes, and genotypes

2.3.2. Genetics features of HLA

1. Haplotype genetic mode: An HLA complex is a group of closely linked genes. Crossing-over between homologous chromosomes rarely occurs in these alleles, which are linked in the same chromosome, i.e., they form a haplotype. During reproduction, the HLA haplotype is inherited from parent to progeny as a complete genetic unit. The progeny can randomly obtain an HLA haplotype from both parents, thereby forming the progeny's new genotype. In the siblings of the same family, the probability of having two identical haplotypes is 25%, the probability of having one identical haplotype is 50%, and the probability of having two different haplotypes is 25%. Therefore, when seeking an appropriate donor for allogeneic organ transplant or transplant of hematopoietic stem cells in clinical practice, it is much easier to find the matched HLA antigen (the matched HLA haplotype in particular) in the patient's family than in nonsibling donors. However, it should be noted that when the haplotype is inherited from parent to progeny, homologous crossing-over between both haplotypes may occur (see details in the recombination section).

2. Codominant inheritance: This means that antigens encoded by each pair of alleles are expressed on the cell membrane, and there is no recessive gene. Allele rejection does not exist. If the haplotypes of an individual's two chromosomes are HLA-A*11:01, B*27:04 and HLA-A*24:01, B*07:02, then four different HLA molecules, A11, A24, B27, and B7, will be expressed on the cytomembrane surface of the individual.

3. Linkage disequilibrium: Various HLA alleles at different loci occur in the group at a specific frequency. In a group, if the frequencies of two alleles at different loci occurring in the same chromosome are higher than the expected random frequencies, i.e.,the haplotype frequency (observed data) is significantly higher or lower than theoretical value (the product of allele frequencies at different loci), then this non-free combination phenomenon is referred to as linkage disequilibrium. For example, A1 and B8 in Caucasians and A2 and B46 in southern Chinese individuals always occur together, and the resulting haplotypes A1-B8 and A2-B46, respectively, exhibit linkage disequilibrium.

3. Estimation of HLA population genetic parameters

3.1. Genetic structure

Studies of the genetic parameters of the HLA system actually start from the loci "HLA-A" and "HLA-B"; these two loci are often used as examples in HLA data analysis. To provide a simple description, we will expand this model to an autosomal double-loci multiple-alleles genetic model and use the following symbols.

Assume that there are two linkage loci (I and J) on a human chromosome; each locus has multiple codominant alleles. The alleles at locus I are labeled as i_1, i_2, i_3, i_n, and i_0. "i_0" represents the undetected blank gene at locus I; therefore, the allele number at locus I is calculated as $l = n + 1$.

Similarly, the alleles at locus J are expressed as $j_1, j_2, j_3, \ldots j_m$ and j_0. "j_0" represents the undetected blank gene at locus J; therefore, the allele number at locus J is calculated as $k = m + 1$.

Because the alleles at loci I and J can randomly combine, the number of all the possible haplotypes is $l*k$. These haplotypes can form various genotypes, calculated as $lk(lk+1)/2$. Considering that the phenotype of genes in a homozygosis state is the same as the phenotype of a gene hybridized with a blank gene, i.e., the phenotype of genotypes i_2i_2 and i_2i_0 is i_2 (+), the number of all possible phenotypes from any allele combination at locus I is $[l+(l-1) \times (l-2)/2]$; similarly, the number of all possible phenotypes from any allele combination at locus J is $[k+(k-1) \times (k-2)/2]$. Thus, the number of all possible phenotypes at loci I and J is $[l+(l-1) \times (l-2)/2] \times [k+(k-1) \times (k-2)/2]$.

Loci I and J are linked, so the gene frequency of each locus correlates to the frequency of haplotypes formed with genes at both loci; the antigen distribution in the population also correlates at both loci. This relation can be fully shown in a 2 × 2 four-space form. Unless specified otherwise, all the populations mentioned in this chapter are Mendelian populations achieving Hardy-Weinberg equilibrium, i.e., this population undergoes completely random mating, and there are no effects of selection, mutation, or migration.

The population distribution of antigens at both loci is presented in the table below. Symbols in the table indicate that in a population with a total number of individuals "N", "a" individuals have antigens i and j, "b" individuals have antigen i but without antigen j, "c" individuals have antigen j but without antigen i, and "d" individuals do not have antigens i and j. The marginal values A, B, C, and D in this table are respectively equal to the sum of the corresponding two spaces, and N is equal to the sum of four spaces.

		Antigen j		**Total**
		+	**-**	
Antigen i	+	a	b	C=a+b
	-	c	d	D=c+d
Total		A=a+c	B=b+d	***N***=a+b+c+d

Table 6. Population distribution of antigens i and j

Table 6 shows the relation between the frequencies of genes i and j and the haplotype frequency. The genes at loci I and J can form four haplotypes, ij, j0, i0, and 00; "0" represents the blank gene. The frequencies of the four genes are expressed as s, t, u, and v respectively. The frequency of gene i is expressed as "p_i", and the frequency sum of the other alleles at locus I is expressed as "q_i"; obviously, $p_i+q_i=1$. Similarly, the frequency of gene j and the frequency sum of the other alleles at locus J are expressed as "p_j" and "q_j", respectively. From the table below, we can see that the frequency of each gene can be expressed as the frequency sum of the corresponding haplotypes.

		Gene j		Total
		+	-	
Gene i	+	s	u	p_i=s+u
	-	t	v	q_i=t+v
Total		p_j=s+t	q_j=u+v	1

Table 7. Relation between the gene frequencies at loci I and J and the haplotype frequencies

3.2. Hardy-Weinberg equilibrium test

According to the gene or haplotype frequency, the expected values of all genotype frequencies and phenotype frequencies can be obtained by combination as per the Hardy-Weinberg equilibrium law; the coincidence degree of the expected value and the corresponding actual observed value is referred to as the Hardy-Weinberg coincidence test. This test is mainly used in two cases: 1) As a prompt for supporting or excluding a certain genetic mode. For example, in an assumed Mendelian genetic system, the gene or haplotype frequency is calculated on the basis of the assumed genetic mode, and recombination is then performed as per the Hardy-Weinberg equilibrium law to obtain the expected value of the phenotype. If the expected value coincides with the observed value of this phenotype, the genetic mode may be true; otherwise, the genetic mode may be excluded. The conclusion obtained by application of the Hardy-Weinberg equilibrium to test a genetic mode cannot be confirmatory because sometimes increasing the assumed loci may give better coincidence results. 2) For reliability estimation of the population survey data. For some genetic systems with well-established genetic modes, such as the HLA system discussed in this book, if the population can perform fully random mating, and there are no effects caused by selection, mutation, or migration, the population distribution should be in good Hardy-Weinberg equilibrium. Poor coincidence of both values shows that the population survey data are not reliable, which can help us identify the causes of errors in aspects sampling, typing technology, etc.

3.2.1. Measuring method for determination of the coincidence degree

The coincidence degree of a phenotype's expected value and observed value is generally measured with χ^2. The χ^2 is calculated for every phenotype, and the values are added to obtain the total χ^2. The P value is calculated by looking up the form. The χ^2 calculation formula is:

$$\chi^2 = \sum \frac{(Expected\ value\ -\ Observed\ value)^2}{Expected\ value}$$

In the Hardy-Weinberg equilibrium test, the expected value of the phenotype is often less than 5. In this case, some authors will incorporate several phenotypes and calculate χ^2 again when the phenotype value is more than 5; however, this method has obvious subjective factors, and the calculated χ^2 value after incorporation will be reduced. In addition, due to variations of incorporation methods, it is difficult to compare data between studies. Therefore, we think that it is unnecessary to incorporate items with the phenotype expected values of less than 5, and the χ^2 should be calculated as in other cases; although this may increase theχ^2 value, the resulting coincidence conclusion is more reliable.

Determination of the degrees of freedom in the χ^2 test: Assume that a genetic system consists of n alleles and Φ phenotypes, and the sample size is N. Because the gene frequencies p_1+p_2+ ......p_n=1, the number of parameters estimated from the sample is (n-1); in addition, a degree of freedom is lost because the sample is too small. Therefore, the degrees of freedom remaining for other tests are:

$$d_f = \Phi - (n-1) - 1 = \Phi - n$$

In the Hardy-Weinberg equilibrium, $p \geq 0.5$ is generally used as the criterion to judge whether there are significant differences between the expected and observed values.

3.2.2. *Hardy-Weinberg equilibrium test for separated loci*

In a genetic system containing one or more loci, the Hardy-Weinberg equilibrium test can be performed for every locus. According to the Hardy-Weinberg equilibrium law, the expected frequency of the homozygous genotype is the product of the corresponding two gene frequencies, and the expected frequency of the heterozygous genotype is twice the product of the corresponding gene frequencies. The expected value of each phenotype is equal to the sum of the expected values of the corresponding genotypes. After multiplying the phenotype frequency by sample size "N" to calculate the expected value of the phenotype, the coincidence degree between this expected value and the observed value of the phenotype can be tested.

The table (Table 8) below shows a Hardy-Weinberg coincidence test of the antigen phenotype at locus HLA-C in Chinese individuals with the Han nationality. The expected values and observed values coincide well, demonstrating that the distribution of these alleles at locus C is in the Hardy-Weinberg equilibrium state. In this table, the HLA-Cw1 phenotype includes two genotypes, "HLA-C*01/HLA-C*01" and "HLA-C*01/blank"; therefore, the expected value of the phenotype is calculated as

$$106 \times (0.1442 \times \ 0.1442 + 0.1442\ 0.3793 \times 2) = 13.5779.$$

The phenotype expected value of HLA-Cw1, 2 is calculated as

$$106 \times 0.1442 \times 0.0143 \times 2 \ = \ 0.4311.$$

3.2.3. *Hardy-Weinberg equilibrium test of haplotypes*

The haplotype Hardy-Weinberg equilibrium test can be performed in a multiple-loci, multiple-alleles genetic system, and the allelic and linkage relationships of all the genes in the system can also be tested. If not considering recombination, haplotypes and alleles also comply with the same genetic rules; therefore, according to Hardy-Weinberg equilibrium, the expected value of the phenotype containing two identical haplotypes should be equal to the square of the haplotype frequency, and the expected value of the phenotype containing two different haplotypes should be equal to twice the product of the frequencies of the two haplotypes. the expected value of the phenotype can be calculated by sorting various haplotype frequencies

Phenotype	Genotype	Observed value	Expected value	Gene frequency
HLA Cw1	HLA-C*01/HLA-C*01 or HLA-C*01/blank	10	13.5779	HLA-C*01=0.1422
HLA Cw1,2	HLA-C*01/HLA-C*02	0	0.4311	HLA-C*02=0.0143
HLA Cw1,3	HLA-C*01/HLA-C*03	17	11.6275	HLA-C*03=0.3857
HLA Cw1,4	HLA-C*01/HLA-C*04	1	2.3665	HLA-C*04=0.0785
HLA Cw1,5	HLA-C*01/HLA-C*05	0	0	HLA-C*05=0
HLA Cw2	HLA-C*02/HLA-C*02 or HLA-C*02/blank	1	1.1716	HLA-C*blank=0.3793
HLA Cw2,3	HLA-C*02/HLA-C*03	1	1.1693	
HLA Cw2,4	HLA-C*02/HLA-C*04	1	0.2380	d_f=16-6=10
HLA Cw2,5	HLA-C*02/HLA-C*05	0	0	P>0.5
HLA Cw3	HLA-C*03/HLA-C*03 or HLA-C*03/blank	43	46.788	
HLA Cw3,4	HLA-C*03/HLA-C*04	5	6.4188	
HLA Cw3,5	HLA-C*03/HLA-C*05	0	0	
HLA Cw4	HLA-C*04/HLA-C*04 or HLA-C*04/blank	9	6.9655	
HLA Cw4,5	HLA-C*04/HLA-C*05	0	0	
HLA Cw5	HLA-C*05/HLA-C*05 or HLA-C*05/blank	0	0	
Blank	Blank/blank	18	15.2501	
Total		106	106.004	

Table 8. Hardy-Weinberg equilibrium test of the antigen phenotype at locus HLA-C in Chinese individuals with the Han nationality

into the corresponding phenotypes, and a coincidence test is then performed with the observed value of the phenotype. Table 9 shows the calculation method for the expected value of phenotype "HLA-A2, B15", where A* is blank, representing the set of all alleles at locus HLA-A except HLA-A*02, and B* is blank, representing the set of all alleles at locus HLA-B except HLA-B*15. Haplotype frequencies would be calculated as HLA-A*02 B*15=0.0113; HLA-A*02 B*blank=0.0559; HLA-A*blank B*15=0.0098; HLA-A*blank B*blank=0.0053.

Haplotype combination mode	Phenotype frequency
A*02 B*blank /A*blank B*15	2 × 0.0559 × 0.0098=0.001096
A*02 B*15 /A*blank B*blank	2 × 0.0113 × 0.0053=0.000120
A*02 B*15 /A*blank B*15	2 × 0.0113 × 0.0098=0.000221
A*02 B*15 /A*02 B*blank	2 × 0.0113 × 0.0059=0.000133
A*02 B*15 /A*02 B*15	0.0113 × 0.0113 × 0.000128

Table 9. The haplotype composition and expected frequency of phenotype "HLA-A2, B15"

3.3. Estimation of genetic parameters

Genetic parameters are estimated by assessing a quantity-limited sample, and thus, sampling error must exist. The size of sampling error is expressed with the standard error σ, where σ is equal to the root extraction of variance "*V*".

3.4. Antigen frequency

Antigen frequency is defined as the ratio or percentage of individuals with the antigen phenotype in the population. If N = total individuals and C = individuals with the antigen phenotype i, then the frequency of antigen i is calculated as:

$$f_i = C / N$$

The frequencies of antigens i and j can be easily obtained from the four-space form above:

$$f_i = (a+b) / N = C / N$$

$$f_j = (a+c) / N = A / N$$

and the standard error is calculated as: $\sigma fi = \frac{1}{N}\sqrt{\frac{CD}{N}} = \sqrt{\frac{fi*(1-fi)}{N}}$

When the antigen frequency f_i is fixed, the greater the sample size N, the lower the standard error.

3.5. Gene frequency

Assuming that i_1 is an allele at locus I, the ratio or percentage of gene i_1 in all the genes of this locus is referred to as the gene or genotype frequency of i_1. The frequency sum of all alleles at a single locus is 1. Gene frequency can be obtained from family or population surveys.

3.5.1. Calculation of gene frequency by direct genotype count

If the genotyping results of N individuals are known, then the frequency of gene i in the population can be obtained by a simple counting method. Assuming that this value is X, the frequency of gene i is:

$$p_i = X / 2N$$

Assume that there are two alleles at autosomal locus I, i_1 and i_2. For diploids, it is possible to form three genotypes: i_1i_1, i_1i_2, and i_2i_2. After surveying 100 individuals, possible count results are presented per genotype in the following table (Table 10). In total, there are 200 genes at locus I: 36 individuals have i_1i_1, and the count of gene i_1 is 72; 48 individuals have i_1i_2, and the count of genes i_1 and i_2 is 48; 16 individuals have i_2i_2, and the count of gene i_2 is 32. Therefore, the gene frequency of i_1 is calculated as (72+48)/200=0.6; similarly, the gene frequency of i_2 is calculated as (32+48)/200=0.4; the sum of both frequencies is 1.

In the HLA system, each locus usually has several alleles. If we want to calculate the frequency of a certain allele at the locus, which can be expressed as i1, then the meaning of i_2 is non-i_1

genes. For example, if we want to calculate the gene frequency of HLA-B*27 at locus HLA-B, which is expressed as i_1, then the frequency sum of all the alleles except HLA-B*27 is expressed as i_2.

Genotype	i_1i_1	i_1i_2	i_2i_2
Observed individuals	36	48	16
Amount of gene i_1	72	48	0
Amount of gene i_2	0	48	32

Table 10. Distribution of genotype I in 100 random individuals

3.5.2. Estimation of gene frequency according to phenotype frequency

Currently, HLA typing technology is developing rapidly. With the popularization of high-throughput sequencing technology, the calculation of HLA gene frequency can be mostly completed using the counting method. However, due to limited technical conditions in some population surveys, we can only obtain the corresponding phenotypes. Therefore, how should be best analyze gene frequency? There are two main methods used in practical work: one is the root method, which involved simple arithmetic and easy to perform; the other is the maximal likelihood algorithm, which is highly efficient in estimating gene frequencies, but required specialized computer software (see details in the next section). A description of how to use the root method for estimation of gene frequency according to phenotype results is given below.

If the frequency of the dominant gene i is p_i, then the frequency sum of all the other alleles at this locus is

$$q_i = 1 - p_i;$$

The relationship between the phenotype frequency and the corresponding genotype frequency can be obtained according to the Hardy-Weinberg law (see the table below).

Phenotype	Phenotype frequency	Corresponding genotype	Frequency of corresponding genotype
I (+)	f_i	i homozygote "ii", i heterozygote "i-"	$p_i^2+2p_iq_i$
I (-)	$1-f_i$	Non-i combination "-/-"	q_i^2

Table 11. Relationship between phenotype and genotype frequencies

We can deduce from the table

$$p_i = 1 - \sqrt{1 - fi}$$

where p_i is the gene frequency of gene I, and f_i is the frequency of the phenotype or antigen containing gene i. This formula is often used for estimation of HLA gene frequency, and its form can be changed.

$$p_i = 1 - \sqrt{1 - C / N}$$

Or $p_i = 1 - \sqrt{D / N}$

The definitions of C, D, and N in the formula are the same as above, and the standard error of p_i is:

$$\sigma p_i = \frac{1}{2}\sqrt{\frac{f_i}{N}} = \frac{\sqrt{N - D}}{2N}$$

It should be noted that when the pi value is small, it can be calculated by the following formula:

$$p_i \approx \frac{f_i}{2}$$

3.6. Haplotype frequency

For double-loci multiple-allele genetic systems, each chromosome has two alleles belonging to two different loci, and the combination of these different alleles forms variant haplotypes. The ratio or percentage of each haplotype in the population is referred to as the frequency of this haplotype. The sum of all haplotype frequencies is 1.

3.6.1. Calculation of haplotype frequency by direct haplotype count

When an individual's haplotype is known, the haplotype frequency can be calculated by a simple counting method, and the calculation method and technology are the same as those for calculation of gene frequency. However, haplotypes can often only be obtained by family surveys, and HLA haplotypes cannot be fully determined in some families. During data analysis, rejection of these individuals may cause error. In this case, the relative haplotype frequency can be estimated by referring to the population survey results. For example, in Table 12 below, whether the mother's haplotype is A9-B13/A2-B13 or A9-B13/A2-B- cannot be fully determined by family analysis. The haplotype can only be determined by estimation of relative frequency. Assume we know that the frequency of haplotype A2-B13 is 0.0356 and that of haplotype A2-B- is 0.0559 from population survey data. Because the mother can only have these two haplotypes, the relative frequency of A2-B13 is 0.0356/(0.0356+ 0.0559)=0.39 and that of A2-B- is 0.0559/(0.0356+ 0.0559)=0.61. During counting, these haplotypes should be counted as 0.39 A2-B13 and 0.61 A2-B-, respectively.

In practical applications, due to advances in HLA genotyping methods, especially the widespread use of sequencing-based typing methods, high-resolution HLA results are comprehensively adopted; when there is only one allele that is detected at the locus of a certain gene, it is often considered a homozygous allele.

	Phenotype	Haplotype combination mode
Father	A10,11; B5,15	A11-B5 & A10-B15
Mother	A2,9; B13	A9-B13 % A2-B13 or A9-B13 % A2-B-
Child 1	A9,11; B5,13	A11-B5 & A9-B13
Child 2	A9,10; B13,15	A10-B15 & A9-B13
Child 3	A9,11; B5,13	A11-B5 & A9-B13

Table 12. A family's HLA typing results

3.6.2. Estimation of haplotype frequency according to phenotype frequency

Assume that codominant genes i and j are located at two different loci, and other blank genes at these two loci are expressed as 0. Therefore, it is possible to have four haplotypes (ij, j0, i0, and 00) in the population, and the frequencies of these four haplotypes are expressed as s, t, u, and v, respectively. The relationship between haplotype frequency and gene frequency is illustrated in Table 7. The actual observed value of the distribution of antigen ij in the population is presented in Table 6.

The expected distribution of antigens i and j in the population can be expressed with the pattern in Table 13, and the expected values in the table are obtained according to Hardy-Weinberg equilibrium. Thus, we can expand $(s+t+u+v)^2$ and then incorporate items with identical phenotypes. N is the sample size.

		Antigen j		Total
		+	-	
Antigen i	+	$(2s-s^2+2tu)N$	$(u^2+2uv)N$	$N[1-(t+v)]^2$
	-	$(t^2+2tv)N$	v^2N	$N(t+v)^2$
Total		$N[1-(u+v)^2]$	$N(u+v)^2$	N

Table 13. Expected values related to the distribution of antigen ij

After changing the formula, the gene frequency is expressed as:

Frequency of haplotype ij, $s = p_j - q_i + \sqrt{d / N}$

Frequency of haplotype j0, $t = q_i - \sqrt{d / N}$

Frequency of haplotype i0, $u = q_j - \sqrt{d / N}$

Frequency of haplotype 00, $v = \sqrt{d / N}$

If expressing as antigen frequency,

$$s=\sqrt{d/N}+1-\sqrt{1-f_j}-\sqrt{1-f_i}$$

$$t=\sqrt{1-f_i}-\sqrt{d/N}$$

$$u=\sqrt{1-f_j}-\sqrt{d/N}$$

$$v=\sqrt{d/N}$$

If expressing as phenotype amount,

$$s=\sqrt{d/N}+1-\sqrt{B/N}-\sqrt{D/N}$$

$$t=\sqrt{D/N}-\sqrt{d/N}$$

$$u=\sqrt{B/N}-\sqrt{d/N}$$

$$v=\sqrt{d/N}$$

The standard error for this equation can be calculated as:

$$\sigma s=\sqrt{\left[\left(1-\sqrt{d/B}\right)\left(1-\sqrt{d/D}\right)+s-s^2/2\right]/2N}$$

$$\sigma t=\sqrt{\left[\left(1-\sqrt{d/D}\right)-t^2/2\right]/2N}$$

$$\sigma u=\sqrt{\left[\left(1-\sqrt{d/B}\right)-u^2/2\right]/2N}$$

$$\sigma v=\frac{1}{2}\sqrt{(1-v^2)/N}$$

and the standard error of "s" can be expressed as:

$$\sigma s=\sqrt{[(1-v/(t+v))(1-v/(u+v))+s-s^2/2]/2}=\sqrt{\left[\left(\frac{p_i-s}{1-p_j}\right)\left(\frac{p_j-s}{1-p_i}\right)+s-s^2/2\right]/2}$$

If a haplotype contains a blank gene, such as A1-B-, then the frequency is equal to the sum of the gene frequency of A1 and the haplotype frequencies of the other alleles at locus B. The haplotype frequency calculated according to the above calculation formula for phenotype data may be a negative value sometimes; this is caused by inadequate sample size and sampling error.

3.7. Linkage disequilibrium parameter

3.7.1. Linkage disequilibrium

Linkage disequilibrium is controlled by inconsistency of the observed and expected values about the appearance of antigens at two linked loci in the same haplotype. Assuming that the genes at two linked loci are i and j, the linkage disequilibrium parameter is defined as the difference between the actual observed haplotype frequency of ij and the product of gene frequencies of i and j, which is expressed as Δ. If the observed frequency of haplotype ij is "s", then $\Delta_{ij}=s-p_ip_j$.

When the genotypes and haplotypes of every individual in the population are known, the Δ value can be easily obtained by the counting method. However, it is generally necessary to estimate the Δ value from population survey data, i.e., $\Delta_{ij}=s-p_ip_j=sv-tu$.

The following formulas are commonly used:

$$\Delta ij=\sqrt{d/N}-q_iq_j$$

$$\Delta ij=\sqrt{d/N}-\sqrt{(1-f_j)(1-f_i)}$$

$$\Delta ij=\sqrt{d/N}-\sqrt{\mathrm{BD}}/N$$

The standard error of Δ can be calculated as:

$$\sigma(\Delta)=\sqrt{\frac{\alpha}{4N^2}-\frac{\Delta}{N}\left(\frac{B+D}{2\sqrt{BD}}-\frac{\sqrt{BD}}{N}\right)}$$

or as:

$$\sigma(\Delta)=\sqrt{\frac{1}{4N}+\frac{1}{4N^2}(\mathrm{B}+\mathrm{D}+\mathrm{d})-\frac{\sqrt{d}}{2\mathrm{N}\sqrt{N}}\left(\sqrt{\frac{D}{B}}+\sqrt{\frac{B}{D}}\right)-\frac{BD}{N^3}+\frac{\sqrt{BDd}}{N^2\sqrt{N}}}$$

$\Delta/\sigma(\Delta)\geq 1.96$ is generally considered to be of significant linkage disequilibrium.

3.7.2. Relative Δ value

There is no comparability among absolute Δ values, so relative Δ values, i.e., "$\Delta_{(r)}$", are generally calculated for comparison.

$$\Delta_{ij(r)}=\Delta_{ij(r)}/\Delta_{ij(Max)}$$

From the calculation formula of

$$\Delta_{ij}=s-p_ip_j=sv-tu$$

we can see:

If tu=0, Δ_{ij} has the maximal value; if t or u is 0, Δ_{ij} is equal to p_jq_i or p_iq_j, and the lower value between p_i and p_j is used to calculate $\Delta_{ij(\mathrm{Max})}$, i.e.:

$$\mathrm{p_i}<\mathrm{q_j}:\Delta_{ij(Max)}=p_i(1-p_j);$$

$$\mathrm{p_i}>\mathrm{q_j}:\Delta_{\mathrm{ij(Max)}}=\mathrm{p_j}(1-\mathrm{p_i});$$

If s = 0, the negative Δ_{ij} has the maximal value, and

$$\Delta_{ij(Max)}=-p_jp_i.$$

3.8. Genetic distance

In order to quantitatively describe the process of generating genetic differences between two populations due to selection, mutation, migration, and random drift, the concept of genetic distance has been introduced.genetic distance is a measure of the gene frequency differences between populations, and it is used to describe interpopulation variance.

In 1977, Cavalli-Sforza and Bodmerthe defined the genetic distance (*d*) as:

$$d = \sqrt{1 - \sum_i \sqrt{p_{i1} p_{i2}}}$$

where p_{i1} and p_{i2} are the frequencies of gene i in populations 1 and 2, respectively.

4. Software analysis of HLA data

To conveniently implement haplotype frequency estimation, linkage disequilibrium, Hardy-Weinberg equilibrium, pairwise genetic distances, etc., of HLA data, computer software is usually required. There are severalprofessional statistical software and genetic analysis software programs.This chapter will introduce some common problems encountered when using software for HLA data analysis.

4.1. The processing method of HLA data analysis using *Arlequin* software

Arlequin is the French translation of "Arlecchino," a famous Italian character from "Commedia dell'Arte." Arlecchinois a multi-faceted character, but he has the ability to switch among his various character assets very easily according to his needs and necessities. This polymorphic ability is symbolized by his colorful costume, from which the *Arlequin* icon was designed (Figure 1).

The goal of *Arlequin* is to provide the average user in population genetics with a large set of basic methods and statistical tests to extract information on genetic and demographic features of a collection of population samples.

Arlequin can handle several types of data either in haplotypic or genotypic form.

- DNA sequences
- RFLP data
- Microsatellite data
- Standard data
- Allele frequency data

HLA data belong to "Standard data" in which the molecular basis of a polymorphism is not defined specifically, or when different alleles are considered mutationally equidistant from

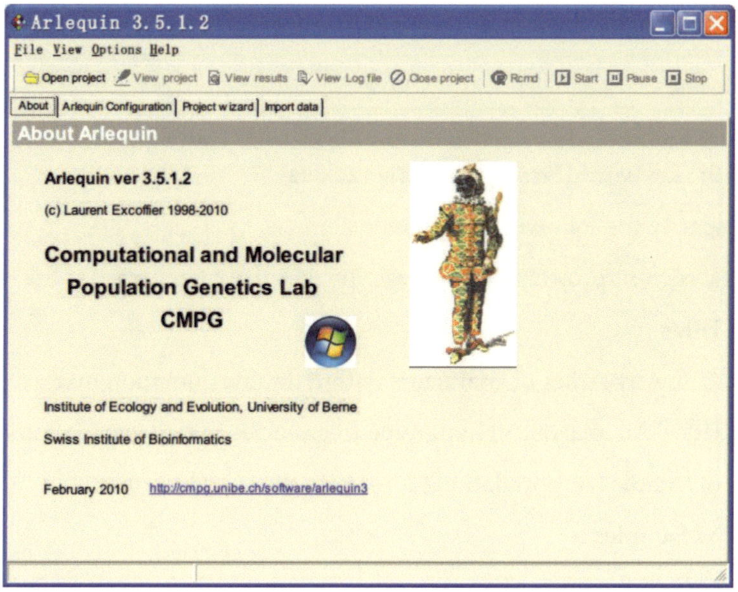

Figure 1. *Arlequin* software

each other. Therefore, standard data haplotypes are compared for their content at each locus, without regarding the nature of the alleles, which can either be similar or different.

4.1.1. Structure of an Arlequin input file

4.1.1.1. Input data file

The first step for the analysis of your data isto prepare an input data file (project file) for *Arlequin*. Because *Arlequin* is a versatile program that is able to analyze several data types, you must include information about the property of your data together with the raw data into the project file. A text editor can be used to define your data using reserved keywords.

Arlequin project files contain a description of the data properties as well as the raw data themselves. The project file may also refer to one or more external data files.

Input files are structured into two main sections with additional subsections that must appear in the following order (Figure 2):

1) Profile section (mandatory)

2) Data section (mandatory)

2a) Haplotype list (optional)

2b) Distance matrices (optional)

2c) Samples (mandatory)

2d) Genetic structure (optional)

2e) Mantel tests (optional)

4.1.1.2. Profile section

The data properties must be described in the profile section. The beginning of the profile section is indicated by the keyword [Profile] (within brackets).

The user must specify the following parameters:

- The title of the current project (used to describe the current analysis)
  - Notation: Title=
  - Possible value: Any string of characters within double quotation marks
  - Example: Title="An analysis of haplotype frequencies in two populations"
- The number of samples or populations present in the current project
  - Notation: NbSamples =
  - Example: NbSamples =3
  - The type of data to be analyzed. Only one type of data isallowed per project.
  - Notation: DataType =
  - Possible values: DNA, RFLP, MICROSAT, STANDARD, and FREQUENCY
  - Example: DataType = DNA
  - The parameter of "STANDARD" is used here when dealing with HLA Data.
- Thetype of data that the project addresses
  - Notation: GenotypicData =
  - Possible values: 0 (haplotypic data), 1 (genotypic data)
  - Example: GenotypicData = 0

This parameter is used to demonstrate whether haplotypic or genotypicdata are being used for the HLA data analysis.Unless specified, the parameter used here is usually "1."

Additionally, the user has the option to specify the following parameters:

- The character used to separate the alleles at different loci (the locus separator)
  - Notation: LocusSeparator =
  - Possible values: WHITESPACE, TAB, NONE, any character other than "#", or a character
  - specifying missing data
  - Example: LocusSeparator = TAB
  - Default value: WHITESPACE

- Thegametic phase of the genotype
  - Notation: GameticPhase =
  - Possible values: 0 (unknown gametic phase), 1 (known gametic phase)
  - Example: GameticPhase = 1
  - Default value: 1
  - For general HLA data analysis, the parameter is "0." If approaches such as pedigree analysis are used, and the HLA haplotype of each individual sample are given, "1" is used as the parameter.In the data input, one haplotype should be entered in the same row.
- Indication of a recessive allele
  - Notation: RecessiveData =
  - Possible values: 0 (co-dominant data), 1 (recessive data)
  - Example: RecessiveData =1
  - Default value: 0

Because the HLA loci are codominant, "1" is used as the parameter when dealing with HLA Data

- The code for the recessive allele
  - Notation: RecessiveAllele =
  - Possible values: Any string of characters within double quotation marks. This character string can be used explicitly in the input file to indicate the occurrence of a recessive homozygote at one orseveral loci.
  - Example: RecessiveAllele ="xxx"
  - Default value: "null"
- The character used to code for missing data
  - Notation: MissingData =
  - Possible values: A character used to specify the code for missing data, which can be
  - entered between single or double quotes.
  - Example: MissingData ='$'
  - Default value: '?'
- The absolute or relative values of haplotype or phenotype frequencies
  - Notation: Frequency =

  - Possible values: ABS (absolute values), REL (relative values: absolute values will be found by multiplying the relative frequencies by the sample sizes)
  - Example: Frequency = ABS
  - Default value: ABS
- The number of significant digits for haplotype frequency outputs
  - Notation: FrequencyThreshold =
  - Possible values: A real number between 1e-2 and 1e-7
  - Example: FrequencyThreshold = 0.00001
  - Default value: 1e-5
- The convergence criterion for the EM algorithm used to estimate haplotype frequencies and linkage disequilibrium from genotypic data
  - Notation: EpsilonValue =
  - Possible values: A real number between 1e-7 and 1e-12.
  - Example: EpsilonValue = 1e-10
  - Default value: 1e-7

4.1.1.3. Data section

In this obligatory subsection, the user defines the haplotypic or genotypic content of the different samples to be analyzed. Each sample definition begins with the keyword Sample-Name and ends after the SampleData have been defined.

The user must specify the following parameters:

- A name for each sample
  - Notation: SampleName =
  - Possible values: Any string of characters within quotation marks
  - Example: SampleName= "A first example of a sample name"
- Thesample size
  - Notation: SampleSize =
  - Possible values: Any integer value
  - Example: SampleSize=732.

    Note: For haplotypic data, the sample size is equal to the haploid sample size. For genotypic data, the sample size should be equal to the number of diploid individuals present in the sample.

- The data
  - Notation: SampleData =
  - Possible values: A list of haplotypes or genotypes and their frequencies contained in the sample, which is entered within braces.
  - Example:

```
    SampleData={
                    MAN0102   1   A33   Cw10   B70    #pseudo-haplotypes
                                  A33   Cw10   B7801  #the second pseudo-haplotype
}
```

If the gametic phase is known, the pseudo-haplotypes are treated as truly defined haplotypes. If the gametic phase is unknown, then only the allelic content of each locus is known.

4.1.1.4. Examples of input files

(1) Example of standard data (genotypic data, unknown gametic phase, recessive alleles)

In this example, the individual genotypes for 5 HLA loci are entered on two separate lines. In this example, the gametic phase between loci is unknown, and the data contains a recessive allele, which has been defined specifically as "xxx". Notably, with recessive data, all of the single locus homozygotes are considered potential heterozygotes with a null allele.

```
[Profile]
Title="Genotypic Data, Phase Unknown, 5 HLA loci"
NbSamples=1
GenotypicData=1
DataType=STANDARD
LocusSeparator=WHITESPACE
MissingData='?'
GameticPhase=0
RecessiveData=1
RecessiveAllele="xxx"
[Data]
[[Samples]]
SampleName="Population 1"
SampleSize=63
SampleData={
MAN0102  12 A33  Cw10  B70   DR1304  DQ0301
            A33  Cw10  B7801  DR1304  DQ0302
MAN0103  22 A33  Cw10  B70   DR1301  DQ0301
            A33  Cw10  B7801  DR1302  DQ0501
MAN0108  23 A23  Cw6  B35  DR1102  DQ0301
```

```
                A29   Cw7   B57   DR1104   DQ0602
MAN0109    6    A30   Cw4   B35   DR0801   xxx
                A68   Cw4   B35   DR0801   xxx
    }
```

(2) Example of standard data (genotypic data, known gametic phase)

In this example, three samples that consist of standard multi-loci data with known gametic phase have been defined. Therefore, the alleles listed on the same line constitute a haplotype on a given chromosome. For example, the genotype G1 consists of the following two haplotypes: A23-Cw6 on one chromosome and A29-Cw7 on the second.

```
[Profile]
Title="An example of genotypic data with known gametic phase"
NbSamples=3
GenotypicData=1
GameticPhase=1
RecessiveData=0
DataType=STANDARD
LocusSeparator=WHITESPACE
[Data]
[[Samples]]
SampleName="standard_pop1"
SampleSize=20
SampleData= {
G1   4   A23   Cw6
         A29   Cw7
G2   5   A30   Cw4
         A68   Cw4
}
```

4.1.2. The calculation of Hardy-Weinberg equilibrium and genetic parameters

4.1.2.1. The calculation of Hardy-Weinberg equilibrium

Performing an exact test of Hardy-Weinberg equilibrium (HWE) tests the hypothesis that the observed diploid genotypes are the product of a random union of gametes. This test is only possible for genotypic data, and separate tests are carried out at each locus. This test is analogous to Fisher's exact test on a two-by-two contingency table but extended to a contingency table of arbitrary size. If the gametic phase is unknown, then the test is only possible locus by locus. For data with a known gametic phase, the association at the haplotypic level within individuals can be tested.

The settings for the Hardy-Weinberg equilibrium test are displayed in Figure 2, and the output results are provided in Figure 3:

http://dx.doi.org/10.5772/57493

Locus by locus: Perform a separate HWE test for each locus.

Whole haplotype: Perform an HWE test at the haplotype level (if the gametic phase is available).

Locus by locus and whole haplotype: Perform both types of tests (if the gametic phase is available)

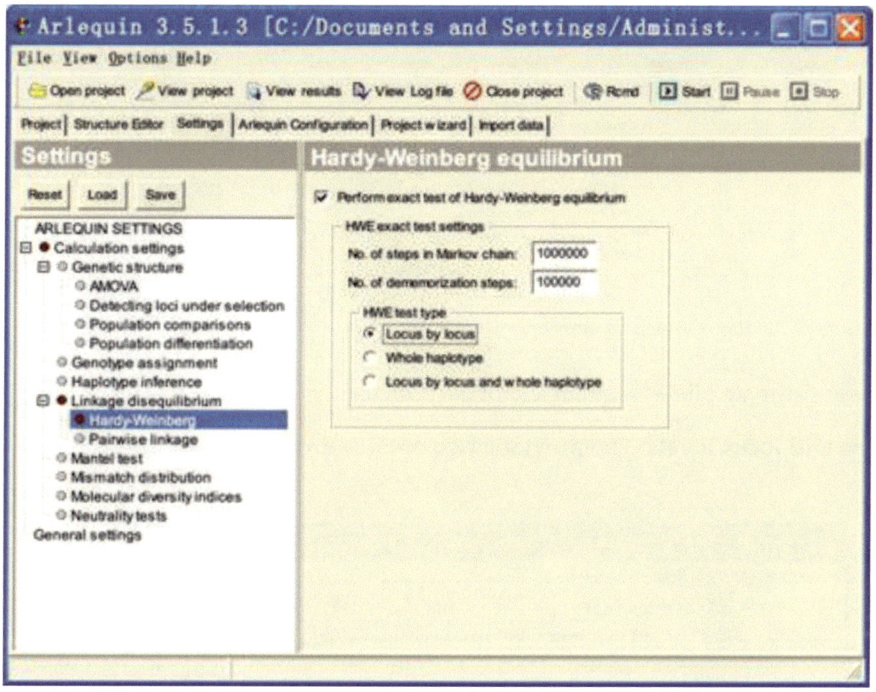

Figure 2. Settings for the Hardy-Weinberg equilibrium test

4.1.2.2. The calculation of genetic parameters

(1) Allele frequency, genotype frequency, and haplotype frequency

When genotypic data with an unknown gametic phase is being processed, two methods can be employed to infer haplotypes: the Expectation-Maximization (EM) algorithm (maximum-likelihood (ML)), which is the most commonly used, or the ELB algorithm (Bayesian).

When the gametic phase is not known or when recessive alleles are present, the ML haplotype frequencies are estimated from the observed data using an EM algorithm for multi-locus genotypic data. The settings are provided in Figure 4, and the results are shown in Figure 5.1, 5.2, and 5.3.

EM algorithms can be performed at the following levels:

Haplotype level: Estimate haplotype frequencies for haplotypes defined by alleles at all loci.

```
=====================================================================================
== Sample :       A test HLA sample
=====================================================================================


===================================
== Hardy-Weinberg equilibrium : (A test HLA sample)
===================================

            Guo, S. and Thompson, E. 1992.
            Levene H. (1949).

Exact test using a Markov chain (for all Loci):
Forecasted chain length        :1000000
Dememorization steps           :100000

------------------------------------------------------------------------------
Locus  #Genot        Obs.Het.      Exp.Het.    P-value      s.d.   Steps done
------------------------------------------------------------------------------
    1      19        0.78947       0.76671     0.13879   0.00037      1001000
    2      19        0.26316       0.80370     0.00000   0.00000      1001000
    3      19        0.84211       0.86486     0.00322   0.00005      1001000
    4      19        0.73684       0.90185     0.00004   0.00001      1001000
    5      19        0.89474       0.70697     0.18591   0.00048      1001000
------------------------------------------------------------------------------
```

Figure 3. Results of the Hardy-Weinberg equilibrium test

Locus level: Estimate allele frequencies for each locus.

Haplotype and locus levels: The previous two options are performed in succession.

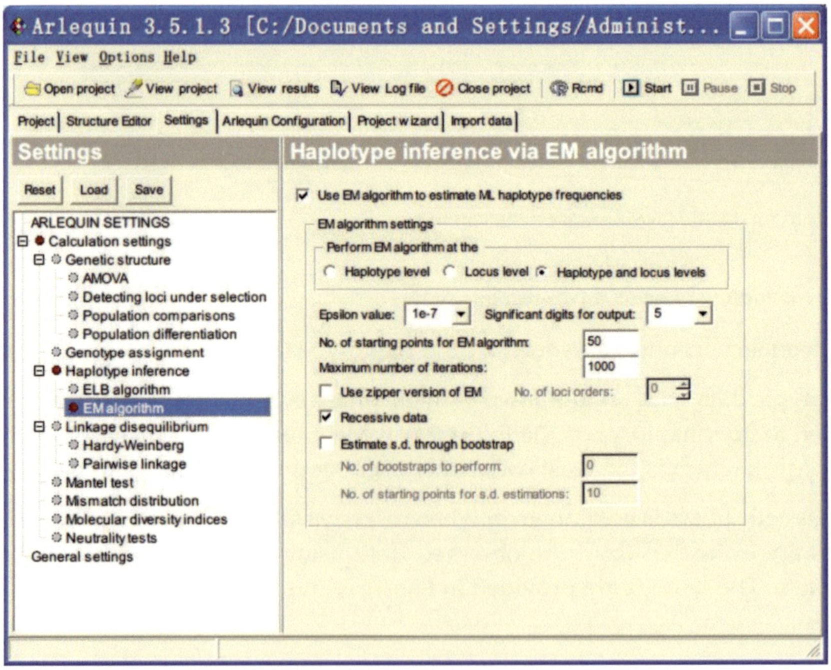

Figure 4. Settings for EM algorithmwith unknown gametic phase

```
===================================
== Haplotypes frequency estimation : (A test HLA sample)
===================================

(1)
-----------------------------------
Conventional EM algorithm  (one pass)
-----------------------------------
No. of gene copies in sample              : 38
No. of random initial conditions for EM   : 50
No. of different maximum likelihoods found : 12
Epsilon value for stopping iterations      : 1.000000e-07
LogLHood  : -99.66905848

Reference: Excoffier, L. and M. Slatkin. 1995.

Standard deviations not computed

-----------------------------------------
Maximum-likelihood haplotype frequencies :
-----------------------------------------

Total number of possible haplotypes     :        410
Minimum frequency to reach for output   :     1.00e-05

-----------------------------------
   #   Haplotype    Freq.      s.d.
-----------------------------------

   1     UNKNOWN  0.052632    0.000000 A2 NULL B7 DR1601 DQ0502
   2     UNKNOWN  0.026316    0.000000 A23 Cw4 B5102 DR0802 DQ0301
   3     UNKNOWN  0.026316    0.000000 A23 Cw6 B35 DR1104 DQ0602
   4     UNKNOWN  0.026316    0.000000 A23 Cw7 B49 DR1304 DQ0301
   5     UNKNOWN  0.026316    0.000000 A23 Cw7 B7 DR1101 DQ0301

-----------------------------------------
(2)  Maximum-likelihood frequencies of genotypes
-----------------------------------------

(Haplotypes that are not listed above have a negative id)

===============
Phenotype #   1
===============
    Name          Abs. Freq.      Rel. Freq.
 MAN0102              1            0.004155

List of genotypes (   30)
-----------------------
Gen. #    Rel. Freq.       Exp. Freq.        Hapl. IDs    Haplotypes
   1      0.990730         0.004117                 25    A33 Cw10 B7801 DR1304 DQ0301
                                                    21    A33 Cw10 B70 DR1304 DQ0302
   2      0.001324         0.000006                 25    A33 Cw10 B7801 DR1304 DQ0301
                                                    47    NULL NULL B70 NULL DQ0302
(3)  Allele frequencies :

(0 bootstrap replicates)
Allele frequencies for the locus 1
--------------------------------

No. of gene copies in sample               : 38
No. of random initial conditions for EM    : 50
No bootstrap confidence interval estimation
No. of different maximum likelihoods found : 1
Epsilon value for stopping iterations       : 1.00000e-07
Logarithm of the sample maximum-likelihood  : -50.3215

-----------------------------------------
Maximum-likelihood haplotype frequencies :
-----------------------------------------

Total number of possible haplotypes     :          8
Minimum frequency to reach for output   :     1.00e-05

-----------------------------------
   #   Haplotype    Freq.      s.d.
-----------------------------------

   1     UNKNOWN  0.052632    0.000000 A2
   2     UNKNOWN  0.105263    0.000000 A23
   3     UNKNOWN  0.052632    0.000000 A29
   4     UNKNOWN  0.263158    0.000000 A30
```

Figure 5. Results of allele frequency, genotype frequencyand haplotype frequency

The settings when process in haplotypic data or genotypic (diploid) data with a known gametic phase are displayed in Figure 6, and the contents of the output results are provided in Figures 5.1, 5.2, and 5.3. The following parameters can be used in the process.

Use original definition: Haplotypes are identified according to their original identifier without considering that haplotype molecular definitions could be identical.

Infer from distance matrix: Similar haplotypes will be identified by computing a molecular distance matrix between haplotypes.

Haplotype frequency estimation:

Estimate haplotype frequencies by mere counting: Estimate the ML haplotype frequencies from the observed data using a mere gene counting procedure.

Estimate allele frequencies at all loci: Estimate allele frequencies at all loci separately.

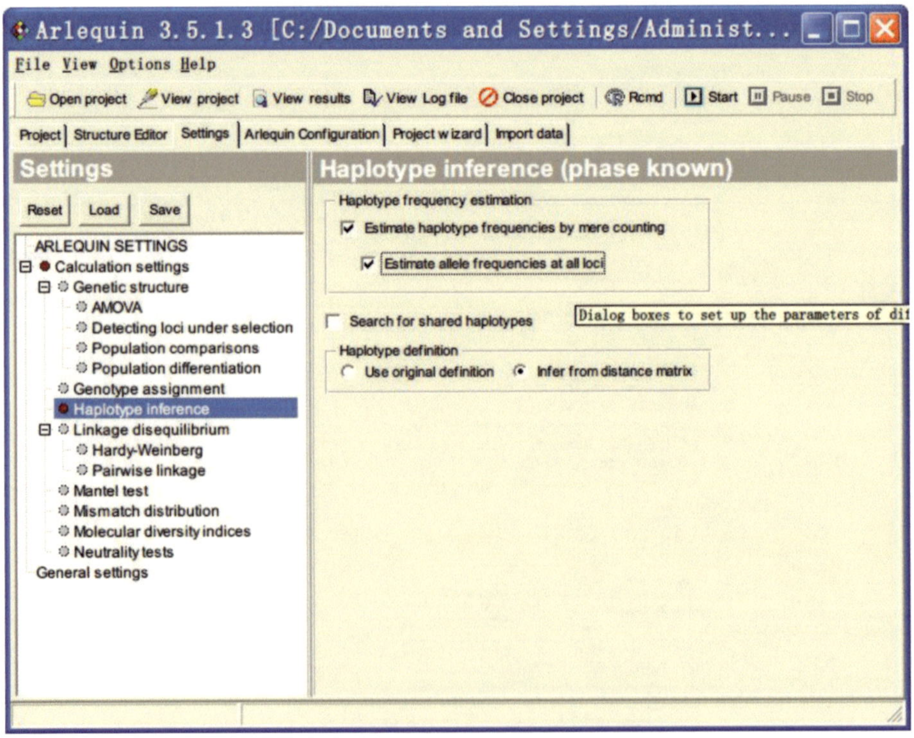

Figure 6. Settings for Haplotype inferencewith a known gametic phase

(2) The estimation of linkage disequilibrium parameters

The settings when processing data where the gametic phase is known are provided in Figure 7, and results of the calculation are shown in Figures 8.1 and 8.2.

Linkage disequilibrium between all pairs of loci: The user can test for the presence of a significant association between pairs of loci based on an exact test of linkage disequilibrium. The number of loci can be arbitrary, but if there are less than two polymorphic loci, this test is not applicable. The test procedure is analogous to Fisher's exact test on a two-by-two contingency table but extended to a contingency table of arbitrary size.

LD coefficients between pairs of alleles at different loci: Using this parameter, the D, D', and r^2 coefficients between all pairs can be calculated. D' is the most commonly used coefficientand represents the above section mentioned relative Δ value.

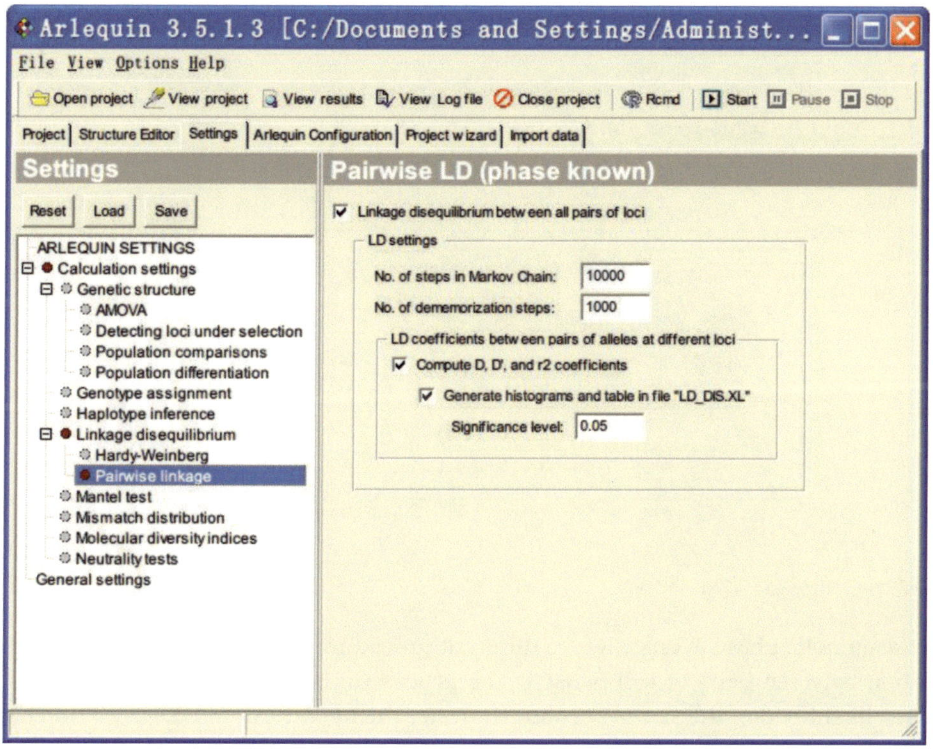

Figure 7. Settings for linkage disequilibrium

(1) == Pairwise linkage disequilibrium : (A test HLA sample)

Slatkin, M. 1994a.
Slatkin, M. and Excoffier, L. 1996.
Lewontin, R. C., and K. Kojima 1960.
Test of linkage disequilibrium for all pairs of loci:

3: Table of disequilibrium values (D=pab-pa*pb) for all two-locus haplotypes

Locus0\Locus1	Cw10	Cw6	Cw7	Cw4	NULL	Cw2	Cw5
A33	0.12	0.02	-0.03	-0.09	-0.01	-0.01	-0.01
A23	-0.03	0.02	0.01	-0.00	-0.02	0.02	-0.00
A29	-0.02	-0.00	0.02	-0.02	-0.01	-0.00	0.02
A30	-0.02	-0.02	0.02	0.06	-0.02	-0.01	-0.01
A68	-0.03	-0.01	-0.01	0.05	0.01	-0.00	-0.00
A2	-0.02	-0.00	-0.01	-0.02	0.04	-0.00	-0.00
A32	-0.01	-0.00	-0.00	0.02	-0.00	-0.00	-0.00

4: Table of standardized disequilibrium values (D'=D/Dmax)

Locus0\Locus1	Cw10	Cw6	Cw7	Cw4	NULL	Cw2	Cw5
A33	0.70	0.45	-0.49	-0.77	-0.16	-1.00	-1.00
A23	-1.00	0.25	0.14	-0.14	-1.00	1.00	-1.00
A29	-1.00	-1.00	0.42	-1.00	-1.00	-1.00	1.00
A30	-0.31	-1.00	0.19	0.30	-0.37	-1.00	-1.00
A68	-1.00	-1.00	-1.00	0.65	0.11	-1.00	-1.00
A2	-1.00	-1.00	-1.00	-1.00	1.00	-1.00	-1.00
A32	-1.00	-1.00	-1.00	1.00	-1.00	-1.00	-1.00

(2) 5: Table of Chi-square values (Chi2=sqr(D)*n/(pa*(1-pa)*pb*(1-pb)))

Locus0\Locus1	Cw10	Cw6	Cw7	Cw4	NULL	Cw2	Cw5
A33	11.62	1.01	0.91	5.98	0.11	0.67	0.67
A23	1.82	1.80	0.55	0.03	0.84	8.73	0.12
A29	0.86	0.18	2.51	0.86	0.40	0.06	18.49
A30	0.53	1.16	0.56	2.92	0.34	0.37	0.37
A68	1.82	0.38	0.68	4.61	0.29	0.12	0.12
A2	0.86	0.18	0.32	0.86	11.26	0.06	0.06
A32	0.42	0.09	0.16	2.52	0.19	0.03	0.03

6: Table of Chi-square P values (1 d.f.)

Locus0\Locus1	Cw10	Cw6	Cw7	Cw4	NULL	Cw2	Cw5
A33	0.00	0.32	0.34	0.01	0.74	0.41	0.41
A23	0.18	0.18	0.46	0.85	0.36	0.00	0.73
A29	0.35	0.67	0.11	0.35	0.53	0.81	0.00
A30	0.47	0.28	0.46	0.09	0.56	0.54	0.54
A68	0.18	0.54	0.41	0.03	0.59	0.73	0.73
A2	0.35	0.67	0.57	0.35	0.00	0.81	0.81
A32	0.52	0.77	0.69	0.11	0.66	0.87	0.87

Figure 8. Results oflinkage disequilibrium

When the gametic phase is unknown, a different procedure for testing the significance of the association between pairs of loci is used. The procedure is based on a likelihood ratio test, where the likelihood of the sample evaluated under the hypothesis of no association between loci (linkage equilibrium) is compared with the likelihood of the sample when association is allowed. The significance of the observed likelihood ratio is found by computing the null distribution of this ratio under the hypothesis of linkage equilibrium, using a permutation procedure. The settings for this procedure are shown in Figure 9, and the output results are provided in Figure 10.

http://dx.doi.org/10.5772/57493

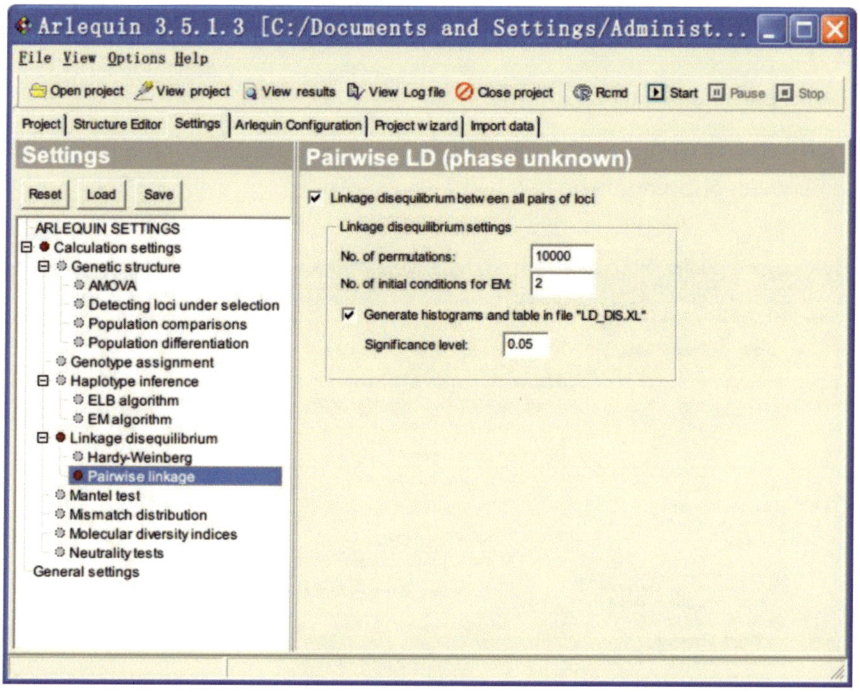

Figure 9. Settings for linkage disequilibrium with unkown phase

```
====================================
== Pairwise linkage disequilibrium : (A test HLA sample)
====================================

          Slatkin, M. 1994a.
          Slatkin, M. and Excoffier, L. 1996.
          Lewontin, R. C., and K. Kojima 1960.

Test of linkage disequilibrium for all pairs of loci:
------------------------------------------------------


Permutation test using the EM algorithm
Number of permutations                 : 10000
Number of initial conditions for EM    : 2

Pair(0, 1)
          LnLHood LD :  -85.13107          LnLHood LE : -110.23678
          Exact P=  0.00129  +-   0.00033 (10100 permutations done)     Chi-square test value=50.21141 (P =  0.05811,  36 d.f.)
Pair(0, 2)
          LnLHood LD :  -86.73838          LnLHood LE : -119.06953
          Exact P=  0.00059  +-   0.00024 (10100 permutations done)     Chi-square test value=64.66230 (P =  0.52355,  66 d.f.)
Pair(1, 2)
          LnLHood LD :  -89.88222          LnLHood LE : -128.66327
          Exact P=  0.00000  +-   0.00000 (10100 permutations done)     Chi-square test value=77.56209 (P =  0.15620,  66 d.f.)
Pair(0, 3)
          LnLHood LD :  -90.92872          LnLHood LE : -127.08772
          Exact P=  0.00010  +-   0.00010 (10100 permutations done)     Chi-square test value=72.31799 (P =  0.27729,  66 d.f.)
```

Figure 10. Results oflinkage disequilibrium with unkown phase

(3) The calculation of genetic distance

Arlequin provides several calculation methods to determine genetic distance, including *Reynolds'* distance, *Slatkin's* linearized coefficient, *Nei's* genetic distance, etc. *Nei's* genetic distance and the *Cavalli-Sforza* genetic distance calculating methods are the most commonly used and produce the most similar results. The settings for calculating genetic distance are shown in Figure 11, and the output results are provided in Figure 12.

The calculation parameters are as follows:

Compute pairwise differences: Computes *Nei's* average number of pairwise differences within and between populations.

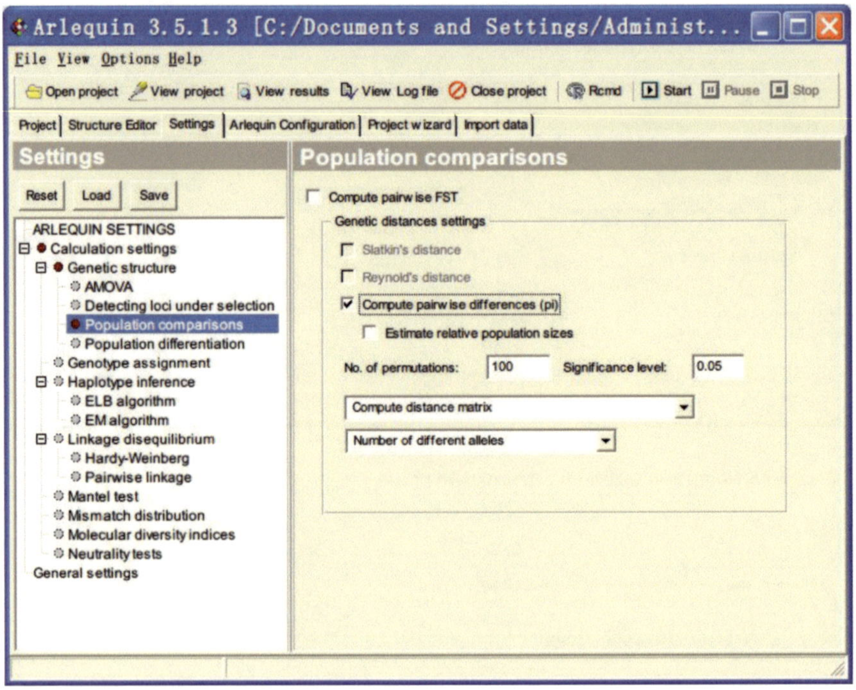

Figure 11. Settings for genetic distance

```
----------------------------------------
Population average pairwise differences
----------------------------------------

Above diagonal    : Average number of pairwise differences between populations (PiXY)
Diagonal elements : Average number of pairwise differences within population (PiX)
Below diagonal    : Corrected average pairwise difference (PiXY-(PiX+PiY)/2)

Distance method: Pairwise differences
```

	1	2	3	4	5	6	7
1	1.77562	1.82713	1.82553	1.80799	1.78133	1.82920	1.86023
2	0.05185	1.77493	1.83481	1.80863	1.76641	1.84444	1.83427
3	0.01880	0.02842	1.83784	1.83406	1.80991	1.85439	1.87138
4	0.02756	0.02855	0.02252	1.78524	1.78046	1.80833	1.85629
5	0.10834	0.09377	0.10581	0.10266	1.57035	1.83631	1.76463
6	0.04114	0.05673	0.03523	0.01547	0.15089	1.80049	1.87949
7	0.13367	0.10806	0.11371	0.12493	0.14071	0.14051	1.67749

Figure 12. Results of genetic distance

http://dx.doi.org/10.5772/57493

4.2. The requirements of data analysis on new-generation HLA typing techniques

HLA data analysis methods have always been closely related to the development of HLA genotyping techniques. In the 1980s and 1990s, HLA serotyping was the preferred technique. HLA phenotypes were determined first, and the square-root method was used commonly to predict HLA genotype frequencies. Currently, HLA genotyping techniques are more prevalent. Researchers tend to use the direct counting method to calculate the genotype. In previous HLA haplotype analyses, the haplotype was predicted using group analysis, and then the individual haplotype frequency was estimated. However, with the considerable cost decrease of genotyping techniques, more pedigree data are available for studies, such as the *Haplomap* program, where haplotypes can be studied directly using pedigree analysis. Moreover, with the development of new-generation gene sequencing techniques and the optimization of large-fragment high-throughput sequencing and fragment (reads) assembly algorithms, individual haplotypes would be distinguished directly. These methods contribute greatly to simplifying the data analyses process.

Currently, HLA data types are no longer limited to allele data. Other types of data, such as SNPs, microsatellite markers, short sequence repeats, etc., could be used for conjoint analysis with HLA data. This chapter has only introduced the application of *Arlequin* software in classic HLA data analysis. However, many other outstanding tools, such as *Phase* are more commonly used in studies of haplotype establishment using group genotype data and hot spot model recombination. *HapView* is more prominent in graphic linkage disequilibrium (LD) and haplotype studies, and the professional statistical software *SAS* is also used commonly for HLA data analysis. With the development of HLA typing techniques and analysis techniques, data processing methods will also become more in-depth and detailed.

Acknowledgements

Supported by grantsfrom the State Key Development Programfor Basic Research of China (No. 2003CB515509 and 2009CB522401) and from National Natural Scientific Foundation of China(No.81070450 and 30470751) to Dr. X.-Y.Z.

Author details

Fang Yuan and Yongzhi Xi*

*Address all correspondence to: xiyz@yahoo.com

Department of Immunology and National Center for Biomedicine Analysis, Beijing Hospital Affiliated to Academy of Medical Sciences, Beijing, PRC

References

[1] Edwards AW. Foundations of Mathematical Genetics, 2nd edition. Cambridge University Press. Cambridge. 2000.

[2] Crow JF. Hardy-Weinberg and Language Impediments. Genetics. 1999, 152: 821.

[3] Masel, Joanna. Rethinking Hardy–Weinberg and Genetic Drift in Undergraduate Biology. BioEssays. 2012, 34: 701.

[4] Cox DR. Principles of Statistical Inference. Cambridge University Press. Cambridge. 2006.

[5] Hu LP. Medical Statistics. People's Military Medical Press. Beijing. 2010.

[6] Xu TH, Wang J. Design of Medical Experiments: Lecture 2, Rules of Randomization and Blinding Method. Chinese Medical Journal. 2005, 40: 54.

[7] Marsh SG, Albert ED, Bodmer WF, et al. Nomenclature for Factors of the HLA System. 2010.

[8] Robinson J, Waller MJ, Fail SC, et al. The IMGT/HLA database. Nucleic Acids Research. 2009,37: 1013.

[9] Sharon L. Sampling: Design and Analysis, 2nd edition. Cengage Learning. 2009.

[10] Tan JM, Tissue Typing Technique and Clinical Application, 1st edition. People's Medical Publishing House. Beijing, 2002.

[11] Wang XZ. Principles of Population Genetics. Sichuan University Press. Chengdu. 1994.

[12] Guo J, Hu LP. Medical Genetics Statistics and SAS Application. People's Medical Publishing House. Beijing. 2012.

[13] Weir BS. Genetic Data Analysis II: Methods for Discrete Population Genetic Data. Sinauer Associates Inc. USA. 1996.

[14] Excoffier L, Slatkin M. Maximum-Likelihood Estimation Of Molecular Haplotype Frequencies In A Diploid Population. Molecular Biology and Evolution. 1995, 12:921.

[15] Excoffier L, Slatkin M. Incorporating genotypes of relatives into a test of linkage disequilibrium. The American Journal of Human Genetics. 1998, 171-180.

[16] Guo S, Thompson E. Performing the Exact Test of Hardy-Weinberg Proportion for Multiple Alleles. Biometrics. 1992, 48:361.

[17] Raymond M, Rousset F. An Exact Test for Population Differentiation. Evolution. 1995,49:1280.

[18] Gaggiotti O, Excoffier L. A Simple Method of Removing the Effect of a Bottleneck and Unequal Population Sizes on Pairwise Genetic Distances. Proceedings of the Royal Society London. 2000, 267: 81.

[19] Dempster A, Laird N, Rubin D. Maximum Likelihood Estimation From Incomplete Data via the EM Algorithm. Journal of the Royal Statistical Society. 1977, 39:1.

[20] Cavalli-Sforza LL, Population structure and human evolution. Proceedings of the Royal Society London, 1966, 164, 362.

[21] Cavalli-Sforza LL, Bodmer WF. The Genetics of Human Populations. W.H. Freeman Publishers. San Francisco. 1971.

[22] Lange K, Mathematical and Statistical Methods for Genetic Analysis. Springer. New York. 1997

[23] Excoffier L, Lischer H. Arlequin Suite ver 3.5: A New Series of Programs to Perform Population Genetics Analyses under Linux and Windows. Molecular Ecology Resources. 2010, 10: 564.

[24] Stephens M, Scheet P. Accounting for Decay of Linkage Disequilibrium in Haplotype Inference and Missing-Data Imputation. American Journal of Human Genetics. 2005, 76:449-462.

[25] Scheet P, Stephens M. A Fast and Flexible Statistical Model for Large-Scale Population Genotype Data: Applications to Inferring Missing Genotypes and Haplotypic Phase. American Journal of Human Genetics. 2006, 78: 629.

Chapter 2

HLA Class I Polymorphism and Tapasin Dependency

Soumya Badrinath, Trevor Huyton,
Rainer Blasczyk and Christina Bade-Doeding

Additional information is available at the end of the chapter

http://dx.doi.org/10.5772/57495

1. Introduction

Human leucocyte antigens (HLA) are highly specialized proteins, expressed on all nucleated cells and platelets, that form stable complexes with peptides of self or pathogenic proteins generated by proteasomal degradation. These peptide-HLA (pHLA) complexes are presented at the cell surface where they are subsequently recognized by T cells. Thus, T cells with their specific antigenic receptor (TCR) continuously scan an array of pHLA complexes which are presented on the cell surface [1]. One of the distinct properties of TCRs is that they can recognize an antigen only when it is associated with a host or "self"-encoded HLA molecule. This property of T cells was discovered by Zinkernagel and Doherty in 1974 and is called ′MHC-restriction′ [2]. The recognition of pHLA complexes by TCRs regulates many immunological responses such as antiviral cytolysis, graft or tumor rejection and regulation of B cell function. The genes encoding for HLA molecules are known to be the most polymorphic genes present in the whole genome. To date more than 9,000 HLA alleles have been identified of which there are ~7,300 HLA class I and ~2,200 class II polymorphic alleles (Figure 1) [3].

These polymorphisms do not occur throughout the HLA molecule, but are confined to specific AA positions in the peptide-binding region (PBR) [4, 5, 6]. They can cause alterations in the conformation of the PBR, thus changing the peptide binding specificities of these molecules [7]. The frequency of HLA alleles varies greatly among different ethnic groups. It has been postulated that evolutionary pressures such as those exerted by epidemics of infectious diseases might lead to the evolution of new HLA alleles having distinct peptide binding properties.

Following hematopoietic stem cell transplantation (HSCT), polymorphic differences between donor and recipient HLA class I molecules can lead to transplant rejection or graft-versus-host disease (GvHD). Extensive clinical data have demonstrated that the risk of GvHD strongly

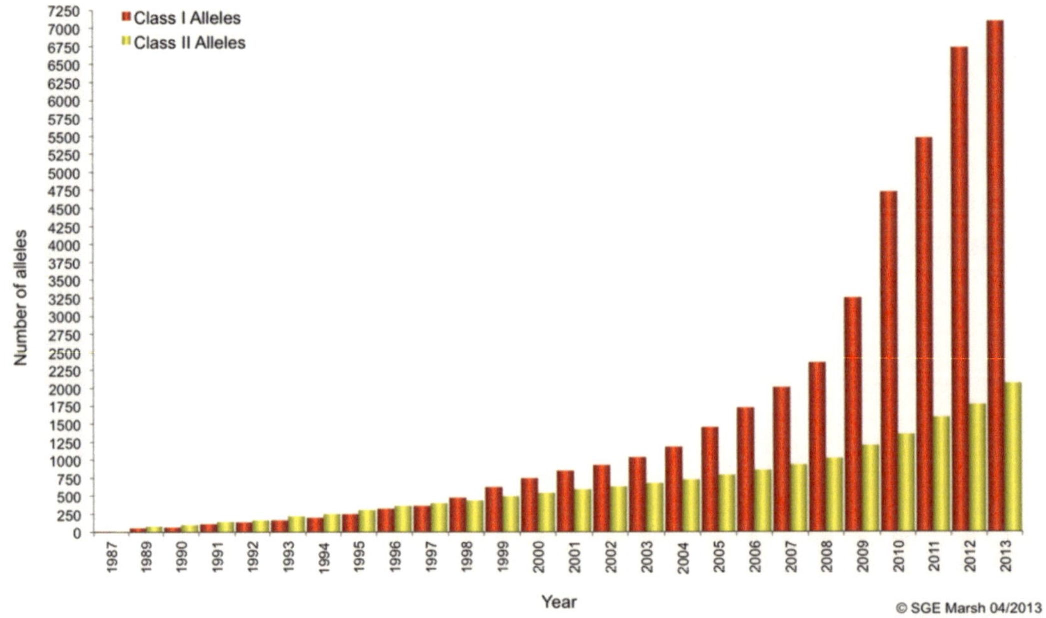

There are currently 9,719 HLA and related alleles described by the HLA nomenclature and included in the IMGT/HLA Database. Red bars represent class I alleles and yellow bards represent class II alleles. As of 2013, there are around 7,353 class I alleles and 2,202 class II alleles that have been identified [3].

Figure 1. Number of HLA alleles that have been identified from the year 1987 until 2013

correlates with the number and kind of HLA mismatches and that both the type of amino acid (AA) substitution and its location within the HLA molecule can directly influence the transplantation outcome. Polymorphisms occurring within the PBR of HLA class I molecules determine which allogenic peptides are selectively bound and subsequently recognized as self or non-self by the effector T-lymphocytes that survey pHLA complexes on antigen presenting cells. Assembly of MHC class I heavy chain (hc) and β2 microglobulin (β2m) subunits with peptides is assisted by the peptide loading complex (PLC). Initially, proteasomally digested peptides are transported into the endoplasmic reticulum (ER) via the transporter associated with antigen processing (TAP) and are then loaded onto HLA class I molecules with the assistance of the PLC. The transmembrane glycoprotein tapasin (TPN) functions within this multimeric PLC as a disulfide-linked heterodimer along with the thiol oxidoreductase ERp57 to stabilize the empty class I molecule and promotes the selection of high affinity peptides. In addition to bridging HLA class I molecules with TAP, TPN was found to stabilize the peptide-receptive state of HLA class I molecules and increased the steady state levels of TAP heterodimers. Certain HLA class I polymorphisms within the PBR appear not only to influence the repertoire of bound peptides, but also determine the requirement for PLC mediated acquisition and optimal loading of peptides for the given HLA class I molecule. Whereas most class I allotypes associate strongly with the PLC and are highly dependent upon TPN for effective presentation of high affinity peptides and cell surface expression, others can acquire peptides even without assistance from the PLC but are then sub-optimally loaded. Due to the crucial role of TPN in selecting peptides, its indirect role in the immunorecognition of pathogens becomes obvious. This makes TPN an ideal target for viruses to interfere with the presentation of viral peptides to CTLs. For instance, US3 protein of HCMV binds to TPN and acts as a TPN inhibitor. This affects the antigen presentation by TPN-dependent HLA class I molecules. However, TPN-independent molecules can selectively escape the US3 mediated class I retention and continue to present the viral peptides.

Given HLA class I polymorphisms affect the generic antigen processing pathway and their dependency on TPN for antigen presentation. TPN-independency is occurring very rarely and might have evolved as an evolutionary trade-off to combat viral infections. However, presentation of unusual ligands by certain HLA class I alleles could be a risk factor during stem cell transplantation and needs to be considered during donor selection process. The future of HSCT relies on our understanding of how successful clinical outcomes can be achieved despite patient-donor allelic mismatches.

2. HLA polymorphisms and transplantation

The HLA system is one of the major barriers in hematopoietic stem cell transplantation (HSCT) and the degree of HLA matching is found to reflect on the outcome following transplantation. The best result following HSCT is achieved when an identical twin or a genotypically HLA identical sibling is used as donor. However, only 30 % of the donors for HSCT have a HLA identical sibling donor available [8]. Therefore, in most of the situations, HLA haplo-identical related, matched unrelated or partially matched related or unrelated donors are considered for transplantation. However, these transplants are associated with high risks of post-transplant complications such as graft failure/rejection or graft-versus-host disease (GvHD), mainly because of undefined or HLA incompatibilities. Many studies have demonstrated the negative impacts of HLA mismatches on the outcome following HSCT [9-11]. To understand the magnitude of distinct mismatches between HLA variants, several studies analyzed allele specific peptide motifs towards a rating of incompatibility [12-21] [22] [23, 24]. The knowledge of the peptide binding motifs of individual alleles and their comparison within allelic groups is the basis for understanding the impact of a given mismatch and is fundamental in predicting the relevance of allelic differences. Since allelic mismatches occurring at critical residues within the class I heavy chain may cause allorecognition, high resolution matching of patients and unrelated donors have been found to significantly improve post-transplant survival [25], lower the incidence and severity of GvHD [26, 27] and improve engraftment [28, 29]. The question whether a mismatch is permissive or not is critical in deciding which individual is the best matched donor. This could be achieved by conducting a systematic study to determine the effect of AA sequence polymorphisms on the function of a particular HLA molecule and on the immune responses post-transplantation.

3. HLA class I molecules and the peptide loading complex

HLA class I molecules loaded with high affinity peptides are essential for efficient immune surveillance and elimination of virally infected cells by CTLs. Newly synthesized class I hc and ß2m are translocated into the ER by their amino terminal signal sequences. Following translocation, HLA class I hcs are glycosylated and folded by the formation of two intra-chain disulphide bonds. Calnexin (CNX) facilitates the stabilization of class I hc and its association with ß2m. Following the formation of class I hc - ß2m heterodimer, CNX is replaced by calreticulin (CRT). Peptides are loaded onto the class I heterodimer by a complex machinery consisting of many chaperons, known as the peptide loading complex (PLC). The PLC consists of the transporter associated with antigen processing (TAP) heterodimers, transmembrane glycoprotein – TPN, lectin like chaperon – CRT, thiol oxidoreductase – Erp57 which is non-covalently associated with CRT and disulphide linked to TPN (Figure 2).

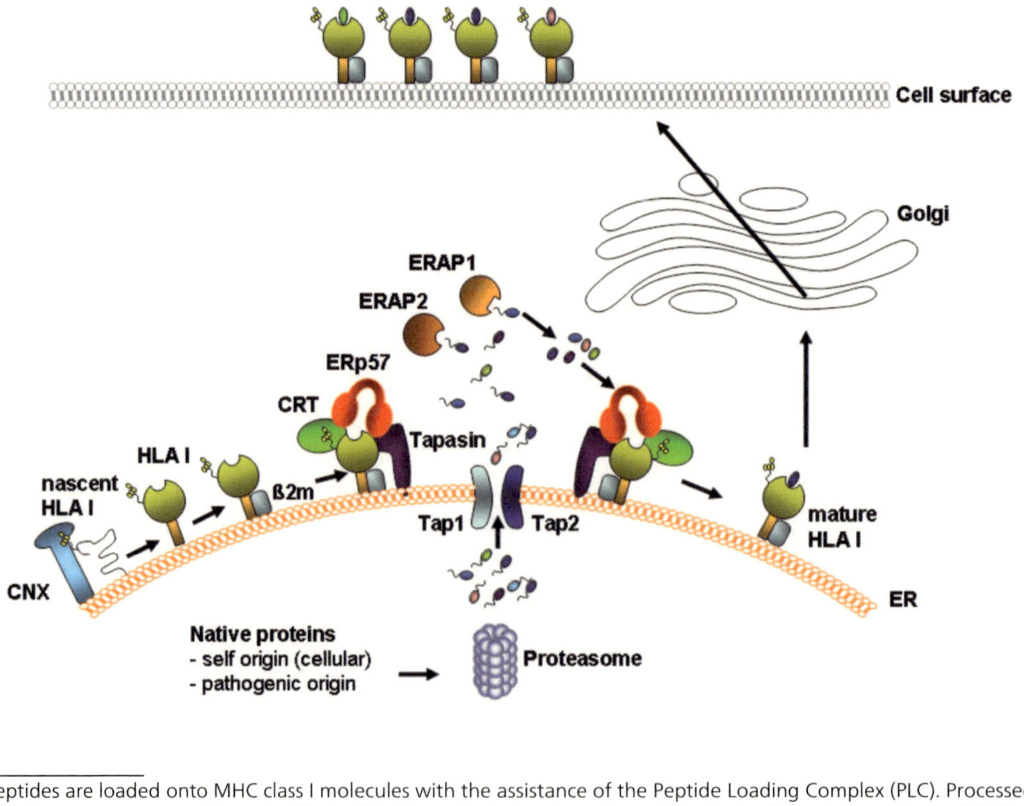

Peptides are loaded onto MHC class I molecules with the assistance of the Peptide Loading Complex (PLC). Processed peptides are transported into the ER via TAP. N-terminal trimming of peptides via the ER aminopeptidases (ERAP) 1 and 2. TPN functions within the multimeric PLC as a disulfide-linked, stable heterodimer with the thiol oxidoreductase ERp57.

Figure 2. Peptide loading complex

Peptides presented by HLA class I molecules originate mostly from cytosolic or nuclear proteins and are processed by the proteasome, a multicatalytic protease complex. TAP helps in the translocation of peptides from cytosol into the ER lumen. TPN bridges class I - ß2m heterodimer to TAP and acts as a peptide editor, facilitating the loading of high affinity peptides onto HLA class I molecules. Stable HLA class I molecules dissociate from TAP heterodimers and are transported through the golgi complex to the cell surface where they present peptides to CD8+ T cells.

4. Tapasin

TPN is a type 1 transmembrane glycoprotein, 428 amino acid long and consisting of three parts: an N-terminal ER luminal region consisting of two domains, a transmembrane domain and a short cytoplasmic tail. TPN has multitudinous roles within the PLC, all of which are directed towards peptide presentation by the class I molecules. The transmembrane domain of TPN interacts with TAP and bridges TAP to class I molecules. TPN facilitates the stabilization of TAP and promotes the binding and translocation of peptides by TAP. Absence of TPN abrogates the binding of class I molecules to TAP. It was also shown that certain class I molecules presented at the cell surface in the absence/independent of TPN were very unstable and dissociated rapidly. The double lysine motif at the C-terminus of the TPN molecule mediates its interaction with coat protein type I (COP I) vesicle and facilitates the recycling of class I molecules which have not been not loaded with optimal peptides. Mutational analysis identified a conserved region on the ER-luminal domain of TPN that interacts with HLA class I molecules and was found to be critical for peptide loading and its editing function. Polymorphisms occurring in HLA class I molecules are found to affect the dependency of these molecules on TPN for antigen presentation and cell surface expression.

5. Inhibitors of TPN

TPN is a critical component of the PLC which plays an important role in optimization and selection of peptides subsequently presented on the cell surface by HLA class I molecules [30, 31]. Transmembrane glycoprotein US3 expressed during the immediate early phase of HCMV infection binds to TPN and inhibits its ability to load kinetically stable peptides onto HLA class I molecules, thus retaining class I molecules in the ER [32]. However, not all HLA class I molecules are equally affected by US3, thus highlighting that not all HLA class I molecules are equally dependent upon TPN for maturation in the ER [33]. US3 and TPN are associated by their ER luminal domains, but the transmembrane domains are also required for the inhibition of TPN [32]. Another transmembrane glycoprotein E3-19K from the adenovirus also inhibits crucial functioning of TPN by blocking its ability to bridge TAP to HLA class I molecules. E3-19K associates with TAP and impairs the formation of TAP-TPN complex and inclusion of TAP in the PLC [34]. This competitive inhibition by E3-19K delays the maturation and assembly of TPN-dependent HLA class I loading complex [34].

Certain other viral proteins prevent surface expression of HLA class I molecules by retention or degradation of HLA molecules in the ER. For example, cowpox virus protein 203 (CPXV 203] causes retention of HLA class I molecules in the ER [35]. US2 and US11 proteins from HCMV and mK3 protein from mouse herpes virus directs HLA class I molecules towards proteasomal degradation [36] [37] [38] [39]. Sorters such as HIV-1 protein Nef and murine CMV protein gp48 averts the trafficking of HLA class I molecules from golgi to lysosomal compartment where they are subsequently degraded [40] [41] [42].

6. Interactions between HLA class I molecules and TPN

In addition to bridging HLA class I molecules to TAP, TPN was found to stabilize the peptide-receptive state of class I molecules [43] and increase the steady state levels of TAP heterodimers [44]. TPN also facilitated the retention of empty class I molecules in the ER of insect cells [30]. Barnden *et al* demonstrated that TPN prevented premature exit of HLA class I molecules from the ER of mammalian cells, thus suggesting a potential role for TPN in the retention of sub-optimally loaded class I molecules in the ER [45]. HLA class I molecules expressed in TPN-deficient cells were found to be unstable and were loaded with a significant proportion of suboptimal ligands [33, 46, 47]. Yu *et al* demonstrated that mutations occurring at residues 128-136 in the $\alpha 2$ helix of class I heavy chain affected the interaction of HLA class I molecules with TPN. These residues are located in the loop region connecting β-pleated sheets below the peptide binding groove with an α-helix reaching above the groove. This region of the heavy which forms a potential interacting site with TPN was found to be sensitive to peptide binding and underwent conformational changes, thus implying the ability of TPN to distinguish between empty and peptide-bound HLA class I molecules [48, 49]. Some groups have speculated about the interaction of TPN with the $\alpha 3$ domain of HLA class I heavy chain [50]. However, given that residues 128–136 in the $\alpha 2$ domain and residues 227–229 in the $\alpha 3$ domain are located on the same plane along the side of class I heavy chain, TPN might be able to interact with both these determinants. Mutations occurring in the HLA class I heavy chain were found to affect the interaction of these molecules with the loading complex components [49, 51-53]. However, precise interacting surfaces/interfaces between the class I molecules and TPN are yet to be defined. To determine the potential interacting surfaces of TPN with HLA class I molecules, Dong *et al* initially compared the sequence of TPN across different species and identified a region in the N terminal domain of TPN that was highly conserved amongst these species [54]. Residues occurring in this region and in other parts of the TPN molecule were mutated and the effect of these mutations on PLC function was tested. Eight different TPN mutants conjugated with ERp57 were incubated with extracts from LCL 721.220/B*08:01 cells that are enriched with empty HLA class I molecules. Co-immunoprecipitation experiments were performed to determine the interaction of HLA class I molecules with these different TPN mutants. HLA class I molecules associated at normal levels with the wild type TPN; with two other TPN mutants in which amino terminal residues (TN1 and TN2) located farthest from the conserved patches were mutated and TPN mutant with a single polymorphism located in the carboxy terminal region (TC1). Mutating the residues in the central, conserved patch of

TPN molecule (TN6 - Glu185Lys, Arg187Glu, Gln189Ser and Gln261Ser) completely abolished its binding with the class I heavy chain. Also, only small amounts of the heavy chain were found to interact with the mutants located in or around the conserved patch. The ability of HLA class I binding to wild type/mutant TPN molecules reflected their relative capacities in mediating peptide loading. TN6 mutant mediated only 8 % of peptide loading activity in. 220.B*08:01 molecules as compared to the activity of wild type TPN. It was also observed that the transduction of TN6 mutant into TPN independent 220.B*44:02 cells did not favour the surface expression of these molecules on the cell surface· The conserved, functionally important central region of TPN was suggested to be responsible for the stabilization of the α2-helix of the PBR. This stabilization was found to maintain the peptide binding groove in an open peptide-receptive conformation until an optimal peptide binds to it [54]. The findings from this study are in agreement with previous studies conducted where Thr134Lys mutation in HLA-A*02:01 was found to disrupt its interaction with TPN [47]. Co-immunoprecipitation experiments performed by Lehner *et al* demonstrated that deletion of the transmembrane region of TPN did not have any effect on the interaction of HLA class I molecules with TPN. However, HLA class I molecules failed to co-precipitate with TPN molecules truncated at the N terminus, suggesting that the residues in this region were important for the interaction of HLA class I molecules with TPN [43].

7. Peptide editing function of TPN

Many studies have highlighted the role of TPN in stabilizing HLA class I molecules [30, 31, 45, 55] and maintaining them in a peptide-receptive conformation [56]. It has also been shown that TPN facilitates peptide optimization, a process in which bound peptides of low affinity are exchanged for the high affinity ones [45, 57-61]. These functions were attributed to TPN based on the findings that the class I-peptide complexes expressed on the surface of cells lacking TPN were less stable than those complexes expressed on normal cells containing TPN. However, analysis of peptides eluted from HLA class I complexes expressed on the cell surface in the presence and absence of TPN demonstrated no co-relation between the decreased stability of HLA class I-peptide complexes and binding of low-affinity peptides in TPN deficient cells [62]. The authors suggested that the plausible ability of TPN to stabilize immature HLA class I molecules in the ER instead broadens the bound peptide repertoire both in terms of complexity of bound peptides and their binding affinities [62]. A more recent study conducted by Howarth *et al* demonstrated key functions of TPN in shaping the peptide repertoire presented to the cell surface based on their intrinsic half-lives [63]. They investigated the effect of TPN on the presentation of a hierarchy of peptides generated based on the H2-K^b-binding peptide SIINFEKL by varying the anchor residues in order to produce peptides having a wide array of binding affinities. These peptides were expressed stably as mini-genes in the cytosol of TPN deficient cell line.220K^b and in.220K^b TPN transfected cell line. Results indicated all the peptides to be presented at high levels in the presence of TPN and their relative expression levels were found to be in accordance to their peptide-half lives. However, in the absence of TPN, this hierarchy was disrupted and a peptide with intermediate half-life was found to be presented more dominantly than the rest of the peptides. Since all the peptides utilized in this study had similar affinities to H2-K^b-binding peptide SIINFEKL, editing function by TPN was suggested to be influenced primarily by the peptide-off rate rather than peptide-affinity per se [63].

Many groups have established *in vitro* assays to provide a molecular understanding of the mechanisms of peptide editing by TPN. However, weak intrinsic interactions between TPN and HLA class I molecules make it difficult to perform *in vitro* experiments using recombinant TPN to assess its functions. In order to overcome this problem, Chen *et al* used leucine zippers to tether soluble TPN together with HLA class I molecules [56]. For this study, they selected HLA-B*08:01 as this allele has earlier shown to be TPN dependent [33] for normal levels of cell surface expression. The results of this study indicated that TPN acts as a chaperon by accelerating the ratio of active to inactive-peptide deficient HLA class I molecules. In addition to stabilizing HLA class I molecules, TPN was also found to increase the association-dissociation rates of peptides with class I molecules owing to its ability to widen the peptide binding groove, thereby enabling a diversified set of peptides to initially bind into the groove. This TPN-assisted mechanism of peptide selection was suggested to be mediated by disruption of the conserved hydrogen bonds at the C terminus of the binding groove [56]. In yet another approach to determine the peptide-editing mechanism of TPN, Wearsch *et al* reconstituted the PLC subcomplex *in vitro* by co-incubating recombinant soluble TPN-ERp57 conjugate with additional cell extracts containing CRT and peptide receptive heavy chain-β2m complex [59]. The results from their study demonstrated that the TPN-ERp57 conjugate promoted rapid exchange of sub-optimal low and intermediate peptides with high affinity ones [59]. Praveen *et al* demonstrated an alternative approach to explore the TPN-mediated peptide editing function in the lumen of ER microsome [60], wherein components of the loading complex can interact with each other with their native affinities. For their experiments, they used the allomorphs K^b wild type (WT) and K^b mutant (T134K) in which the replacement of Thr134Lys abolished the interaction of these molecules with TPN. They found that when these allomorphs were incubated with a mixture of high affinity peptides and a 100-fold excess of a low affinity peptide or alternatively with the low affinity peptides and a 100-fold reduced concentration of a high affinity peptide, the high affinity peptide was predominantly bound by wild type K^b while K^b mutant (T134K) mostly bound the low affinity ones [60].

8. TPN dependence/ independence of HLA class I molecules

Polymorphisms occurring at specific AA positions within the HLA class I hc are found to influence the dependency of these molecules on TPN for efficient cell surface expression and peptide presentation. It has been hypothesized that the nature of AAs occurring at the bottom of the F pocket influences the conformational flexibility of empty class I molecules [55, 64], which could in turn determine the ability of a particular allotype to bind peptides in the presence or absence of TPN [65]. It has been shown that in the TPN dependent alloforms, the region around the F pocket of the peptide binding groove is in a disordered conformation due to a partially open disulphide bond in the α2 domain [66] and that TPN facilitates the conversion of this disordered conformation into a stable, peptide-receptive conformation [55].

Studies performed using TPN deficient cell lines (LCL 721.220] transfected with various HLA-A and B allotypes demonstrated an altered dependency of these class I variants on TPN for their cell surface expression [33, 67, 68] [18]. HLA-B*27:05 molecules showed high levels of surface expression and were able to present specific viral peptides even in the absence of TPN. On contrary, HLA-B*44:02 molecules were found to be highly dependent upon TPN for these functions and HLA-B8 molecules showed intermediate dependency on TPN [33]. It has also been observed that while HLA-A1 molecules fail to present antigens in the absence of TPN [31], HLA-A2 molecules present peptides very efficiently on the surface of these cells [69].

Many studies have highlighted the importance of AAs occurring at position 114 of class I hc in determining their dependency on TPN for efficient antigen processing and presentation [33, 55, 64, 70, 71]. Park *et al* demonstrated that the class I molecules having an acidic AA at position 114 such as HLA-B*44:02$^{\text{114Asp}}$ or HLA-A*30:01$^{\text{114Glu}}$ are highly dependent upon TPN for their cell surface expression, alleles with neutral AAs such as HLA-B*08:01$^{\text{114Asn}}$ or HLA-B*54:01$^{\text{114Asn}}$ are weakly dependent while alleles with basic AAs such as HLA-B*27:02$^{\text{114His}}$, HLA-B*27:05$^{\text{114His}}$, HLA-A*02:10$^{\text{114His}}$ or HLA-A*24:01$^{\text{114His}}$ are independent of TPN for their surface expression [71]. However, both HLA-B*44:02 and HLA-B*44:05 are found to have an acidic AA at position 114 and yet show opposite ends of the TPN dependency spectrum. In the absence of TPN, HLA-B*44:02 fails to bind high affinity peptides and is prone to intracellular degradation. In contrast, HLA-B*44:05 shows efficient cell surface expression both in the presence and absence of TPN [58]. These two allotypes differ exclusively at AA position 116 which is located in the F pocket of the peptide binding groove and contacts C terminus of the bound peptide. HLA-B*44:02 has an Asp while B*44:05 has a Tyr at position 116. While HLA-B*44:02 binds very efficiently to TAP and undergoes significant optimization of its peptide cargo, B*44:05 molecules are not incorporated in the PLC and undergo only partial optimization of their peptide cargo in the presence of TPN [58]. Asp116His mutation in HLA-B*44:02 resulted in a TPN-independent molecule [55]. Sieker *et al* hypothesized that the presence of two acidic residues at positions 114 and 116 in HLA-B*44:02 hc resulted in the disruption of the F-pocket conformation due to excessive hydration [65] and that the ability of HLA-B*44:05 to acquire limited peptides without being incorporated into the PLC was due to the aspartic acid to tyrosine exchange at residue 116 which decreased the electronegativity and increased the hydrophobicity around the F pocket [64]. Experiments performed by Neisig *et al* demonstrated that among the HLA-B allotypes investigated, those containing an aromatic AA at position 116 bound efficiently to TAP while the others did not [70]. HLA-B*35:02 and B*35:03 having aromatic AAs Tyr and Phe respectively at position 116 demonstrated strong associations with TAP while B*35:01 and B*35:08 both containing Ser at position 116 showed no significant association with TAP [70]. Similarly, among the HLA-B*15 allotypes, B*15:10 having a Tyr at position 116 showed stronger association not only to TAP but also to TPN and CRT when compared to B*15:18 or B*15:01 having Ser at this position [72]. It was also observed that HLA-B*68:07$^{\text{116His}}$ associated much stronger with TAP than B*68:03$^{\text{116Asp}}$ [73]. The authors pointed out that residue 116 pointing upwards from the F pocket into the binding groove might be involved in the association of TPN with the class I heavy chain, which in turn regulates the differential binding of position 116 variants with TAP. However, it is seen that HLA-B*44:02 and B*44:03 both have an Asp at position 116 and yet associate differentially with TAP. These two alleles differ from each other by a single AA at position 156. While HLA-B*44:02 binds efficiently to TAP, B*44:03 is found to be a weak TAP binder. The authors pointed out that the AA at position 156 located at the centre of the $\alpha 2$ helix of class I heavy chains might determine the strong and the weak binding of HLA-B*44:02 and B*44:03 respectively to TAP [70].

Some of the more recent studies have shed light on the functional consequences of HLA class I polymorphisms in modulating the presented peptide repertoire. It could be demonstrated that the TPN dependent B*44:02^{116Asp} and TPN-independent variant B*44:05^{116Tyr} differed in their preference at the PΩ anchor residue [64]. Binding preference of HLA-B*44:05 at P9 was restricted to Phe while B*44:02 showed preference for both Phe and Tyr at this position, largely due to the ability of Asp116 in B*44:02 to make hydrogen bond with Tyr at P9 [64]. In yet another study, it was demonstrated that although the surface expression of HLA-B*27:05 was similar both in the presence and absence of TPN, there was a difference in the cytotoxic lysis of B*27:05 targets upon infection with recombinant vaccina viruses under these two circumstances. Measurement of cytotoxicity at four hours post infection demonstrated that the lysis of B*27:05/TPN negative targets was only half the cytotoxicity level observed for B*27:05/TPN positive target cells. At 12 hours post infection, the cytotoxic lysis of B*27:05/TPN negative targets was similar to B*27:05/TPN positive target cells. However, this study pointed out an impairment in the presentation of specific viral peptides by B*27:05 in the absence of TPN. Although there was some overlap in the peptides presented in the presence and absence of TPN, unique set of peptides were selected and presented by B*27:05 under these two conditions. B*27:05 molecules on the surface of cells lacking TPN are more unstable probably owing to the nature of peptides selected and bound by them in the absence of TPN [33].

Studies examining single AA exchanges within the hc of naturally occurring HLA class I alleles have identified some of the residues in the $\alpha 2$ domain which are of critical importance for the interaction of class I molecules with the PLC components. Elliott *et al* demonstrated that the replacement of Thr with Lys at residue 134 (T134K) in HLA-A2 resulted in disruption of the interaction between class I and the PLC components [47, 52]. In contrast, replacement of Ser with Cys at residue 132 (S132C) in these molecules resulted in prolonged association of class I molecule with the PLC components, slower maturation of the complex and binding of optimal high-affinity ligands [52].Yu *et al* have shown that residues 128-136 occurring in the $\alpha 2$ domain play an important role in peptide loading and formation of the class I loading complex [49]. These studies have led to the identification of a putative PLC binding surface of the class I heterodimer that is located on the $\alpha 2$ domain of the molecule. The surface on the class I molecule that these regions contribute to defines a pronounced groove which might form a docking structure for one or more components of the PLC. Also, the conserved disulphide bond between AAs Cys101 and Cys164 are located within this region of the $\alpha 2$ domain. This disulphide bond is responsible for linking the $\alpha 2$ helix to the peptide binding floor and isomerisation of this bond has been implicated during peptide binding [74].

Previous studies have demonstrated that the nature of AAs occurring at residues 114 or 116 determine the interaction of these different class I allotypes with the PLC components [64]. These two residues are located in the F pocket of the PBR, that interacts with the C-terminal peptide residue and thus determine the nature of a bound peptide. It is found that certain AA polymorphisms occurring at these positions result in loading and presentation of peptides independent of the loading complex (TAP/ TPN) [64, 71] via a non-classical pathway resulting in the presentation of pHLA complexes, that might be poorly tolerated by the self immune system.

9. Impact of mismatch at residue 156 in B*44 allotypes

Recently the association of TPN with HLA subtypes featuring micro-polymorphisms at AA position 156 was discovered [18]. This position is part of the pockets D and E within the peptide binding region and contacts peptide of canonical length at positions p3 and p7 [75], explaining its distinct structural role in influencing the conformation of the pHLA complex [76] [77]. Polymorphisms at residue 156 represent one of the most non-permissive transplantation scenarios and are associated with acute GvHD for HLA-A, -B and -C alleles [58] [78] [76] [77] [79] [80].

The HLA-B*44 allelic group occurring in approximately 25 % of the Caucasian population has four naturally occurring variants (B*44:02^{156Asp}, 44:03^{156Leu}, 44:28^{156Arg}, 44:35^{156Glu}), which exclusively differ by just one single AA at residue 156. The mismatch B*44:02^{156Asp} / B*44:03^{156Leu} e.g. is described to represent a non-permissive transplantation scenario. The association with strong alloreactive T-cell responses due to distinct structural differences between B*44:02 and B*44:03 pHLA complexes leads to acute GvHD [79]. It has also been demonstrated that the resulting mismatch leads to a disparity in the derived peptide repertoire, which explains the cytotoxic T-lymphocyte recognition of different pHLA landscapes between B*44:02 and B*44:03. Structural involvement of position 156 in influencing the conformation of PBR was demonstrated by comparing the crystal structures of HLA-B*44:02 and HLA-B*44:03 complexed with the same, natural high affinity ligand [18]. In order to determine if position 156 is also involved in the PLC/HLA association and if polymorphism at this position affect TPN dependency through alteration of the structure and property of the PBR and subsequently the peptide repertoire, we investigated the mode of peptide loading for the B*44/156 mismatched variants.

Our data demonstrates that exclusively HLA-B*44:28^{156Arg} variant can acquire peptides independently of TPN and that AA position 156 is unambiguously responsible for the HLA/TPN interaction within B*44 subtypes. Based on its position and orientation, residue 156 is unlikely to contact TPN directly. Similarly, TPN-dependent B*44:02 and TPN-independent B*44:05 alleles with a micropolymorphic difference at residue 116 also appear unlikely to contact TPN directly. Although AA residue 156 is not a part of the first segment of α2-helix, it is likely that it influences the strand/loop region that TPN interacts with and in a similar manner to residue 116 affects the stability/dynamics of the unloaded HLA molecule.

By systematically analysing the influence of residue 156 in B*44 variants and their interaction with TPN could clearly be demonstrated. Using mass spectrometry we sequenced those peptides derived from B*44:02 aquired with the assistance of TPN and hence through the optimization machinery of the PLC and compared those with peptides bound to B*44:28 aquired in a TPN-independent manner. Significant differences between these sets of peptides could be observed, both in their attributed binding affinity and in the length of the derived peptides. The peptide repertoires of sHLA-B*44:02 and sHLA-B*44:28 display subtle differences, suggesting an alternate antigen presentation pathway, the core binding motifs are strongly retained [18]. The results from the structural insight through computational analysis indicated a role for 156Arg in increasing the stability of the pHLA complex through contacts to both Asp114 and to peptide backbone at P5 (Figure 3).

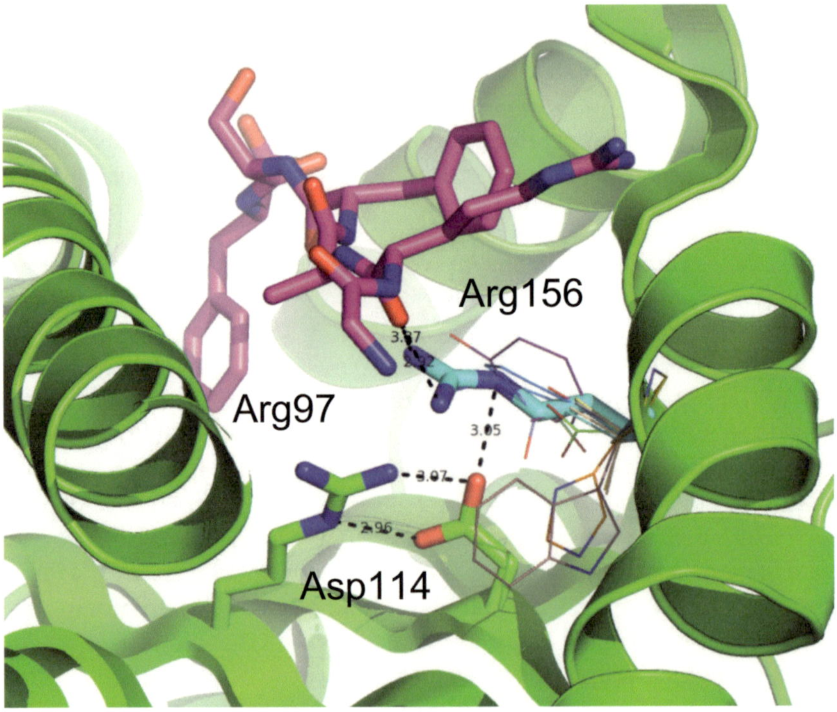

Based on the B*44:02 structure (1M6O) [76] all 20 AAs were modelled at position 156 fitting the best side chain rotamer. Arg156 shows increased hydrogen bonding both to residue Asp114 and to peptide backbone. This is likely to increase stability of the HLA-peptide complex.

Figure 3. B*44/156 substitution model

Our results indicate that the HLA-B*44:28^{156Arg} variant stabilises the binding groove in its empty state, thus negating the contribution of the PLC and allowing independent loading of high affinity peptides. The interaction between Arg156 and Asp114 on the floor of the peptide binding groove seems to be able to generate a stable peptide receptive state.

10. Conclusion

TPN independency offers flexibility on one hand, because it provides an effective pathogen evasion, however peptides are loaded suboptimally and that might influence the immunogenicity and half-life time of pHLA complexes and this might result in autoimmunity.

The question whether TPN-dependency or TPN-independency is advantageous or not is likely to depend on the combination of HLA-A, -B, and C- alleles of an individual. An appreciation of the interaction between TPN, HLA class I molecules and peptide loading may therefore be important not only during viral infections, but also while considering transplantation scenarios.

Nomenclature

- Human leucocyte antigens (HLA)
- Major Histocompatibility Complex (MHC)
- T cell receptor (TCR)
- peptide-HLA complexes (pHLA)
- peptide-binding region (PBR)
- hematopoietic stem cell transplantation (HSCT)
- graft-versus-host disease (GvHD)
- amino acid (AA)
- heavy chain (hc)
- β2 microglobulin (β2m)
- peptide loading complex (PLC)
- endoplasmic reticulum (ER)
- transporter associated with antigen processing (TAP)
- tapasin (TPN)
- cytotoxic T lymphocyte (CTL)
- human cytomegalie virus (HCMV)
- Calnexin (CNX)
- Calreticulin (CRT)

Acknowledgements

The authors would like to thank Heike Kunze-Schumacher for excellent technical assistance.

Author details

Soumya Badrinath, Trevor Huyton, Rainer Blasczyk and Christina Bade-Doeding

*Address all correspondence to: bade-doeding.christina@mh-hannover.de

Institute for Transfusion Medicine, Hannover Medical School, Hannover, Germany

References

[1] Germain RN, Margulies DH. The biochemistry and cell biology of antigen processing and presentation. Annu Rev Immunol. 1993;11:403-50.

[2] Zinkernagel RM, Doherty PC. Restriction of in vitro T cell-mediated cytotoxicity in lymphocytic choriomeningitis within a syngeneic or semiallogeneic system. Nature. 1974 Apr 19;248(450):701-2.

[3] Marsh SG, Albert ED, Bodmer WF, Bontrop RE, Dupont B, Erlich HA, et al. An update to HLA nomenclature, 2010. Bone Marrow Transplant. May;45(5):846-8.

[4] Bjorkman PJ, Saper MA, Samraoui B, Bennett WS, Strominger JL, Wiley DC. Structure of the human class I histocompatibility antigen, HLA-A2. Nature. [Research Support, Non-U.S. Gov't Research Support, U.S. Gov't, P.H.S.]. 1987 Oct 8-14;329(6139):506-12.

[5] Bjorkman PJ, Parham P. Structure, function, and diversity of class I major histocompatibility complex molecules. Annu Rev Biochem. 1990;59:253-88.

[6] Klein J, Sato A. The HLA system. First of two parts. N Engl J Med. 2000 Sep 7;343(10): 702-9.

[7] Falk K, Rotzschke O, Stevanovic S, Jung G, Rammensee HG. Allele-specific motifs revealed by sequencing of self-peptides eluted from MHC molecules. Nature. 1991 May 23;351(6324):290-6.

[8] Zuckerman T, Rowe JM. Alternative donor transplantation in acute myeloid leukemia: which source and when? Curr Opin Hematol. 2007 Mar;14(2):152-61.

[9] Mickelson EM, Petersdorf E, Anasetti C, Martin P, Woolfrey A, Hansen JA. HLA matching in hematopoietic cell transplantation. Hum Immunol. 2000 Feb;61(2): 92-100.

[10] Ottinger HD, Ferencik S, Beelen DW, Lindemann M, Peceny R, Elmaagacli AH, et al. Hematopoietic stem cell transplantation: contrasting the outcome of transplantations from HLA-identical siblings, partially HLA-mismatched related donors, and HLA-matched unrelated donors. Blood. 2003 Aug 1;102(3):1131-7.

[11] Schaffer M, Aldener-Cannava A, Remberger M, Ringden O, Olerup O. Roles of HLA-B, HLA-C and HLA-DPA1 incompatibilities in the outcome of unrelated stem-cell transplantation. Tissue Antigens. 2003 Sep;62(3):243-50.

[12] Bade-Doeding C, Cano P, Huyton T, Badrinath S, Eiz-Vesper B, Hiller O, et al. Mismatches outside exons 2 and 3 do not alter the peptide motif of the allele group B*44:02P. Hum Immunol. Nov;72(11):1039-44.

[13] Bade-Doeding C, DeLuca DS, Seltsam A, Blasczyk R, Eiz-Vesper B. Amino acid 95 causes strong alteration of peptide position Pomega in HLA-B*41 variants. Immunogenetics. 2007 Apr;59(4):253-9.

[14] Bade-Doeding C, Eiz-Vesper B, Figueiredo C, Seltsam A, Elsner HA, Blasczyk R. Peptide-binding motif of HLA-A*6603. Immunogenetics. 2005 Jan;56(10):769-72.

[15] Bade-Doeding C, Elsner HA, Eiz-Vesper B, Seltsam A, Holtkamp U, Blasczyk R. A single amino-acid polymorphism in pocket A of HLA-A*6602 alters the auxiliary anchors compared with HLA-A*6601 ligands. Immunogenetics. 2004 May;56(2):83-8.

[16] Bade-Doeding C, Huyton T, Eiz-Vesper B, Blasczyk R. The composition of the F pocket in HLA-A*74 generates C-terminal promiscuity among its bound peptides. Tissue Antigens. Nov;78(5):378-81.

[17] Badrinath S, Huyton T, Schumacher H, Blasczyk R, Bade-Doeding C. Position 45 influences the peptide binding motif of HLA-B*44:08. Immunogenetics. Mar;64(3): 245-9.

[18] Badrinath S, Saunders P, Huyton T, Aufderbeck S, Hiller O, Blasczyk R, et al. Position 156 influences the peptide repertoire and tapasin dependency of human leukocyte antigen B*44 allotypes. Haematologica. Jan;97(1):98-106.

[19] Elamin NE, Bade-Doeding C, Blasczyk R, Eiz-Vesper B. Polymorphism between HLA-A*0301 and A*0302 located outside the pocket F alters the POmega peptide motif. Tissue Antigens. Dec;76(6):487-90.

[20] Huyton T, Ladas N, Schumacher H, Blasczyk R, Bade-Doeding C. Pocketcheck: updating the HLA class I peptide specificity roadmap. Tissue Antigens. Sep;80(3): 239-48.

[21] Huyton T, Schumacher H, Blasczyk R, Bade-Doeding C. Residue 81 confers a restricted C-terminal peptide binding motif in HLA-B*44:09. Immunogenetics. Sep;64(9): 663-8.

[22] Krausa P, Munz C, Keilholz W, Stevanovic S, Jones EY, Browning M, et al. Definition of peptide binding motifs amongst the HLA-A*30 allelic group. Tissue Antigens. 2000 Jul;56(1):10-8.

[23] Prilliman K, Lindsey M, Zuo Y, Jackson KW, Zhang Y, Hildebrand W. Large-scale production of class I bound peptides: assigning a signature to HLA-B*1501. Immunogenetics. 1997;45(6):379-85.

[24] Prilliman KR, Jackson KW, Lindsey M, Wang J, Crawford D, Hildebrand WH. HLA-B15 peptide ligands are preferentially anchored at their C termini. J Immunol. 1999 Jun 15;162(12):7277-84.

[25] Bray RA, Hurley CK, Kamani NR, Woolfrey A, Muller C, Spellman S, et al. National marrow donor program HLA matching guidelines for unrelated adult donor hematopoietic cell transplants. Biol Blood Marrow Transplant. 2008 Sep;14(9 Suppl):45-53.

[26] Morishima Y, Kawase T, Malkki M, Petersdorf EW. Effect of HLA-A2 allele disparity on clinical outcome in hematopoietic cell transplantation from unrelated donors. Tissue Antigens. 2007 Apr;69 Suppl 1:31-5.

[27] Morishima Y, Sasazuki T, Inoko H, Juji T, Akaza T, Yamamoto K, et al. The clinical significance of human leukocyte antigen (HLA) allele compatibility in patients receiving a marrow transplant from serologically HLA-A, HLA-B, and HLA-DR matched unrelated donors. Blood. 2002 Jun 1;99(11):4200-6.

[28] Petersdorf EW. Optimal HLA matching in hematopoietic cell transplantation. Curr Opin Immunol. 2008 Oct;20(5):588-93.

[29] Petersdorf EW, Hansen JA, Martin PJ, Woolfrey A, Malkki M, Gooley T, et al. Major-histocompatibility-complex class I alleles and antigens in hematopoietic-cell transplantation. N Engl J Med. 2001 Dec 20;345(25):1794-800.

[30] Schoenhals GJ, Krishna RM, Grandea AG, 3rd, Spies T, Peterson PA, Yang Y, et al. Retention of empty MHC class I molecules by tapasin is essential to reconstitute antigen presentation in invertebrate cells. Embo J. 1999 Feb 1;18(3):743-53.

[31] Ortmann B, Copeman J, Lehner PJ, Sadasivan B, Herberg JA, Grandea AG, et al. A critical role for tapasin in the assembly and function of multimeric MHC class I-TAP complexes. Science. 1997 Aug 29;277(5330):1306-9.

[32] Lee S, Yoon J, Park B, Jun Y, Jin M, Sung HC, et al. Structural and functional dissection of human cytomegalovirus US3 in binding major histocompatibility complex class I molecules. J Virol. 2000 Dec;74(23):11262-9.

[33] Peh CA, Burrows SR, Barnden M, Khanna R, Cresswell P, Moss DJ, et al. HLA-B27-restricted antigen presentation in the absence of tapasin reveals polymorphism in mechanisms of HLA class I peptide loading. Immunity. 1998 May;8(5):531-42.

[34] Bennett EM, Bennink JR, Yewdell JW, Brodsky FM. Cutting edge: adenovirus E19 has two mechanisms for affecting class I MHC expression. J Immunol. 1999 May 1;162(9): 5049-52.

[35] Byun MW, Kim JH, Kim DH, Kim HJ, Jo C. Effects of irradiation and sodium hypochlorite on the micro-organisms attached to a commercial food container. Food Microbiol. 2007 Aug;24(5):544-8.

[36] Lilley BN, Ploegh HL. Viral modulation of antigen presentation: manipulation of cellular targets in the ER and beyond. Immunol Rev. 2005 Oct;207:126-44.

[37] Lybarger L, Wang X, Harris M, Hansen TH. Viral immune evasion molecules attack the ER peptide-loading complex and exploit ER-associated degradation pathways. Curr Opin Immunol. 2005 Feb;17(1):71-8.

[38] Wiertz EJ, Jones TR, Sun L, Bogyo M, Geuze HJ, Ploegh HL. The human cytomegalovirus US11 gene product dislocates MHC class I heavy chains from the endoplasmic reticulum to the cytosol. Cell. 1996 Mar 8;84(5):769-79.

[39] Wiertz EJ, Tortorella D, Bogyo M, Yu J, Mothes W, Jones TR, et al. Sec61-mediated transfer of a membrane protein from the endoplasmic reticulum to the proteasome for destruction. Nature. 1996 Dec 5;384(6608):432-8.

[40] Schwartz O, Marechal V, Le Gall S, Lemonnier F, Heard JM. Endocytosis of major histocompatibility complex class I molecules is induced by the HIV-1 Nef protein. Nat Med. 1996 Mar;2(3):338-42.

[41] Collins KL, Chen BK, Kalams SA, Walker BD, Baltimore D. HIV-1 Nef protein protects infected primary cells against killing by cytotoxic T lymphocytes. Nature. 1998 Jan 22;391(6665):397-401.

[42] Reusch U, Muranyi W, Lucin P, Burgert HG, Hengel H, Koszinowski UH. A cytomegalovirus glycoprotein re-routes MHC class I complexes to lysosomes for degradation. Embo J. 1999 Feb 15;18(4):1081-91.

[43] Lehner PJ, Surman MJ, Cresswell P. Soluble tapasin restores MHC class I expression and function in the tapasin-negative cell line.220. Immunity. 1998 Feb;8(2):221-31.

[44] Li S, Paulsson KM, Chen S, Sjogren HO, Wang P. Tapasin is required for efficient peptide binding to transporter associated with antigen processing. J Biol Chem. 2000 Jan 21;275(3):1581-6.

[45] Barnden MJ, Purcell AW, Gorman JJ, McCluskey J. Tapasin-mediated retention and optimization of peptide ligands during the assembly of class I molecules. J Immunol. 2000 Jul 1;165(1):322-30.

[46] Purcell AW, Kelly AJ, Peh CA, Dudek NL, McCluskey J. Endogenous and exogenous factors contributing to the surface expression of HLA B27 on mutant APC. Hum Immunol. 2000 Feb;61(2):120-30.

[47] Lewis JW, Elliott T. Evidence for successive peptide binding and quality control stages during MHC class I assembly. Curr Biol. 1998 Jun 4;8(12):717-20.

[48] Yu YY, Myers NB, Hilbert CM, Harris MR, Balendiran GK, Hansen TH. Definition and transfer of a serological epitope specific for peptide-empty forms of MHC class I. Int Immunol. 1999 Dec;11(12):1897-906.

[49] Yu YY, Turnquist HR, Myers NB, Balendiran GK, Hansen TH, Solheim JC. An extensive region of an MHC class I alpha 2 domain loop influences interaction with the assembly complex. J Immunol. 1999 Oct 15;163(8):4427-33.

[50] Suh WK, Derby MA, Cohen-Doyle MF, Schoenhals GJ, Fruh K, Berzofsky JA, et al. Interaction of murine MHC class I molecules with tapasin and TAP enhances peptide loading and involves the heavy chain alpha3 domain. J Immunol. 1999 Feb 1;162(3): 1530-40.

[51] Carreno BM, Schreiber KL, McKean DJ, Stroynowski I, Hansen TH. Aglycosylated and phosphatidylinositol-anchored MHC class I molecules are associated with calnexin. Evidence implicating the class I-connecting peptide segment in calnexin association. J Immunol. 1995 May 15;154(10):5173-80.

[52] Lewis JW, Neisig A, Neefjes J, Elliott T. Point mutations in the alpha 2 domain of HLA-A2.1 define a functionally relevant interaction with TAP. Curr Biol. 1996 Jul 1;6(7):873-83.

[53] Peace-Brewer AL, Tussey LG, Matsui M, Li G, Quinn DG, Frelinger JA. A point mutation in HLA-A*0201 results in failure to bind the TAP complex and to present virus-derived peptides to CTL. Immunity. 1996 May;4(5):505-14.

[54] Dong G, Wearsch PA, Peaper DR, Cresswell P, Reinisch KM. Insights into MHC class I peptide loading from the structure of the tapasin-ERp57 thiol oxidoreductase heterodimer. Immunity. 2009 Jan 16;30(1):21-32.

[55] Garstka MA, Fritzsche S, Lenart I, Hein Z, Jankevicius G, Boyle LH, et al. Tapasin dependence of major histocompatibility complex class I molecules correlates with their conformational flexibility. Faseb J. Nov;25(11):3989-98.

[56] Chen M, Bouvier M. Analysis of interactions in a tapasin/class I complex provides a mechanism for peptide selection. EMBO J. [Research Support, N.I.H., Extramural Research Support, Non-U.S. Gov't]. 2007 Mar 21;26(6):1681-90.

[57] Garbi N, Tan P, Diehl AD, Chambers BJ, Ljunggren HG, Momburg F, et al. Impaired immune responses and altered peptide repertoire in tapasin-deficient mice. Nat Immunol. 2000 Sep;1(3):234-8.

[58] Williams AP, Peh CA, Purcell AW, McCluskey J, Elliott T. Optimization of the MHC class I peptide cargo is dependent on tapasin. Immunity. 2002 Apr;16(4):509-20.

[59] Wearsch PA, Cresswell P. Selective loading of high-affinity peptides onto major histocompatibility complex class I molecules by the tapasin-ERp57 heterodimer. Nat Immunol. [Research Support, Non-U.S. Gov't]. 2007 Aug;8(8):873-81.

[60] Praveen PV, Yaneva R, Kalbacher H, Springer S. Tapasin edits peptides on MHC class I molecules by accelerating peptide exchange. Eur J Immunol. Jan;40(1):214-24.

[61] Barber LD, Howarth M, Bowness P, Elliott T. The quantity of naturally processed peptides stably bound by HLA-A*0201 is significantly reduced in the absence of tapasin. Tissue Antigens. 2001 Dec;58(6):363-8.

[62] Zarling AL, Luckey CJ, Marto JA, White FM, Brame CJ, Evans AM, et al. Tapasin is a facilitator, not an editor, of class I MHC peptide binding. J Immunol. 2003 Nov 15;171(10):5287-95.

[63] Howarth M, Williams A, Tolstrup AB, Elliott T. Tapasin enhances MHC class I peptide presentation according to peptide half-life. Proc Natl Acad Sci U S A. 2004 Aug 10;101(32):11737-42.

[64] Zernich D, Purcell AW, Macdonald WA, Kjer-Nielsen L, Ely LK, Laham N, et al. Natural HLA class I polymorphism controls the pathway of antigen presentation and susceptibility to viral evasion. J Exp Med. 2004 Jul 5;200(1):13-24.

[65] Sieker F, Straatsma TP, Springer S, Zacharias M. Differential tapasin dependence of MHC class I molecules correlates with conformational changes upon peptide dissociation: a molecular dynamics simulation study. Mol Immunol. 2008 Aug;45(14): 3714-22.

[66] Fussell HE, Kunkel LE, Lewy CS, McFarland BH, McCarty D. Using a standardized patient walk-through to improve implementation of clinical trials. J Subst Abuse Treat. 2008 Dec;35(4):470-5.

[67] Greenwood R, Shimizu Y, Sekhon GS, DeMars R. Novel allele-specific, post-translational reduction in HLA class I surface expression in a mutant human B cell line. J Immunol. 1994 Dec 15;153(12):5525-36.

[68] Grandea AG, 3rd, Androlewicz MJ, Athwal RS, Geraghty DE, Spies T. Dependence of peptide binding by MHC class I molecules on their interaction with TAP. Science. 1995 Oct 6;270(5233):105-8.

[69] Lewis JW, Sewell A, Price D, Elliott T. HLA-A*0201 presents TAP-dependent peptide epitopes to cytotoxic T lymphocytes in the absence of tapasin. Eur J Immunol. 1998 Oct;28(10):3214-20.

[70] Neisig A, Wubbolts R, Zang X, Melief C, Neefjes J. Allele-specific differences in the interaction of MHC class I molecules with transporters associated with antigen processing. J Immunol. 1996 May 1;156(9):3196-206.

[71] Park B, Lee S, Kim E, Ahn K. A single polymorphic residue within the peptide-binding cleft of MHC class I molecules determines spectrum of tapasin dependence. J Immunol. 2003 Jan 15;170(2):961-8.

[72] Turnquist HR, Thomas HJ, Prilliman KR, Lutz CT, Hildebrand WH, Solheim JC. HLA-B polymorphism affects interactions with multiple endoplasmic reticulum proteins. Eur J Immunol. 2000 Oct;30(10):3021-8.

[73] Turnquist HR, Schenk EL, McIlhaney MM, Hickman HD, Hildebrand WH, Solheim JC. Disparate binding of chaperone proteins by HLA-A subtypes. Immunogenetics. 2002 Feb;53(10-11):830-4.

[74] Cresswell P, Bangia N, Dick T, Diedrich G. The nature of the MHC class I peptide loading complex. Immunol Rev. 1999 Dec;172:21-8.

[75] Chelvanayagam G. A roadmap for HLA-A, HLA-B, and HLA-C peptide binding specificities. Immunogenetics. 1996;45(1):15-26.

[76] Macdonald WA, Purcell AW, Mifsud NA, Ely LK, Williams DS, Chang L, et al. A naturally selected dimorphism within the HLA-B44 supertype alters class I structure, peptide repertoire, and T cell recognition. J Exp Med. 2003 Sep 1;198(5):679-91.

[77] Archbold JK, Macdonald WA, Gras S, Ely LK, Miles JJ, Bell MJ, et al. Natural micropolymorphism in human leukocyte antigens provides a basis for genetic control of antigen recognition. J Exp Med. 2009 Jan 16;206(1):209-19.

[78] Park B, Kim Y, Shin J, Lee S, Cho K, Fruh K, et al. Human cytomegalovirus inhibits tapasin-dependent peptide loading and optimization of the MHC class I peptide cargo for immune evasion. Immunity. 2004 Jan;20(1):71-85.

[79] Fleischhauer K, Kernan NA, O'Reilly RJ, Dupont B, Yang SY. Bone marrow-allograft rejection by T lymphocytes recognizing a single amino acid difference in HLA-B44. N Engl J Med. 1990 Dec 27;323(26):1818-22.

[80] Fleischhauer K, Avila D, Vilbois F, Traversari C, Bordignon C, Wallny HJ. Characterization of natural peptide ligands for HLA-B*4402 and -B*4403: implications for peptide involvement in allorecognition of a single amino acid change in the HLA-B44 heavy chain. Tissue Antigens. 1994 Nov;44(5):311-7.

Chapter 3

HLA-E, HLA-F and HLA-G — The Non-Classical Side of the MHC Cluster

Iris Foroni, Ana Rita Couto, Bruno Filipe Bettencourt,
Margarida Santos, Manuela Lima and
Jácome Bruges-Armas

Additional information is available at the end of the chapter

http://dx.doi.org/10.5772/57507

1. Introduction

Traditionally, the MHC is divided into the classes containing groups of genes with related functions; the MHC class I and II genes encode for human leukocyte antigens (HLA), proteins that are displayed on the cell surface. In humans, MHC class I molecules comprise the classical (class I-a) HLA-A, -B, and -C, and the non-classical (class I-b) HLA-E, -F, -G and – H (HFE) molecules (Pietra et al., 2009). Both categories are similar in their mechanisms of peptide binding and presentation and in the induced T-cell responses (Rodgers and Cook, 2005). The most remarkable feature of MHC class I-b molecules is their highly conserved nature (van Hall et al., 2010). In contrast with class Ia molecules they have been under a distinct selective pressure, exhibiting very low levels of allelic polymorphism (Strong et al., 2003). Classical MHC class I gene transcription is mediated by several cis-acting regulatory elements, in the proximal promoter region (Gobin and van den Elsen, 2000). Those elements determine the constitutive and cytokine induced expression levels of the molecule (Gobin and van den Elsen, 2000).

The literature on the different roles played by class I-b molecules is in rapid expansion and focus in pathogen recognition, virus-induced immunopathology, tumor immunosurveillance and regulation of autoimmunity (Hofstetter et al., 2011). The HLA-G, HLA-E and HLA-F genes encode for molecules that have been shown to be involved in regulation of autoimmune disease (Donadi et al., 2011; Kim et al., 2008). HLA-G biological features include: restricted tissue expression, the presence of membrane bound and soluble isoforms, generated by alternative splicing, limited protein variability, unique molecular structure, with a reduced citoplasmic tail and modulation of the immune response. The presence of HLA-G molecules in both membranes bound and soluble forms was associated with tolerogenic functions (Baricordi et al., 2008). HLA-E is the best characterized MHC Class Ib molecule. With a low level of polymorphism its role is thought to be confined to the regulation of NK cell function (Pietra et al., 2009). The HLA-F gene was first identified in 1990 by Geraghty et al. (Geraghty et al., 1990; Ishitani et al., 2006). So far it is the nonclassical class I molecule least characterized and neither its native structure nor function is known (Boyle et al., 2006; Goodridge et al., 2010; Lee et al., 2010). Several studies confirmed HLA-F protein expression in a number of diverse tissues and cell lines, including bladder, skin and liver cell lines, but no surface expression was detected in the majority of them (Lee et al., 2010). Just like other class Ib molecules, HLA-F restrictive tissue expression suggests specialized functions and tight transcriptional control of the gene (Gobin and van den Elsen, 2000). Furthermore, unique potential regulator motifs were identified consistent with tissue-specific expression (Geraghty et al., 1990).

In this chapter we aim to provide a wide view about:

1. The characteristic of non-classical HLA-E, F and G molecules based on the data available in scientific literature;
2. The polymorphism of HLA-E, HLA-F, and HLA-G in the world populations;
3. The association of non-classical HLA-E, F and G alleles and disease.

2. Morfo-functional description of HLA-E molecule

In humans, the major histocompatibility complex (MHC) class I molecules include the classical (class Ia) human leukocyte antigens (HLA)-A, -B, and -C, and the non-classical (class Ib) HLA-E, -F, -G and -H (HFE) molecules. HLA-E is the best-characterized MHC class Ib molecule, defined by a limited polymorphism and a restricted pattern of cellular expression (Iwaszko and Bogunia-Kubik, 2011; Pietra et al., 2009).

The HLA-E gene is situated in the MHC cluster on cromossome 6, about 650 kb from HLA-C, and consists of seven exons. The first one encodes the leader peptide. The next three exons encode a1, a2 and a3 domains, respectively. Exon 5 encodes the transmembrane region and the last two, the intracellular tail (Iwaszko and Bogunia-Kubik, 2011). HLA-E promoter regulatory sequence is divergent from other MHC class Ib molecules, determining differential transcription factor binding and transcriptional regulation. HLA-E is induced by CIITA through the SXY module. This is in line with the conserved sequences for the S, X, and Y boxes in the SXY module and shows that the divergent Y box (AATGG) does not influence the complex formation and transactivation by CIITA. However, this gene is not regulated by its upstream module. In fact, is strongly responsive to IFN-γ through a further upstream STAT1 binding site (Gobin and van den Elsen, 2000).

The HLA-E protein is the least polymorphic, one of the most studied and, unlike other MHC class Ib molecules, is transcribed in practically all human tissues (Braud et al., 1997). Ten alleles

http://dx.doi.org/10.5772/57507

in the human population encoding for three different peptides have been reported. Only two of these alleles, HLA-E*0101 and HLA-E*0103, are widely distributed (approximately 50% each). The proteins encoded by these alleles differ from each other in one amino acid (non-synonymous mutation), in the $\alpha2$ heavy chain domain, where an arginine in position 107 in HLA-E*0101 is replaced by a glycine in HLA-E*0103. The difference between these proteins manifests itself in surface expression levels, affinities to leader peptides and thermal stabilities of their complexes (Iwaszko and Bogunia-Kubik, 2011).

Like classical class I molecules, the complex stability on the cell surface requires a peptide, but unlike classical MHC-I proteins binding sites, which are typically limited at two or three positions, HLA-E has five anchor residues. This imposes strict restrictions on the sequence of peptides capable of binding to HLA-E (Sullivan et al., 2008). Five conserved hydrophobic pockets in the groove of HLA-E anchor the peptides in residues P2, P3, P6, P7, and P9; a wide hydrogen-bonding network between the heavy chain and the peptide main chain, as well as conserved charged interactions, further stabilize the peptides; these peptides derive from leader sequences of classical MHC proteins and provides a link to the primary function of HLA-E in the innate immune response as ligands for the family of CD94/NKG2 receptors expressed by natural killer (NK) and T cells (Braud et al., 1998).

The leader peptides originate in signal sequences of transmembrane proteins. HLA-E preferentially present peptides derived from leader sequences of other classical class I molecules (Aldrich et al., 1994; Braud et al., 1997). The signal sequence is cut during translocation of the protein by a signal peptidase; it remains in the membrane, where it is cleaved and its hydrophilic N-part is released into the cytosol (Lemberg et al., 2001). The hydrophilic oligopeptide is processed further by the proteasome, resulting in a leader peptide (Bland et al., 2003). Transporters associated with antigen processing (TAP), in cooperation with tapasin, transfer leader peptides to the endoplasmic reticulum (ER), where they can be associated to HLA-E molecules permitting their surface expression (Braud et al., 1997; Braud et al., 1998; Lee et al., 1998). HLA-E–peptide complex is then transported via Golgi apparatus to the cell surface where it interacts with CD94/NKG2A receptor expressed on NK cell or CTL (Iwaszko and Bogunia-Kubik, 2011). The availability of leader sequences is compromised by downregulation of classical class I protein production, thus interfering with the expression of HLA-E on the cell surface. Without the inhibitory signal that these molecules provide for the CD94/NKG2A receptor, cytolytic cells such as NK cells can detect and eliminate compromised host cells (Adams and Luoma, 2013).

Unlike other highly conserved systems, there is no cross-reactivity between human and mouse CD94/NKG2 receptors. This is likely due to a cluster of species-specific residues present near the peptide-binding region (Zeng et al., 2012) that constitutes part of the CD94/NKG2- binding site as revealed in the HLA-E/CD94/NKG2A complex crystal structures (Kaiser et al., 2008; Petrie et al., 2008). The correspondence of the CD94/NKG2A receptor on HLA-E covers the peptide-binding groove, with the CD94 and NKG2A subunits binding almost exclusively to the $\alpha1$- and $\alpha2$- helices, respectively (Adams and Luoma, 2013). This places the receptor over the P5, P6, and P8 positions of the peptide and explains the extreme sensitivity of CD94/NKG2 binding to subtle changes in peptide conformation at these positions (Adams and Luoma, 2013).

HLA-E was first described as a non-polymorphic ligand of the CD94/NKG2 receptors expressed mainly by natural killer (NK) cells and its role was thus limited to the regulation of NK cell function (Pietra et al., 2009). At present it is known that HLA-E molecule is a ligand for CD94/NKG2 receptors on NK cells and TCR receptors on NK-CTL (NK-cytotoxic T lymphocyte) cells, so it plays a double role in both innate and adaptive immunity (Iwaszko and Bogunia-Kubik, 2011). In fact, it has been shown that this ubiquitously expressed molecule plays a dual role as a modulator of NK cell activity in the innate immune pathway interacting with CD94/NKG2 receptors (Borrego et al., 2002; Braud et al., 1998; Lopez-Botet and Bellon, 1999; Shawar et al., 1994), as well as a molecule presenting antigens to αβ T cells in a specific immune response (Heinzel et al., 2002; Tomasec et al., 2000; Ulbrecht et al., 1998).

The interaction of HLA-E with the CD94/NKG2 receptors can result in either inhibition or activation of NK cells, depending on the peptide presented and on the association of the NKG2 receptor CD94. So, the association CD94/NKG2A functions as an inhibitory receptor, whereas CD94/NKG2C functions as an activating receptor. However, recent evidences showed that HLA-E represents a novel restriction element for αβ T-cell receptor (TCR)-mediated recognition. Although HLA-E displays a selective preference for nonameric peptides derived from the leader sequences of various HLA class I alleles, several reports showed that, in specific situations, it can also present other peptides derived from both stress-related and pathogen-associated proteins. Since HLA-E displays binding specificity for innate CD94/NKG2 receptors but also has the features of an antigen-presenting molecule, including the ability to be recognized by αβ T cells, it seems that this MHC class Ib molecule is implicated in both natural and acquired immune responses (Pietra et al., 2009).

In stress conditions, such as malignant cell transformation or intracellular infection with chronic pathogens, HLA-E has an alternative role. In such conditions the bound signal peptides are replaced by a novel much more diverse collection of peptides, which can be identified by αβ TCRs. It was recently described two such novel peptide repertoires, presented by HLA-E molecules to specific $CD8^+$ T cells, related to the detection of intracellular infection with mycobacteria, or to antigen processing defects in tumors (Joosten et al., 2010; Oliveira et al., 2010). These two situations of intracellular stress show that HLA-E probably serves a much wider function in adaptive immunity than thus far anticipated (van Hall et al., 2010). The peptides characterized from these responses can differ markedly in sequence from the established leader peptide sequence or can be highly similar. The human CMV UL40 is identical in sequence to some HLA leader sequences. This way, the expression of HLA-E on the cell surface is maintained and avoided the CD94/NKG2 detection of downregulated classical class I. This peptide can cause a strong CD8+ Tcell response in individuals lacking the identical endogenous leader sequence because these T cells have escaped negative selection. They can go on to make up a significant proportion of the CD8+ T cell memory pool in some immune individuals (Adams and Luoma, 2013; Hoare et al., 2006). The crystal structure of a αβ TCR interacts with HLA-E/UL40 peptide complex (Hoare et al., 2006; Adams and Luoma, 2013).

http://dx.doi.org/10.5772/57507

3. Morfo-functional description of HLA F molecule

The human MHC-F class Ib was the third non-classical HLA loci identified by Geraghty et al. in 1987 (Geraghty et al., 1987; Geraghty et al., 1990). HLA-F gene is located at the terminal end of the chromosome 6 and contains eight exons: exon 1 encodes the leader peptide; exons 2, 3, and 4 encode the alpha1, alpha2, and alpha3 domains; exons 5 and 6 encode the transmembrane region; and exons 7 and 8 encode the cytoplasmic tail. The intron/exon organization of the HLA-F is very similar to the HLA I class, except for the in-frame translation termination codon located at codon 2 in exon 6 (Geraghty et al., 1987). Thus the entire seventh and eight exons are not translated. The HLA-F gene is expressed as transmembrane heavy chain (HC) associated noncovalently on the cell surface with an invariant light chain β2-microglobulin (β2m). The glycoprotein is approximately 42 kDa, two KDa shorter than typical HLA class I, due to the exclusion of exons 7 and 8 from the mature mRNA. The leader peptide consists of 21 amino acids present at the N-terminus of the HLA-F protein. The extracellular domain consists of the heavy chain folded into three globular domains plus the light chain β2m. The $\alpha 1$, $\alpha 2$, and $\alpha 3$ regions together with β2m form a peptide binding groove. Most polymorphisms are located in this region influencing the peptide binding and the T-cell recognition (Howcroft and Singer, 2003). The transmembran spanning domain consists of a hydrophobic region of 26 amino acid of heavy chain. The carboxy-terminal cytoplasmic segment consists of only six amino acids: the COOH-terminal, plus five amino acids encoded by exon 5 and the aspartic acid residue encoded by exon 6.

The expression pattern of HLA-F molecule is generally tissue-restricted and cell specific. It can be detected in a number of diverse tissue and cell lines, including tonsil, bladder, liver, skin, and spleen. Predominantly it is express in an intracellular, unstable, and immature form in monocytes and most lymphocyte subsets, including NK cells, B cells, and T cells, except T reg cells (Lee et al., 2010).

The expression of HLA-F molecules is regulated at transcriptional level. The most of the regulatory elements reside in the 5′ proximal promoter regions. Those regulating elements are determinant for the tissue-specific expression and for the response to hormones and cytokines (Girdlestone, 1996; Le Bouteiller, 1994; Singer and Maguire, 1990). Additional sequence elements, like distal flanking regions and core promoter sequences, are also important in determining an appropriate expression. The main regions within the core promoter are the CCAAT box, G/C-rich region, TATA box, and the Initiator (INR) (Howcroft and Singer, 2003). The CCAAT box is a distinct pattern of nucleotides with GGCCAATCT consensus sequence that occur upstream to the initial transcription site. It represents a binding site for various transcription factors and it facilities the proper positioning of RNA polymerase. The G/C-rich region is located between CCAAT box and TATA box. It is still unknown its contribution to HLA class I genes. The TATA box is the binding site of the general transcription factors TFIID and is involved in the process of transcription by RNA polymerase. The INR element overlaps the transcript start site and facilitates the binding of transcription Factor II D (TBP). The principal modules that drive the HLA-F expression in the proximal promoter region are the upstream module consisting of the Enhancer A and ISRE element and the downstream module consisting of the SXY regions. The Enhancer A and ISRE element modulate the transactivation by two kB sites that bind nuclear (NF)-kB family factors and one binding site for IFNs. The SXY module consists of S, X, and Y box sequences. The X_1 and X_2 boxes are binding sites for RFX transcription factor and CREB/ATF family factors. The Y box is recognized by NF-Y factors. The SXY module is necessary to the activation of the HLA-F promoter by the CIITA master control factor induced by γINF.

HLA-F is currently the most enigmatic of the HLA molecules, as its function (mainly intracellular) is not clear. Human HLA Ia class molecules posses ten highly conserved amino acids responsible for the Ag recognition (Wainwright et al., 2000). The class Ib HLA-E and HLA-G present eight and nine amino acids of ten characteristic of HLA Ia, respectively. Instead HLA-F highly conserves only 5 residues of ten, suggesting a different biological function than a general peptide presentation to the T cells (Ishitani et al., 2006).

Although HLA-F is intracellular expressed in normal lymphocytes, under specific circumstances such protein can reach the cell surface (Lee et al., 2010). High level of HLA-F surface expression was observed in activated B, T, and NK cells (Lee et al., 2010). It appears that HLA-F is express in conjunction with the activated immune response, very early after the lymphocytes activation. An unusual property of HLA-F expressed on activated B and T cells is the high-mannose hybrid-type glycosilation. The glycosilation is a post-translational modification common to all the proteins transported from ER, through the Golgi, to cell surface. Similarly, CD1d protein is expressed in cell surface as 45 kDa endo-H-sensisitive glycoprotein (Kim et al., 1999). The endosomal localization of CD1d is mediated by its cytoplasmatic tail. The key residues for the signaling mechanism present on the CD1d tail are shared with HLA-F cytoplasmatic tail (Lawton et al., 2005). The HLA-F cytoplasmic tail shows a C-terminal valine essential for the ER export and the R x R motif responsible for the Golgi localization (Boyle et al., 2006; Iodice et al., 2001; Nufer et al., 2002). In different studies HLA-F was found associated with TAP but its surface expression was not reduced in TAP-mutant lines, but there was a low reduction in Tapasin-deficent lines (Lee and Geraghty, 2003). Moreover, a classical 10 amino acid-peptide has never been eluted from the peptide binding groove of HLA-F protein. These results could suggest that such glycoprotein is capable to escape the ER lumen and reaching the cell surface independently from TAP, Tapasina, and peptide binding, but using an alternative ER signal encoded in its cytoplasmic tail.

Some studies on molecular modeling of HLA-F reported a particular peptide binding groove conformation defined "open-ended" (Goodridge et al., 2010). It is well known that HLA I proteins binds 8-10 aa peptides and the end of the pocket is closed (Peaper and Cresswell, 2008). Theoretically, the peptide opened ended binding groove is able to include large peptides of up to 25 amino acids in length. It was demonstrated that HLA-F could be found in multiple conformational forms, at least three: complexed with the light chain β2m, in open conformation, and complexed with a HLA I heavy chain (HC). In a recent studies Goodridge et al. demonstrated that HLA-F expression was not only coincident with HLA I HC expression but also that HLA-F expression was downregulated after modification of HLA I HC structure (Goodridge et al., 2010). They also demonstrated that HLA I HC interacted only with HLA-F in open conformation (OC) and not in peptide bound complex (Goodridge et al., 2010).

Normally, MHC I molecules in open conformation are instable while HLA-F showed enough stability to enter into Golgi traffic and to reach and remain on the cell surface. It is possible that after immune response activation, HLA-F OC binds free forms of HLA I and as heterodimer reaches the cell surface (Goodridge et al., 2010). This data suggests that in absence of peptide bound complex HLA-F OC acts as chaperone to stabilize HLA I HC and to transport the free HLA I to, on, and from the cell surface (Goodridge et al., 2013). It was observed that after addition of free Ag, expressed HLA-F molecules were internalized through the endosomal pathway into lysosomes, where proteins are degradated to produce new peptides for Ag presentation in TAP independent way. Besides, the internalization and localization of Ag were coincident with the internalization and localization of HLA I HC and HLA-F (Goodridge et al., 2013). In addition, the downmodulation of HLA-F was coincident with the downmodulation of HLA I and in interference with Ag binding and presentation (Goodridge et al., 2013). On the base of these recent reports, HLA-F appears to cooperate with free HLA I molecules in a novel pathway for Ag cross-presentation on activated lymphocytes and monocytes (Goodridge et al., 2013).

It is known that HLA-F glycoproteins interacts with killer-cell immunoglobulin-like receptor (KIR) inhibiting their cytotoxic response. KIR receptors show a very high ability to differentiate between different allotypes (Parham et al., 2012). Considering the high expression of HLA-F on activated cells, its ability to form heterodymers with free forms of HLA I, and the alternative pathway of Ag cross presentation, Goodridge et al. supposed that the interaction between HLA-F-HLA I HC complex with KIRs may represent a new class of ligands (Goodridge et al., 2013). Clearly, this new relation receptor-ligand suggests a deeper function of KIR-HLA-F in the activated immune response (Goodridge et al., 2013). It has been found that the LILRB2 receptor binds peptide-free HLA I molecules in both folder and open conformation forms (Jones et al., 2011). Moreover in inflammatory conditions, KIR3DL2 and KIR3DL1 receptors expression highly increases early after NK cells activation (Chrul et al., 2006). The coincident upregulation of KIR receptors with the upregulation of the HLA-F-HLA I HC complex suggests an immunoregulatory role of HLA-F in inflammatory response.

4. Morfo-functional description of HLA-G molecule

The alternate splicing of HLA-G primary transcript generates seven different mRNAs. Thus, the same number of isoforms is encoded, and are divided into four membrane-bound (HLA-G1, G2, G3 and G4) and three soluble proteins (HLA-G5, G6 and G7) (Carosella et al., 2003). The alternative splicing that occurs in the primary transcripts is noteworthy not only because it is directly related to the production of soluble and truncated proteins, but specially because it can be regulated and, consequently, the expression of a specific HLA-G isoform will depend on the cell type and location (Le Rond et al., 2004; LeMaoult et al., 2005; Morales et al., 2003). Despite this alternate splicing of the mRNAs, the gene structure of HLA-G is homologous to other HLA class I genes, the so called classic HLA genes.

The extracellular structure of HLA-G1 and HLA-G5 is identical to the well described structure of classic HLA class I molecules. They are composed by three globular domains heavy-chain non-covalentely bound to beta2-microglobulin and a nonapeptide (Carosella et al., 2008). The other isoforms are simpler structures with only one or two globular domains, not binding to beta2-microglobulin neither presenting peptides (figure 1) (Carosella et al., 2008; Clements et al., 2005). The presence of an alpha-3 domain represents a binding site for HLA-G receptors, being consensual that this domain has an important role in the molecule function (Clements et al., 2005). HLA-G1 and HLA-G5 are the most described isoforms in healthy tissue, as well as shed HLA-G1, a soluble HLA-G1 isoform. This soluble shed HLA-G1 derives from the proteolytic shedding of the membrane HLA-G1. This process is dependent on metalloproteinase activity, at post-translational level, and is regulated by different levels of nitric oxide concentration and the activation of Tumor Necrosis Factor – alpha/NFkB pathway (Diaz-Lagares et al., 2009; Park et al., 2004; Zidi et al., 2006).

The HLA-G capability to form dimmers is one of its main features, since they bind to HLA-G receptors, showing higher affinity and slower dissociation rates, when compared to the monomers (Boyson et al., 2002; Shiroishi et al., 2006). Accordingly, it is thought that dimmers are responsible for the majority of HLA-G functions (Gonen-Gross et al., 2003). The dimerization of HLA-G, by intramolecular disulfide bonds, is a result of the presence of two unique cysteine residues, located in the position 42 of the alpha-1 domain and in the position 147 of the alpha-2 domain (Boyson et al., 2002).

The HLA-G molecules do not seem to have significant functions at immune response level, unlike classic HLA class I molecules (Carosella et al., 2008). However, they have the same capability to bind inhibitory receptors, just like the HLA class I molecules (Colonna et al., 1997; Colonna et al., 1998; Rajagopalan and Long, 1999). Three HLA-G receptors have been described, namely: immunoglobulin-like transcript 2 (ILT2) (CD8 5j/LILRB1), ILT4 (CD85d/LILRB2) and the killer cell immunoglobulin-like receptor (KIR) 2DL4 (CD1 58d) (Colonna et al., 1997; Colonna et al., 1998; Rajagopalan and Long, 1999).

ILT2 is expressed by B cells, some T cells (both CD4+ and CD8+), some NK cells and all monocytes/dendritric cells (Colonna et al., 1997). On the contrary, ILT4 is myeloid-specified and is only expressed by monocytes/dendritric cells (Colonna et al., 1998). The higher affinity of HLA-G for LILR1 and, consequently, ILT2, may result from the presence of phenylalanine and tyrosine in the positions 195 and 197 of the alpha-3 domain, respectively. This altered structured, when compared with other HLA class I molecules, increase hydrophobicity, which seems to be the basis of this affinity increased level (Clements et al., 2005). Both ILT receptors are able to recognize different HLA-G structures. ILT2 binds only to beta-2m-associated HLA-G1/G5 isoforms, while ILT4 is also able to recognize the beta-2m-free counter parts from this isoforms (Gonen-Gross et al., 2005; Shiroishi et al., 2006). The presence of antibodies reactive with ILT receptors revealed that the interaction of HLA-G tetramers with blood monocytes was largely due to binding to ILT4, so, higher expression of ILT2 was necessary for efficient HLA-G tetramer binding (Allan et al., 1999). This suggests that the interaction of ILT2 has lower affinity, compared to that of ILT4.

The other ligand, KIR2DL4, is expressed by some CD8+ T and NK cells (Goodridge et al., 2003). These subsets of NK cells (CD56) are a minority of peripheral NK cells, but a majority of uterine NK cells (Goodridge et al., 2003; Kikuchi-Maki et al., 2003). While ILT2 and ILT4 are clearly described as inhibitory receptors, the same cannot be said about KIR2DL4, in such an absolute way. Despite the capacity of KIR2DL4 of sending inhibitory signals, it can send also activatory signals. This receptor has a single immunoreceptor tyrosine-based inhibitory motif in its cytoplamsatic tail and a positively charged arginine in the transmembrane region (Selvakumar et al., 1996; Yusa et al., 2002). Finally, this receptor also differentiates from ILTs because these ones bind classic HLA molecules, whereas HLA-G molecules are the only ligands of KIR2DL4 (Colonna et al., 1997; Colonna et al., 1998).

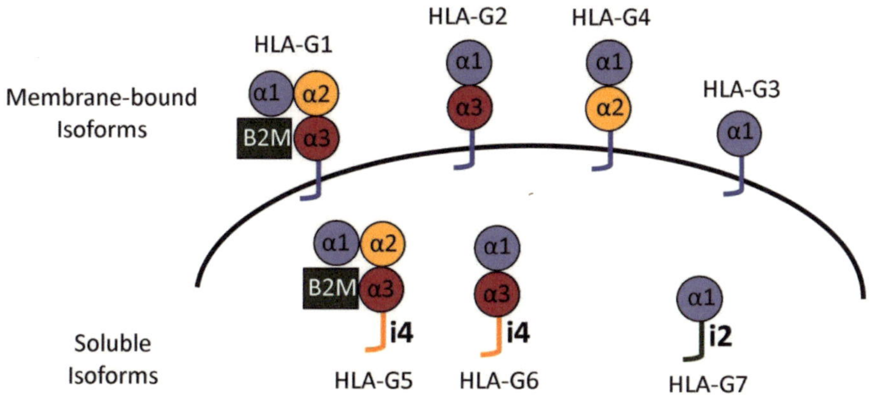

Figure 1. HLA-G isoforms. The alternate splicing of HLA-G primary transcript generates seven different mRNAs. The same number of isoforms is encoded, divided into four membrane-bound and three soluble proteins. Truncated isoforms are generated by excision of one or 2 exons encoding globular domains, whereas translation of intron 4 or intron 2 yields soluble isoforms that lack the transmembrane domain.

5. The HLA-E, HLA-F, and HLA-G polymorphism in world populations

The Human Major Histocompability Complex (MHC) consists of 224 genes encoding proteins controlling cell-to-cell interactions. These genes include the classical class Ia and the non classical class Ib loci. The Ia class is involved in immunological recognition and the Ib class is associated with modulation of the immune system (Hviid, 2006; Townsend and Bodmer, 1989). Each of the nonclassical molecules can be distinguished by well identified biological features: low expression levels, restricted tissue expression, reduced cytoplasmatic tail, unique molecular structure, limited protein variability, and modulation of the immune response cells (Carosella et al., 2008; Diehl et al., 1996; Ishitani et al., 2003; Kovats et al., 1990; Lee et al., 1998). Although the Ia class genes are the most polymorphic known in human, the Ib class genes show a low level of polymorphism. Such variation can be explained by different evolutionary forces acting on HLA family genes. It is believed that the nonclassical gene have been maintained under a distinct selective pressure while the classical gene have been characterized by overdominant selection (Little and Parham, 1999). The polymorphisms of the Ib class do not involve the peptide binding groove (unlike the classical HLA Ia) but it is distributed among the $\alpha1$, $\alpha2$, and $\alpha3$ domains (van der Ven et al., 1998). The limited polymorphism of nonclassical HLA has long been believed to reflect the functional diversity required of these molecules (Little and Parham, 1999). The low variability is probably due to a very limited repertoire of peptides presented to T cells (Castro et al., 2000). In fact, HLA-E proteins exhibit on the cell surface a restricted subset of peptides derived from other HLA sequences (Braud et al., 1998; Llano et al., 1998). Moreover, a non variable molecule structure allows an opportune modulation of the immune response in vital situations. HLA-G proteins act as mediator of maternal-fetal tolerance, in order to anergizing the maternal allo-response to antigens. Lack of polymorphism ensures that the paternally derived HLA-G molecules are similar to those of the mother (Le Bouteiller, 1997; Ober, 1998). On the other side, a variation concentrated at the peptide binding groove let the Ia class bind diverse and overlapping sets of peptides. This way, their high polymorphism permits the exhibition as many different peptides as possible to the αβ T-cell receptors (TCR).

Compared to classical HLA class I that exhibit hundreds of alleles, the HLA Ib present only few variants. With the increasing number of HLA alleles identified, much effort has been devoted to standardize HLA nomenclature. Currently an allele name may be composed by HLA prefix, following by the name of the gene and four, six, or eight digits. Longer names with more digits are only assigned when necessary. A separator (*) is necessary to clearly separate the name of the gene from the number identifying the allele and a colon (:) is necessary to delimit each single fields. The first two digits refer to the allele family, which often corresponds to the serological specificity. The third and the fourth assign the order in which the sequence were determined (Marsh et al., 2010). Alleles whose names differ in the first four digits must have at least one non-synonymous nucleotide substitution that changes the amino acid sequence of the encoded protein. Exemplifying, the HLA G*01:03 allele differs from HLA G* 01:01 allele by a non-synonymous substitution (A-T) at codon 31 in exon 2, exchanging a threonine for serine. Alleles showing synonymous substitution within the coding sequence are distinguished by the use of the fifth and sixth digits (Marsh et al., 2010). For instance the HLA E*01:03:01 allele differs from HLA E* 01:03:02 allele by a silent substitution (C-T) at codon 77 in exon 2. Finally, nucleotide modification observed in introns and in 3′ or 5′ untranslated regions are distinguished by the use of the seventh and the eight digits (Marsh et al., 2010). In addition, an optional suffix may be added to the end of the allele name to indicate its expression status. For example, the HLA G*01:05N (null) allele shows a cytosine deletion at the codon 130 in exon 3 that changes the reading frame and creates a premature stop at codon 171.

5.1. HLA-E polymorphism

HLA-E loci are the most conserved of all the HLA system (Grimsley and Ober, 1997). Currently, 11 HLA-E alleles have been identified in worldwide human populations, encoding three distinct functional proteins (HLA E*01:01, E*01:02, E*01:03) (http://www.ebi.ac.uk/ipd/imgt/hla., Ocober 2013; Robinson et al., 2013). The HLA E*01:03 allele differs from HLA E* 01:01 allele by a non-synonymous substitution (A-G) at codon 107 in exon 3, exchanging arginine/glycine. In spite of its limited polymorphism, the major two alleles showed different biological properties and expression patterns (Tripathi et al., 2006). HLA E*01:04 allele is characterized by two non-synonymous substitutions: the first is the (A-G) mutation at codon 107 in exon 3 and the second is a (A-G) mutation at codon 157 in exon 3, exchanging arginine /glycine (Strong et al., 2003). Previously, another HLA-E allele has been identified (HLA E*01:02), but this sequence has been deleted from IMGT/HLA database because it was identical to HLA E*01:01:01:01 allele (Lauterbach et al., 2012). Until now the existence of the HLA E*01:04 allele has been subject of many controversy. In 1990, the HLA E*01:04 was originally identified in 1 Japanese out of 22 individuals (Ohya et al., 1990). In 2000, the allele was found in an English population with a low allele frequency (Hodgkinson et al., 2000). Thereafter, the E*01:04 allele has not been identified in any other population so far studied. Some authors speculated that such allele could represent a consequence of a sequencing artifact (Antoun et al., 2009; Grimsley et al., 2002; Park et al., 2007; Romero et al., 2007).

HLA-E polymorphism has been already well studied in several populations and clinical cohorts. Table 1 lists the HLA-E distribution in different ethnic populations. Although several alleles were found among the ethnic groups, the two major alleles (HLA E*01:01 and HLA E*01:03) have been always reported with high frequencies, suggesting a balancing selection operating in order to maintain the two sequences unaltered (Grimsley and Ober, 1997). In 1992 four ape species sequences were examined and the mutation A107G was found in all genomes. This implies that HLA E*01:03 is the original allele and the mutation occurred during the human evolution, probably before the *H. sapiens* expansion, as the two alleles are present in worldwide populations (Grimsley and Ober, 1997).

The geography and the ethnicity were associated to HLA-E variation. In occidental populations the HLA E*01:01 allele was the predominant, while in oriental populations the allele frequency of *01:03 was equal or higher than HLA E*01:01 frequency. The only exceptions were two population of South America (Wayu Indian and Afro-Colombian) where *01:03 was found more frequently than *01:01 (Arnaiz-Villena et al., 2007). It is possible that in these cases the high frequency of the *01:03 allele derives from Caucasian admixture where such allele is the second most common (Arnaiz-Villena et al., 2007). In North America, the Caucasian populations presented the two alleles at nearly equal proportions while the Afro-Americans presented a pattern more similar to that one from African populations, with *01:01 more frequent than *01:03 (Ferguson et al., 2011; Geraghty et al., 1992; Grimsley and Ober, 1997). Furthmore, higher variability was found inside the HLA E*01:03 group. A silent substitution (C-T) at codon 77 in exon 2 distinguished HLA E*01:03:01 from HLA E*01:03:02. In Africa and in Asia the two variants showed nearly equal frequencies. In Europe and in South America populations the *01:03:02 allele was more common than *01:03:01 allele. An exception was an Afro-Caribbean study where the two alleles showed the same frequencies, like in African populations (Antoun et al., 2009). The similarity in the allelic pattern of Afro-Americans and Afro-Caribbean with African population probably reflects their ethnic history, composition and evolution.

5.2. HLA-F polymorphism

There is very little information about HLA-F allelic polymorphism among worldwide populations. Only two studies on HLA-F investigating multiple human populations exist so far (Pan et al., 2013; Pyo et al., 2006). Currently, 22 distinct HLA-F alleles encoding for four distinct proteins (HLA F*01:01, HLA F*01:02, HLA F*01:03, HLA F*01:04) are currently described in human populations (http://www.ebi.ac.uk/ipd/imgt/hla., Ocober 2013; Robinson et al., 2013). The HLA F*01:02 allele differs from HLA F* 01:01 allele by a (C-T) mutation at codon 13 in exon 1, exchanging alanine /valine. The HLA F*01:03 allele is characterized by a (C-A) mutation at codon 71 in exon 2, exchanging a proline for a glutamine. HLA F*01:04 contains a (T-C) substitution at codon 272 in exon 4, exchanging a serine for a proline. Table 2 lists the HLA-F distribution in different ethnic populations studied so far. The HLA-F polymorphism differed among the ethnic groups. The HLA F*01:01 was the most common with a frequency always up to 90% (Pan et al., 2013). HLA F*01:03 was the second most common but with a low frequency (4-6%) and with even lower frequency in two populations of South China (1-2%) (Pan et al., 2013). The HLA F*01:04 and *01:02 were rare (Pan et al., 2013; Pyo et al., 2006). It is reasonable to consider HLA F*01:01 the ancestral allele considering the strong predominance of HLA F*01:01 and the rarity of other HLA-F alleles (Pan et al., 2013).

5.3. HLA-G polymorphism

HLA-G polymorphism has been extensively analyzed (Hviid, 2006; Morales et al., 1993; Ober et al., 1996). According to the international ImmunoGeneTics Database, 50 HLA-G alleles are currently described, generating 16 distinct functional proteins (HLA G*01:01, *01:02, *01:03, *01:04, *01:06, *01:07, *01:08, *01:09, *01:10, *01:11, *01:12, *01:14, *01:15, *01:16, *01:17 *01:18) and two null alleles (*01:05N, *01:13N) (http://www.ebi.ac.uk/ipd/imgt/hla., Ocober 2013; Robinson et al., 2013). Table 3 lists the HLA-G distribution in different ethnic populations. Beside the original allele HLA G*01:01, only four variations related to amino acid exchange in the coding regions were frequent in worldwide populations (HLA G*01:03, *01:04, *01:05N, and *01:06) (Castelli et al., 2007). The HLA G*01:04 allele differs from HLA G* 01:01 allele by a non-synonymous substitution (C-A) at codon 110 in exon 3, exchanging leucine/isoleucine. The HLA G*01:06 allele is characterized by a C-T mutation at codon 258 in exon 4, exchanging a threonine for a methionine. HLA-G alleles frequencies vary among different ethnic groups, but an accurate comparison among populations is difficult, as there are not many reports using a high resolution data and each study was performed at different time (Park et al., 2012).

The distribution of the HLA-G was not significantly different among populations with respect to HLA G*01:01 group. HLA G*01:01:01 was the predominant allele with a frequency of 60% in Europe, 50% North America, 40% in South America and Africa, and 30% in Asia. It was originally described in 1987 and probably it is the wild-type sequence as it is present in other primate genomes (Geraghty et al., 1987). The frequency of HLA G*01:01:02 was high, constituting approximately 50% in Europe populations, 30% in North America, 20% in South America and Africa, and 15 % in Asia. This allele is characterized by a nonsynonymous C-T mutation at codon 142 in exon 3. HLA G* 01:01:08 was a rare allele in most populations with exception of Brazil (8 and 15%), Zimbabwe (6%), and Poland (5%) (Simoes et al., 2009; Sipak-Szmigiel et al., 2008). This allele is characterized by a nonsynonimous G-A mutation at codon 57 in exon 2.

The HLA G*01:02 allele was found only in South America while it was completely absent in other populations (Arnaiz-Villena et al., 2013). This allele is characterized by a nonsynonimous mutation at codon 54 in exon 2, exchanging a glycine for an arginine.

The HLA G* 01:04:01 allele was found with high frequencies in Canadian, Asian, and Africa populations while it was low in Brazil and Caucasian population. The population of Nunavik in Canada presented the highest level of frequency with 50%, followed by Singapore (45%), Japan (38%), Korea (34%), and Iran (29%) (Ishitani et al., 1999; Metcalfe et al., 2013; Park et al., 2012; Tan et al., 2008). This allele is characterized by a synonymous G-A mutation at codon 57 in exon 2 and a nonsynonymous C-A mutation at codon 110 in exon 3 exchanging a leucine for an isoleucine.

The null allele HLA G*01:05N was detected with high frequency in Spanish (6%) and in Africa-Americans (7%) and with even higher frequency in Iraqi (8%), Indians (14%), and Iranians (18%) (Abbas et al., 2004; Ishitani et al., 1999; Jassem et al., 2012; Rahimi et al., 2010; Suarez et al., 1997). The frequency of the null allele among Caucasian from Europe and South America was low. In Brazil the prevalence of the allele varied from 1% to 3%, while in Europe from 1% to 6%. In Singapore, China, and in some populations of USA the null allele was rare (Abbas et al., 2004; Aldrich et al., 2001; Lin et al., 2006; Yan et al., 2006). In Peru, Guatemala, Japan, and Portugal the allele was completely absent (Alvarez et al., 1999; Arnaiz-Villena et al., 2013; Ishitani et al., 1999). Those reports suggest that the null mutation arose recently in the human population, probably in Africa. Considering the role of HLA-G in the placenta and the selective pressures operating at this stage of development, a new allele could be easily fixed in a population (Ishitani et al., 1999). Then, from Africa it could be introduced into the Spanish population by Arab invaders and into African America population with the slave deportation (Ishitani et al., 1999).

The distribution of the HLA G* 01:06 allele revealed some differences among the populations. This allele contains a nonconservative amino acid substitution (C-T) at codon 258 in exon 4, exchanging threonine/methionine. It occurred with frequencies minor then 8% in Europe, Canada, and Brazil. It showed low frequencies in Asia, and it is completely absent in Africa.

Nine alleles exhibited a point substitution detected only in a single study: the HLA G*01:07, *01:12, *01:13N, *01:14, *01:16, and *01:18 alleles were detected only in one population in Canada (Lajoie et al., 2008; Roger et al., 2012); the HLA G*01:10, *01:11, *01:17 alleles were detected only in Kenia (Luo et al., 2013); and HLA G*01:15 was detected only in Kenya and Canada (Alvarez et al., 1999; Lajoie et al., 2008; Roger et al., 2012).

Country	Reference	HLA E alleles									
		01:01	01:01:01	01:02	01:03	01:03:01	01:03:02	01:03:03	01:03:04	01:03:05	01:04
Spain	(Gomez-Casado et al., 1997)	•		•		o	•				
Spain	(Guzman-Fulgencio et al., 2013)	•			•						
England	(Hodgkinson et al., 2000)	•		•	•						•
Germany	(Furst et al., 2012)	•			•						
Italy	(Paladini et al., 2009)		•			•	•				
South France	(Di Cristofaro et al., 2011)	•				•	•	•	•		
The Neitherland	(Paquay et al., 2009)	•			•						
France	(Tamouza et al., 2006)				*						

Country	Reference	HLA E alleles									
		01:01	01:01:01	01:02	01:03	01:03:01	01:03:02	01:03:03	01:03:04	01:03:05	01:04
Austria	(Danzer et al., 2009)				*						
Caucasian	(Grimsley et al., 2002)	•				•	•				
Caucasian	(Pyo et al., 2006)		•			•	•		•		
Euro-Caucasian	(Antoun et al., 2009)		•			•	•	•	•		
Hispanic	(Grimsley and Ober, 1997)	•			•						
Caucasian	(Grimsley and Ober, 1997)	•			•						
Caucasian	(Arnaiz-Villena et al., 2007)	•				•	•				
Canada	(Ferguson et al., 2011)	•			•						
USA	(Geraghty et al., 1992)	•			•						
Hutterites	(Grimsley and Ober, 1997)	•			•						
Afro-American	(Grimsley and Ober, 1997)	•			•						
Afro-American	(Pyo et al., 2006)		•			•	•		•		
Afro-American	(Grimsley et al., 2002)	•				•	•				
Mazatecan	(Arnaiz-Villena et al., 2007)	•				•	•				
Mexico	(Arnaiz-Villena et al., 2007)	•				•	•				
Wayu	(Arnaiz-Villena et al., 2007)	•				•	•				
Colombia	(Arnaiz-Villena et al., 2007)	•				•	•				
Afro-Colombia	(Arnaiz-Villena et al., 2007)	•				•	•				
Afro-Carabbean	(Antoun et al., 2009)		•			•	•	•	•		
Mapuche	(Arnaiz-Villena et al., 2007)	•				•	•				
Brazil	(Veiga-Castelli et al., 2012)		•			•	•				
Brazil	(Veiga-Castelli et al., 2012)									o	
South Brazil	(Carvalho dos Santos et al., 2013)	•				•	•	•	•		
Negroids	(Arnaiz-Villena et al., 2007)	•				•	•				
Tunisia	(Hassen et al., 2011)	•			•						
Egypt	(Mosaad et al., 2011)	•			•						
Mapuche	(Arnaiz-Villena et al., 2007)	•				•	•				
Teke Congolese	(Di Cristofaro et al., 2011)	•				•	•	•	•		
Tswa Pygmies	(Di Cristofaro et al., 2011)	•				•	•	•	•		
Zimbawe	(Lajoie et al., 2006)	•			•						
Africa (Shona)	(Matte et al., 2000)	•				•	•				
Japan	(Grimsley et al., 2002)	•				•	•	•			
Japan	(Pyo et al., 2006)		•			•	•		•		
Shangai Han	(Zhao et al., 2001)	•				•	•				
Thailand	(Kimkong et al., 2003)	•				•	•				
Thai -China	(Kimkong et al., 2003)	•				•	•				

http://dx.doi.org/10.5772/57507

Country	Reference	HLA E alleles									
		01:01	01:01:01	01:02	01:03	01:03:01	01:03:02	01:03:03	01:03:04	01:03:05	01:04
Thailand	(Hirankarn et al., 2004)	•			•						
Korea	(Park et al., 2007)	•				•	•				
India	(Arnaiz-Villena et al., 2007)	•				•	•				
India	(Tripathi et al., 2006)	•				•	•				
China (Hunan han)	(Liu et al., 2012)	•			•						
China (Mongolia Han)	(Liu et al., 2012)	•			•						
China (Mongolia Mongol)	(Liu et al., 2012)	•			•						
China (Guangdong Han)	(Liu et al., 2012)	•			•						
China	(Zhen et al., 2013)	•				•	•				
China	(Grimsley and Ober, 1997)	•			•						
Indo-Asian	(Antoun et al., 2009)	•				•	•	•	•		
Orientals	(Arnaiz-Villena et al., 2007)	•				•	•				
Australia	(Hosseini et al., 2013)	•			•						

*: HLA E 01:03 specific study

o New allele identification

Table 1. HLA E distribution in different ethnic populations.

Country	Reference	HLA F Alleles																						
		01:01	01:01:01:01	01:01:01:02	01:01:01:03	01:01:01:04	01:01:01:05	01:01:01:06	01:01:01:07	01:01:02	01:01:02:01	01:01:02:02	01:01:02:03	01:01:02:04	01:01:02:05	01:01:03:01	01:01:03:02	01:01:03:03	01:01:03:04	01:02	01:03	01:03:01:01	01:03:01:02	01:04
Japan	(Uchigiri et al., 1997)	•																						
Japan	(Pyo et al., 2006)		•	•	•	•	•	•	•		•	•	•	•	•	•	•	•	•	•		•	•	•
Japan	(He et al., 2004)									o														
Hunana-Han	(Pan et al., 2013)	•																			•			•
Mongolia-Han	(Pan et al., 2013)	•																			•			•
Mongolia-Mongol	(Pan et al., 2013)	•																			•			•
Guangdong-Han	(Pan et al., 2013)	•																			•			•
Caucasian	(Pyo et al., 2006)		•	•	•	•	•	•	•		•	•	•	•	•	•	•	•	•	•		•	•	•
Afro-American	(Pyo et al., 2006)		•	•	•	•	•	•	•		•	•	•	•	•	•	•	•	•	•		•	•	•

o New allele identification.

Table 2. HLA F distribution in different ethnic populations.

Country	Reference	HLA G alleles																																				
		01:01	01:01:01	01:01:02	01:01:03	01:01:04	01:01:05	01:01:06	01:01:07	01:01:08	01:01:09	01:01:10	01:01:11	01:01:12	01:01:14	01:01:15	01:01:17	01:01:20	01:02	01:03	01:03:01	01:04	01:04:01	01:04:02	01:04:03	01:04:04	01:04:05	01:05N	01:06	01:07	01:09	01:10	01:11	01:12	01:13N	01:14	01:15	01:16	01:17	01:18
Quebec (Inuit)	(Metcalfe et al., 2013)		•	•	•					•										•			•							•										
Quebec	(Metcalfe et al., 2013)		•	•	•																		•						•											
Quebec	(Ferguson et al., 2011)		•	•	•		•		•	•										•			•		•			•												
Canada	(Lajoie et al., 2008)																																	o	o	o	o	o		
Canada	(Roger et al., 2012)																																							o
Canada	(Ferguson et al., 2012)		•	•	•					•										•			•			•		•	•											
Caucasian	(Warner et al., 2002)		•	•	•															•			•					•	•											
USA - Canada	(Aldrich et al., 2001)		•	•	•		•	•	•	•										•			•	•	•			•												
Africa - America	(Ishitani et al., 1999)		•	•	•																	•						•												
Guatemala	(Arnaiz-Villena et al., 2013)	•	•	•	•														•		•		•						•		•									
Peru	(Arnaiz-Villena et al., 2013)	•	•	•	•														•		•		•						•		•									
Euro-Brazilian	(Nardi Fda et al., 2012)		•	•	•			•	•	•				•	•			•			•		•		•	•		•	•											
Brazil	(Castelli et al., 2011)	•	•	•	•		•				•									•		•	•			•	•	•	•		•									
Brazil	(Simoes et al., 2009)	•																		•		•						•												
Brazil	(Castelli et al., 2008)	•	•	•	•	•	•	•		•			•							•		•	•			•		•	•		•									
Brazil	(Pirri et al., 2009)	•			•	•				•										•			•					•												
Brazil	(Castelli et al., 2007)		•	•	•	•		•		•										•			•			•		•	•											
France	(Di Cristofaro et al., 2011)	•																		•		•						•	•											
Poland	(Sipak-Szmigiel et al., 2009)		•	•	•			•		•	•									•			•					•	•											
Poland	(Sipak-Szmigiel et al., 2008)		•	•	•	•	•	•		•		•								•			•					•												
Italy	(Rizzo et al., 2008)			•	•															•								•												
Italy	(Moreau et al., 2008)	•																		•		•						•	•											
Denmark	(Hviid et al., 2002)		•	•	•		•			•										•			•		•			•	•											
Germany	(Pfeiffer et al., 2001)		•	•	•																		•	•				•												
Portugal	(Alvarez et al., 1999)		•	•	•															•		•																		
Finland	(Karhukorpi et al., 1996)		•	•	•																																			
Spain	(Suarez et al., 1997)		•	•	•																	•						o												
Caucasian	(van der Ven et al., 1998)	•	•	•	•																•	•	•					•												
Kenia	(Luo et al., 2013)		•	•	•					•	•					•	•				•		•				•	•				•	•						•	
Teke Congo	(Di Cristofaro et al., 2011)	•																		•		•						•									•			
Tswa Pygmie	(Di Cristofaro et al., 2011)	•																		•		•						•												
Zimbabwe	(Matte et al., 2004)		•	•						•										•			•					•												
Tunisia	(Ghandri et al., 2011)	•																				•						•												
Ghana	(Ishitani et al., 1999)		•	•																		•						•												
East Africa	(Matte et al., 2002)		•	•						•										•			•					•												
Iraq	(Jassem et al., 2012)	•	•	•	•															•		•						•	•											
Korea	(Park et al., 2012)		•	•	•					•										•			•					•	•											
Iran	(Rahimi et al., 2010)		•	•	•		•		•	•													•		•			•												
Singapore	(Tan et al., 2008)	•	•	•	•					•										•			•					•	•											
India	(Abbas et al., 2004)		•	•	•	•	•			•									•	•		•						•	•											
Japan	(Ishitani et al., 1999)		•	•	•																	•																		
China Han	(Yan et al., 2006)		•	•	•					•										•			•	•	•			•												
China Han	(Lin et al., 2006)		•	•	•					•										•			•	•	•			•												

o New allele identification.

Table 3. Table 3. HLA G distribution in different ethnic populations.

6. HLA-G and disease association

Since its cloning and sequencing, in 1987 (Geraghty et al., 1987), and the discovery of HLA-G expression in early gestation human cytotrophoblasts (Kovats et al., 1990) that this locus has been investigated for its tolerogenic function. The maternal-fetal interface is known to protect the fetus from destruction by the immune system of its mother (Loustau et al., 2013). Besides this function, HLA-G and its pathological relevance have long been investigated, in several areas of research, and it has already been associated with numerous conditions (Carosella et al., 2008; Donadi et al., 2011).

As previously mentioned, HLA-G gene exhibits several distinctive biological features that differ from other HLA Class I molecules: 1) limited protein variability due to low number of polymorphic sites within the coding region, 2) presence of several membrane-bound and soluble isoforms (G1-G5), generated by alternative splicing, 3) unique molecular structure with a reduced cytoplasmic tail due to a STOP codon in exon 6, 4) modulation of the immune response, being a potent tolerogenic molecule with known inhibitory functions, 5) and restricted tissue expression to trophoblast cells (Kovats et al., 1990), adult thymic medulla (Mallet et al., 1999) and stem cells (Selmani et al., 2008). However, HLA-G neo expression can be induced in several pathological conditions such as cancers, transplantation, multiple sclerosis, inflammatory diseases and viral infections.

The association of the HLA-G molecule and diseases/conditions is obviously related to its function (Table 4) and many studies provide evidence of this association. The objective of this section is not to review all of those studies but to highlight the most recent and significant.

Action	Cells	Activity	References
inhibits	NK cell and cytotoxic T lymphocyte	cytolytic activity	(Riteau et al., 2001; Rouas-Freiss et al., 1997)
inhibits	CD4+ T cell	alloproliferative responses	(LeMaoult et al., 2004)
inhibits	T cell and NK cell	ongoing proliferation	(Bahri et al., 2006; Caumartin et al., 2007; LeMaoult et al., 2004)
inhibits	dendritic cell	maturation	(Gros et al., 2008; Liang et al., 2008)
induces	suppressive T cells	generation	(Agaugue et al., 2011; Gros et al., 2008)

Table 4. The association of the HLA-G molecule with diseases/conditions and its function.

6.1. HLA-G and pregnancy related problems

Human leukocyte antigen (HLA)-G has long been considered an important participant on the fetal-maternal tolerance and is thought to play a crucial role in ensuring a successful pregnancy. A vast number of studies have suggested that the expression of HLA-G, influenced by the genetic variation in the gene, is associated with pregnancy related problems. However, there is no actual consensus about the real clinical value of specific genetic variations. Furthermore, some authors stress out that most of the studies on this topic assessed the role of HLA-G taking into account only the maternal genotype and ignored the contribution of the fetus. The authors suggest that studies on placental diseases should address HLA-G expression and genetic variations also to the fetus/placenta (Cecati et al., 2011).

In the latest published studies there is a special interest in the 14bp insertion(ins)/deletion(del), which may have an effect on the HLA-G protein stability and soluble HLA-G quantity. A meta-analysis study was recently performed to evaluate the association of this polymorphism with unexplained recurrent spontaneous abortions (URSA). 14 studies with 1464 cases and 1247 controls were included. Significant associations between 14 bp ins/del polymorphism and risk of URSA were observed in both dominant and codominant models, suggesting that this polymorphism is indeed associated with increased risk of URSA (Wang et al., 2013). Another study investigated the homozygous carriage of the 14 base pair (bp) insertion and recurrent miscarriage (RM). The authors investigated the G14bp insertion(ins)/deletion(del) polymorphism in 339 women with unexplained RM and 125 control women. The authors observed that homozygosity for G14bp ins predisposes to RM. The combination of G14 ins homozygosity and carriage of an HLA class II (HYrHLA) allele restricting immunity against male-specific minor HY antigens predisposes to secondary RM in women with a firstborn boy and negatively affects birth weight in these boys (Christiansen et al., 2012).

A recent case-control study, investigated the association between the genetic variability of the HLA-G gene and serum levels of soluble HLA-G in cases of embryo implantation failure (IF). 40 couples with implantation failure and 83 fertile couples were investigated. HLA-G alleles were typed (SBT) and the quantification of soluble HLA-G (sHLA-G) was performed by ELISA. There was a significant difference between the HLA-G allelic distributions between IF couples and the control couples. The HLA-G*01:03:01 allele was increased in the IF couples. There were no significant differences in the serum levels of sHLA-G in the IF and control groups. The authors suggest that the distribution of HLA-G products may play a significant role in the modulation of maternal-fetal immune response (Nardi Fda et al., 2012).

Another study shows evidence of HLA-G regulation at the post-transcriptional level. The authors investigated the role of a specific micro RNA (miR-133a) in regulating HLA-G expression and the pathogenesis of recurrent spontaneous abortion (RSA). Twelve patients with RSA at 7 gestational weeks were screened by array-based comparative genome hybridization. The villi of RSA with normal karyotype were further screened by miRNA microarrays. Multi-software prediction and real-time PCR confirmed that miR-133a was most likely to bind to HLA-G 3' untranscribed region (UTR). Relevance analysis showed that, compared with IA villi, miR-133a was greatly overexpressed in RSA villi with normal karyotype ($P<0.01$), but not in abnormal RSA villi. A luciferase reporter assay suggested that miR-133a interacted with HLA-G 3' UTR. Overexpression of miR-133a in JEG-3 cells decreased HLA-G expression at the protein level, with no effect on mRNA. These findings provide strong evidence that miR-133a regulates HLA-G expression by reducing translation and is involved in the pathogenesis of RSA (Wang et al., 2012).

There is still much to be learnt about the HLA-G and pregnancy related topics. The interest of HLA-G in Assisted Reproduction Technology (ART) has been growing since the existence of markers to determine a successful pre-implantation embryo would definitely minimize the negative outcomes of In vitro fertilization (IVF) techniques. A multicenter retrospective study was recently undertaken to determine whether the presence of soluble human leukocyte antigen G (sHLA-G) affects implantation and pregnancy outcomes *in vitro*. Embryos obtained

http://dx.doi.org/10.5772/57507

from 2,040 patients from six different IVF clinics were investigated. Soluble HLA-G determination on day-2 embryos after intracytoplasmic sperm injection, with embryos transferred on day 3 using the sHLA-G data. All embryos were individually cultured, and a chemiluminescence enzyme-linked immunosorbent assay was used to detect the presence of sHLA-G in the culture medium surrounding the embryos. Embryos were selected based on a positive sHLA-G result and a graduated embryo scoring (GES) score >70, or on embryo morphology if the test was negative. In all centers, a positive sHLA-G result was associated with an increase in the odds of an ongoing pregnancy. The incidence of an ongoing pregnancy was 2.52 times greater in embryos transferred on day 3 with a positive sHLA-G test result than the incidence of an ongoing pregnancy in embryos with a negative sHLA-G test result. As a conclusion, data from this multicenter study confirm that sHLA-G expression is a valuable noninvasive embryo marker to assist in improving pregnancy outcomes (Kotze et al., 2013).

The results of this study are promising but further confirmation is needed.

6.2. HLA-G and cancer

Cancer cells exhibit tumor-associated antigens which are coded by mutated or normal deregulated genes that, once presented by classical MHC class I molecules, may be recognized by host immune system, being frequently eliminated. Neoplastic cells are capable of growing and evolving, by tumour immunoediting, to aggressive malignant lesions (Carosella and Horuzsko, 2007; Donadi et al., 2011; Dunn et al., 2004). Tumor immunoediting consists of three major steps based on the elimination, equilibrium and escape (Dunn et al., 2004):

1. Most immunogenic tumor cells are eliminated by cytotoxic T and NK cells;
2. Tumour cells with reduced immunogenicity are selected;
3. Variants that no longer respond to the host immune system are maintained.

The ectopic expression of HLA-G in cancer occurs in several types of primary tumors, metastases and malignant effusions and can be found in tumour cells and tumour infiltrating cells. This expression has been shown important for the first step of the immunoediting process as it inhibits the cytotoxic function of T and NK cells (Carosella and Horuzsko, 2007).

A recent review paper written by Curigliano and colleagues highlights the underlying molecular mechanisms of impaired HLA-G expression, the immune tolerant function of HLA-G in tumors, and the potential diagnostic use of membrane-bound and soluble HLA-G as a biomarker to identify tumors and to monitor disease stage. The authors stress out the importance of HLA-G as an attractive therapeutic strategy against cancer (Curigliano et al., 2013).

A recent study made the evaluation of plasma soluble HLA-G (sHLA-G) concentrations and the 14-bp insertion/deletion polymorphism of the HLA-G gene in patients with papillary thyroid carcinoma (PTC) or Hashimoto's thyroiditis (HT) to assess the possible association of these parameters with PTC aggressiveness. Besides the confirmation of the frequent association between PTC and chronic autoimmune thyroiditis, this study suggests that elevated circulating sHLA-G levels, can be an important signal of alterations of immune homeostasis that can possibly be considered a potential novel marker of PTC histopathological aggressiveness at diagnosis. However, additional studies are needed to confirm the actual role and clinical relevance of the HLA-G complex in PTC development and progression (Dardano et al., 2012).

An interesting study investigated whether or not HLA-G expression is associated with breast cancer molecular subtypes. HLA-G expression was immunohistochemically investigated in 104 patients with invasive ductal breast carcinoma, in which 56 were luminal A, 17 were luminal B, 19 were HER-2, and 12 were basal-like/normal breast-like subtype classified according to immunohistochemical staining results of ER, HER-2, CK5/6, and EGFR. Host immune response status was assessed by estimating the density of tumor infiltrating lymphocytes (TIL). The authors reported that there were more cases with high expressions of HLA-G in non-luminal than in luminal subtypes (P=0.035). In contrast, more cases with high density of TIL was found in luminal than in non-luminal subtypes (P=0.023). Compared to all the biomarkers studied, only HLA-G expression was found to be inversely associated with the density of TIL (P=0.004). Furthermore, patients with HLA-G(high)/TIL(low) status had a higher risk of recurrence than those with HLA-G(low)/TIL(high) status, regardless of the molecular subtypes. The authors suggest that a combination of the status of HLA-G and TIL could improve the prognostic prediction for patients with various molecular subtypes of breast cancer (Dong et al., 2012). HLA-G expression has also been recently investigated in acute lymphoblastic leukemia (ALL) patients. HLA-G showed a negative correlation with NK cells confirming its importance in tumor escape through down-regulation of NK cells. The authors suggest that HLA-G expression could be used as a prognostic tumor marker to monitor disease state and improvement in ALL (Alkhouly et al., 2013).

There has been considerable interest on the association of HLA-G and cervical neoplasia as well as HPV infection. HLA-G expression was recently examined by immunohistochemistry in 22 normal cervical tissues, 14 cervical intraepithelial neoplasia (CIN) patients and 129 patients with squamous cell cervical cancer. It was found that HLA-G expression was absent in normal cervical tissues, and that HLA-G expression was increased from patients with CIN III (35.7%, 4/14) to patients with cervical cancer (62.8%, 81/129). Among the cervical cancer patients, HLA-G expression in FIGO stage I, II, and stage III+IV was 53.6% (45/84), 76.3% (29/38), and 100.0% (7/7), respectively. This study gives a clear indication that HLA-G expression is associated with the disease progression in patients with cervical cancer (Li et al., 2012).

6.3. HLA-G and viral infections

Viruses have developed numerous strategies to sabotage host immune surveillance and responses. The immune-inhibitory functions of HLA-G, elect this molecule as a potential immune escape strategy that would protect virus infected cells against immune effectors, thus facilitating viral progression (Gonzalez et al., 2012). Given the HLA-G role in immune tolerance, its function in viral infections has been increasingly investigated.

A recent study investigated the association between HLA-G polymorphisms and human papillomavirus (HPV) infection and squamous intraepithelial lesions (SIL). The results suggest that HLA-G polymorphisms may play a role in the natural history of HPV infection, likely at the stage of host immune recognition. The authors conclude that HLA-G polymorphisms interacted differently with the three alpha papillomavirus groups (Metcalfe et al., 2013). Another study investigated the possible influence of two HLA-G polymorphisms located on the 3'UTR, 14 bp In/Del and +3142C/G, on the susceptibility to cervical cancer. The authors conclude that the 3'UTR of HLA-G is associated with an increased risk of developing cervical cancer, especially in smokers (Silva et al., 2013).

The association of HLA-G polymorphisms and HCV infection has previously been reported (Cordero et al., 2009; Martinetti et al., 2006) however, the reason why HLA-G is up regulated and expressed in the presence of different viruses is still not clear. It is thought that cytokines such as IFNs or IIL-10 are involved in this expression. The specific role of HLA-G molecules was recently investigated in chronic hepatitis C. For the first time, the HLA-G^{+} cells were identified as being mast cells. HLA-G secretion was significantly induced in human mast cells stimulated by IL-10 or interferons of class I. The transcriptome of the secretome of this cell line stimulated by IFN-α revealed that i) the HLA-G gene is upregulated late, ii) T lymphocytes and NK cells are recruited. Based on this study the authors suggest an autocrine loop in the genesis of HCV liver fibrosis, based on mast cells expressing HLA-G (Amiot et al., 2013).

The first evidence of an association between HLA-G polymorphisms and malaria infection was recently provided (Garcia et al., 2013). However, further investigations will have to be undertaken before establishing this possible involvement of the HLA-G molecule in the control of *P. falciparum* infection.

HLA-G polymorphism and expression are also associated with the risk of human immunodeficiency virus (HIV) infection (Lajoie et al., 2006; Matte et al., 2004). A recent study showed that non-classical HLA-G-expressing CD4 Treg are highly susceptible to HIV-1 infection and significantly reduced in persons with progressive HIV-1 disease courses. In addition, the authors found that the proportion of HLA-G^{+} CD4 and CD8 T cells was inversely correlated to markers of HIV-1 associated immune activation. Mechanistically, this corresponded to an increased ability of HLA-G^{+} Treg to reduce bystander immune activation, while only minimally inhibiting the functional properties of HIV-1-specific T cells. This study suggests an important role of HLA-G^{+} Treg; the loss of these cells, during advanced HIV-1 infection, may contribute to immune dysregulation and HIV-1 disease progression (Li et al., 2013). The role of HLA-G in mother-to-child HIV transmission (MCHT) was also recently investigated in Kenya. HLA-G was sequenced and genotyped in 266 mothers and 251 children. Among 14 HLA-G alleles identified, only 4 alleles have a phenotype frequency above 10%. Correlation analysis showed that HLA-G(∗)01:03^{+} mothers were less likely to perinatally transmit HIV-1 to their children (p=0.038, Odds ratio:0.472, 95%CI:0.229-0.973). Mother-child HLA-G concordance was not associated with the increased perinatal HIV transmission. There was no significant difference in the general health between the transmitting mothers and the mothers who did not transmit HIV to their children (Luo et al., 2013).

The association between HLA-G and cytomegalovirus infection has been long investigated. In 2000, Onno and colleagues investigated the hypothesis that HLA-G molecules could be induced during HCMV reactivation in activated macrophages to favor virus dissemination. The authors suggested that the modulation of HLA-G protein expression during HCMV replication occurs at a post-transcriptional level and that this could be an additional mechanism that helps HCMV to subvert host defenses (Onno et al., 2000). A study found evidences that support a potential role of HLA-G 14 bp insertion/deletion polymorphism as a susceptible factor for the active hCMV infection (Zheng et al., 2009). The same polymorphism (14bp in/del) was recently investigated in the risk of acute rejection (AR) and CMV infection. Multivariate analysis demonstrated that HLA-G homozygous +14 bp and -14 bp genotypes were an independent risk factor for allograft rejection and CMV infection, respectively (Jin et al., 2012).

6.4. HLA-G and autoimmune diseases

HLA-G has been associated to several autoimmune and inflammatory diseases. The implication of HLA-G in the development of autoimmune diseases is probably related to its suppressive effect of the immune response in these diseases.

HLA-G role in ankylosing spondylitis (AS) is poorly understood since it has not been thoroughly studied. It has been shown that lower serum levels of sHLA-G contribute to susceptibility to AS, and predispose to poor spinal mobility. The expression of HLA-G on PMBCs is up-regulated in AS, which is correlated with acute phase reactants, decreasing after TNF-alpha blocker therapy (Chen et al., 2010). A recent study investigated the role of HLA-G in sacroiliitis of Ankylosing spondylitis (AS) and concluded that there is a significant association between HLA-G expression and the AS sacroiliitis stages suggesting that HLA-G is possibly involved in the pathology of the disease. The authors suggest that detection of HLA-G expression may be a useful laboratory test to reveal disease progress in AS patients (Zhang et al., 2013). HLA-G has also been recently investigated in rheumatoid arthritis patients. The authors report that sHLA-G, mHLA-G and ILT2 expression were inversely correlated with DAS28 disease scores. The frequency of 14 bp deletion allele was increased in patients with disease remission. Thus, HLA-G is suggested to be a candidate biomarker to evaluate early prognosis and disease activity in rheumatoid arthritis patients (Rizzo et al., 2013). However, discrepant results about the association of HLA-G and rheumatoid arthritis have also been presented (Kim et al., 2012). HLA-G has been investigated in another inflammatory autoimmune disease, systemic lupus erythematosus (SLE), with unknown etiology. The influence of two HLA-G polymorphisms, 14bp indel polymorphism and the +3142 C>G, was investigated in European patients with SLE. The authors report a significant increase of the +3142G allele frequency among patients as compared with controls (0.58 vs 0.47, $P = 0.011$). Also, patients presented a higher frequency of the GG genotype (OR = 1.90, 95% CI: 1.08-3.42). Double heterozygotes for the two polymorphisms presented a milder mean systemic lupus erythematosus disease activity index (SLEDAI) than heterozygotes for only one of the variants or non-heterozygous individuals (1.56 vs 3.15 and 3.26, respectively, corrected $P = 0.044$). These results suggest the involvement of the HLA-G molecule on SLE susceptibility and outcome (Consiglio et al., 2011). The interest of HLA-G in multiple sclerosis (MS) has been growing in the last decade. Original findings suggested a potential immunoregulatory role for IL-10 in the control of MS disease activity by shifting the sHLA-I/sHLA-G balance towards sHLA-G response (Fainardi et al., 2003). Furthermore, HLA-G and its receptor ILT2 has been identified on CNS cells and in areas of microglia activation. These findings further implicated HLA-G as a contributor to the fundamental mechanisms regulating immune reactivity in the CNS. The authors postulated that this pathway may act as an inhibitory feedback aimed to downregulate the deleterious effects of T-cell infiltration in neuroinflammation (Wiendl et al., 2005). Several HLA-G polymorphisms have been thoroughly investigated; some were shown to be associated with MS in different populations (Rizzo et al., 2012; Wisniewski et al., 2010). A recent genome wide association study opened new perspectives on MS pathogenesis and further implicated HLA loci, in particular HLA-G, in the genetic susceptibility (Song et al., 2013).

7. HLA-E and HLA-F disease association

HLA class Ib family members include HLA-E, -F, -G, and HFE (HLA-H). They are poorly polymorphic, have a lower surface expression when compared with the classic MHC class Ia molecules, and have a narrow tissue distribution. They are best known for their capability of regulating innate immune responses (Rodgers and Cook, 2005). However, there is also evidence that, like the MHC class Ia molecules, certain class Ib can participate in the regulation of acquired immune responses to bacteria and viruses (Lenfant et al., 2003; Rodgers and Cook, 2005).

7.1. HLA-E and HLA-F in cancer and infection

Downregulation of MHC class Ia molecule expression is a mechanism used by tumor cells to escape antitumor T-cell-mediated immune responses. However, it was not known why tumors escape from NK cells activity, and it was postulated that the aberrant expression of nonclassical HLA class Ia molecules could provide the required inhibitory signal to NK cells. The possible role of HLA-E molecules in providing tumor cells with an NK escape mechanism was analyzed, through the investigation of this class Ib molecule in a variety of tumor cell lines (Marin et al., 2003). The result of this investigation showed that further to HLE-E expression in leukemia-derived cell lines, this allele was detected in tumor cells of different origin.

HLA-E is involved in the regulation of NK cell function (Pietra et al., 2009), and is the only known ligand for the lecitin receptor CD94 combined with different NKG2 subunits (Kaiser et al., 2005; Lee et al., 1998), expressed on NK and CD8+ $\alpha\beta$ T cells. This interaction may augment (CD94/NGK2C), or inhibit (CD94/NGK2A) NK cell mediated cytotoxicity and cytokine production. HLA-E, unlike other MHC class Ib molecules is transcribed in virtually all human tissues and cell lines, although at lower levels than MHC class Ia (Braud et al., 1997; Wei and Orr, 1990) and bind nonamer peptides derived from other HLA class I signal sequences with a high restricted repertoire (Lee et al., 1998). As stated in previous sections of this chapter, the coding variation of HLA-E is mainly limited to two alleles, with similar frequencies in most populations. These alleles probably are the result of balancing selection and although there are few specific coding variants, they may have functional consequences affecting quantitatively or qualitatively protein expression. The non-synonymous alleles of HLA-E are referred as HLA-E^r (E*0101) and HLA-E^g (E*0103) since they are distinguished by having either an arginine or a glycine at position 107 of the protein. Clear differences exist between the two alleles in relative peptide affinity, which correlated with and may be explained by differences between their thermal stabilities. (Strong et al., 2003). The functional diferences between the two HLA-E alleles also correlates with the expression levels which has been shown to affect inhibitory activity (Lee et al., 1998). According to several reports the increased inhibitory activity may be involved in increasing inhibitory signals to NK cells, allowing tumor escape. A recent manuscript, investigating HLA-E gene polymorphisms expression in colorectal cancer tissue of two hundred thirty patients, using immunohistochemistry, found that patients with overexpression exhibited the lowest long-term survival rate. Interestingly the authors found out that the type of HLA-E polymorphism did not had an impact on HLA-E expression or prognosis in patients with stage III colorectal cancer (Zhen et al., 2013). A previuos report on colorectal cancer had demonstrated, in situ, that HLA-E/beta2m overexpression on tumor cells was a factor for unfavorable prognosis and that the overexpression was associated with celular infiltration with intraepithelial tumor infiltrating lymphocytes (IEL – TIL) (Wischhusen et al., 2005). Cetuximab, an anti-epidermal growth factor receptor monoclonal antibody which renders cancer cells more sensitive to antibody–dependent cellular toxicity (ADCC), has increased activity if cells are treated previously with an anti-NKG2A monoclonal antibody, that restored the ability of immune cells to kill their target. This result demonstrates that HLA-E at the cell surface can reliably suppress the ADCC effect (Levy et al., 2009).

Using an immunohistochemistry approach, a correlation was also found in early breast cancer between increased expression of HLA-E, loss of classical HLA class I and a worse relapse-free period (de Kruijf et al., 2010). Using the same technique, increased in vivo expression of HLA-E in lower grade gliomas and a massive overexpression in grade IV glioblastomas compared with normal CNS tissue and, siRNA-mediated silencing of HLA-E or blocking of CD94/NKG2A, enabled NKG2D-mediated lysis of 51Cr-labeled tumor cells by NK cells, provided the first evidence that expression and interaction of HLA-E on cancer cells with CD94/NKG2A expressed on lymphocytes compromises innate anti-tumor immune responses (Wischhusen et al., 2005). The overexpression of HLA-E was again detected in WHO grade IV glioblastoma, and a correlation with the identification of immune cell infiltration (NK and Tcells) was established (Mittelbronn et al., 2007). The expression of HLA-G and HLA-E by neoplastic cells in 39 cases of glioblastoma was recently evaluated, and a positive correlation between the expression of HLA-E and length of survival was found (Kren et al., 2011). It was also demonstrated that HLA-E expression at the cell surface of melanoma and ovarian carcinoma cell lines decreased their susceptibility to CTL lysis. (Derre et al., 2006; Malmberg et al., 2002). Both studies also shows that IFN-gamma modulation of target cells, although facilitates the T-cell receptor-mediated recognition by CD8+ T cells, by increasing the expression of HLA class I molecules, decreases target cell sensitivity to lysis by NK cells, a phenomenon that is dependent on enhanced inhibitory signaling via CD94/NKG2A receptors expressed on the effector cells. Recently another study showed that overall survival of ovarian cancer patients is strongly influenced by HLA-E, and that CTL infiltration in ovarian cancer is associated with better survival only when HLA-E expression is low, and that intratumoral CTLs are inhibited by CD94/NKG2A receptors in the tumor microenvironment (Gooden et al., 2011).

Recent evidence revealed that several proteins other than MHC class I molecules encode peptides that can bind to HLA-E. These peptides may be derived from pathogens, stress-related or from normal proteins, and they markedly differ in sequence from the canonical MHC class I-derived leader sequence peptides. The best characterized peptides are derived from the gpUL40 leader sequence of two cytomegalovirus (CMV) strains, and are assembled with HLA-E via a TAP independent mechanism. Other peptides are derived from the human heat shock protein 60 (hsp60) (Michaelsson et al., 2002), the multidrug resistance-associated protein 7 (MRP7) (Wooden et al., 2005), the human immunodeficiency virus (HIV) gag protein (HIV p24) (Nattermann et al., 2005), the Salmonella entérica serovar Typhi GroEL protein (GroEL) (Salerno-Goncalves et al., 2004), and gliadin (gliadin α2 chain) (Terrazzano et al., 2007).

Other viral proteins previously shown to bind MHC class I molecules, may also bind HLA-E, like peptides from the Epstein Barr virus (EBV) BZLF-1 protein, the influenza matrix protein (InflM) (Ulbrecht et al., 1998), and the Hepatitis C vírus (HCV) core protein (HCV Core) (Nattermann et al., 2005). EBV vírus has been associated with nasopharyngeal carcinoma (NPC), a geographically restricted tumor of epitelial cell lining nasopharynx, with several MHC class I associations reported in the literature (Ren and Chan, 1996). The NPC susceptibility is associated with HLA-E*0103 allele, suggesting that this allele may be one of several causes contributing to NPC development. (Hirankarn et al., 2004). A genome-wide association study on NPC found significant association within the HLA region at chromosome 6p21.3, with HLA-A, gamma aminobutyric acid 1 (GABBR1), and HLA-F (Tse et al., 2009). HIV down-regulates the expression of MHC class I proteins H, but not HLA-C, HLA-E and HLA-G molecules on the surface of infected cells via the action of Nef protein. Women who are homozygous for the HLA-E*0103 allele have a 4.0-fold decreased risk of human immunodeficiency vírus 1 (HIV-1) infection in Zimbabwean women. This protection increased to 12.5-fold in women carrying the combination of the protective HLA-E*0103 genotype and HLA-G*0105N heterozygote genotype. The authors of these findings speculate that the differential regulation of HLA molecular expression may modulate mucosal imune response to HIV facilitating or preventing the establishment of disease in the female genital tract (Lajoie et al., 2006).

Further to its important role in innate immunity functioning as a ligand for the CD94/NKG2 receptors, expressed by NK cells and a subset of CTLs (Braud et al., 2003), HLA-E can present peptide antigens for $\alpha\beta$ TCR-mediated recognition (Li et al., 2001) (Li J et al 2001). HLA-E dependent presentation of bacteria-derived antigens to human CD8+ T cells has been reported particularly in bacteria, like Mycobacterium tuberculosis (Mtb)(Heinzel et al., 2002) and Salmonella enterica serovar Typhi GroEL (Salerno-Goncalves et al., 2004). It was also demonstrated that an HLA-E-restricted CD8+ T cells subset represents a significant component of the adaptive immune response to CMV in genetically predisposed individuals (Mazzarino et al., 2005). Furthermore, recent findings demonstrated that HCV gives rise to a peptide that is recognized by CD8+ T cells via their TCR. The same authors also demonstrated that chronic hepatitis C is associated with increased intrahepatic HLA-E expression (Schulte et al., 2009). More recently, however, HLA-E allelic variant HLA-E*0101, was associated with increased odds of HCV clearance and may help to predict sustained virological response among HIV/HC-coinfected patients under therapy with pegylated-interpheron-alpha and ribavirin (Guzman-Fulgencio et al., 2013). These patients have a high level of antiviral HLA-E CD8+ Tcells with a high degree of antiviral HLA-E restricted IFN-gama secretion which is associated with low HCV viral load. HLA-E*0101 has lower affinity to their natural ligands when compared to HLA-E*0103, and possibly is more available to bind the HCV peptides facilitating HLA-E-restricted CD8+ T-cell responses (Schulte et al., 2009).

HLA-F shows limited polymorphism, and the function of its mainly intracellular protein is not clear. The key residues of the peptide-binding region are highly conserved in all primate studies, suggesting an importante role in cellular physiology (Moscoso et al., 2007). HLA-F is the nonclassical class I molecule least characterized. (Boyle et al., 2006; Lee et al., 2010). Several studies confirmed HLA-F protein expression in diverse tissues and cell lines including B cell, monocytes, bladder, skin, liver, tonsils, spleen and thymus, but no surface expression was detected in the majority of them. Unique potential regulator motifs were identified in HLA-F consistent with tissue specific expression and suggesting specialized functions and tight transcriptional control of the gene (Geraghty et al., 1990; Gobin and van den Elsen, 2000)). No data have been reported regarding peptide or other ligand-binding properties of HLA-F, although the predicted dimensions of the grove are similar to class I molecules which bind peptides (Braud et al., 1998). There are few reports in the literature about the association of HLA-F with disease. Lin A et al (Lin et al., 2011) investigated HLA-F expression in non small-cell lung cancer (NSCLC), and found out that the expression identified in a significant number of câncer cells was not associated with the clinical parameters such as grade of tumor differentiation and disease stage, but NSCL patients with high expression had a poor prognosis. Esophageal câncer was investigated by the same group, and the authors found that patients with upregulated HLA-F expression (lesion vs normal tissue), had significantly worse survival, than those with HLA-F unchanged and downregulated (Zhang et al., 2013).

7.2. HLA-E and autoimmune disease

Behçet disease (BD) is a chronic inflammatory disorder characterized by recurrent genital and oral aphtous ulcers, uveitis, skin lesions and arthritis. Association with variants of candidate genes were reported - HLA-B51, MICA-A6 and MICA-009 (Mizuki et al., 1999). However, the genetic mechanisms underlying this disease are still unrecognized and other genetic variants are under investigation. A study performed in 312 patients with BD and 486 controls, in Korea, reported an association of HLA-E*0101 and HLA-G*010101 and reduced risk of BD. In contrast, the variants HLA-E*010302, HLA-G* 010102, G*0105N and 3741_3754ins14bp were all associated with increased BD risk. The authors conclude that HLA-E and –G appear to function independently and synergistically, increasing BD risk through an imbalance of lymphocyte functions (Park et al., 2007). A report associates HLA-E gene polymorphism with Ankylosing Spondylitis (AS) in Sardinia. The authors genotyped 120 patients with AS, 175 HLA-B27 positive controls and 200 random controls, for six single nucleotide polymorphisms (SNPs) spanning the HLA region between the HLA-E and HLA-C loci. The strongest association was found with the HLA-E functional polymorphism rs1264457, raising the possibility that natural killer cells tmay have a possible role in the pathogenesis of AS (Paladini et al., 2009).

Although the genetic susceptibility of Type I Diabetes Mellitus reside in the major histocompatibility complex (MHC) (Todd, 1995), particularly with the class II DQA1 and DQB1 loci, other alleles have been investigated inside the HLA region. An association between HLA-E locus and age at onset and susceptibility to type 1 diabetes mellitus was reported (Hodgkinson et al., 2000). The authors speculate that abnormal expression or presentation of leader sequences by HLA-E may lead to an autoagressive act by NK cells on self tissue, although the role of these cells in the autoimmune destruction of islet B-cells is poorly understood.

In a recent study on Multiple Sclerosis (MS). Serum and cerebrospinal fluid (CSF) samples from MS patients were compared with other inflammatory disorders and non-inflammatory neurological disorders. The data obtained suggest that soluble HLA-E may have a protective role in MS patients, contributing to the inhibition of the intrathecal inflammatory response (Morandi et al., 2013). Another study in Juvenile Idiopathic Arthritis detected higher concentrations of soluble HLA-E (sHLA-E) in the synovial fluid (SF) in extended oligoarticular/ polyarticular than in limited articular disease; the higher concentrations correlated with the number of affected joints. The authors speculate that higher SF HLA-E concentrations may protect against cytolysis (Prigione et al., 2011).

Author details

Iris Foroni[1,2], Ana Rita Couto[1,2], Bruno Filipe Bettencourt[1,2], Margarida Santos[1,2], Manuela Lima[2,3] and Jácome Bruges-Armas[1,2]

1 Serviço Especializado de Epidemiologia e Biologia Molecular, Hospital de Santo Espírito de Angra do Heroísmo, Portugal

2 Genetic and Arthritis Research Group (GARG), Institute for Molecular and Cell Biology (IBMC), University of Porto, Portugal

3 Departamento de Biologia, Universidade dos Açores, Portugal

References

[1] Abbas, A. Tripathi, P. Naik, S. and Agrawal, S. (2004). Analysis of human leukocyte antigen (HLA)-G polymorphism in normal women and in women with recurrent spontaneous abortions. *Eur J Immunogenet*, Vol. 31, (6), pp. 275-278

[2] Adams, E. J.Luoma, A. M. (2013). The adaptable major histocompatibility complex (MHC) fold: structure and function of nonclassical and MHC class I-like molecules. *Annu Rev Immunol*, Vol. 31, pp. 529-561

[3] Agaugue, S. Carosella, E. D. and Rouas-Freiss, N. (2011). Role of HLA-G in tumor escape through expansion of myeloid-derived suppressor cells and cytokinic balance in favor of Th2 versus Th1/Th17. *Blood*, Vol. 117, (26), pp. 7021-7031

[4] Aldrich, C. J. DeCloux, A. Woods, A. S. Cotter, R. J. Soloski, M. J. and Forman, J. (1994). Identification of a Tap-dependent leader peptide recognized by alloreactive T cells specific for a class Ib antigen. *Cell*, Vol. 79, (4), pp. 649-658

[5] Aldrich, C. L. Stephenson, M. D. Karrison, T. Odem, R. R. Branch, D. W. Scott, J. R. Schreiber, J. R. and Ober, C. (2001). HLA-G genotypes and pregnancy outcome in couples with unexplained recurrent miscarriage. *Mol Hum Reprod*, Vol. 7, (12), pp. 1167-1172

[6] Alkhouly, N. Shehata, I. Ahmed, M. B. Shehata, H. Hassan, S. and Ibrahim, T. (2013). HLA-G expression in acute lymphoblastic leukemia: a significant prognostic tumor biomarker. *Med Oncol*, Vol. 30, (1), pp. 460

[7] Allan, D. S. Colonna, M. Lanier, L. L. Churakova, T. D. Abrams, J. S. Ellis, S. A. McMichael, A. J. and Braud, V. M. (1999). Tetrameric complexes of human histocompatibility leukocyte antigen (HLA)-G bind to peripheral blood myelomonocytic cells. *J Exp Med*, Vol. 189, (7), pp. 1149-1156

[8] Alvarez, M. Santos, P. Martinho, A. Simoes, O. Abade, A. and Breda-Coimbra, H. (1999). HLA-G genetic polymorphism in 57 Portuguese white families studied by PCR-RFLP and PCR-SSOP. *Transplant Proc*, Vol. 31, (4), pp. 1829-1831

[9] Amiot, L. Vu, N. Rauch, M. Helgoualc'h, A. L. Chalmel, F. Gascan, H. Turlin, B. Guyader, D. and Samson, M. (2013). Expression of HLA-G by mast cells is associated with hepatitis C virus-induced liver fibrosis. *J Hepatol*, Vol., pp.

[10] Antoun, A. Jobson, S. Cook, M. Moss, P. and Briggs, D. (2009). Ethnic variability in human leukocyte antigen-E haplotypes. *Tissue Antigens*, Vol. 73, (1), pp. 39-45

[11] Arnaiz-Villena, A. Enriquez-de-Salamanca, M. Areces, C. Alonso-Rubio, J. Abd-El-Fatah-Khalil, S. Fernandez-Honrado, M. and Rey, D. (2013). HLA-G(*)01:05N null allele in Mayans (Guatemala) and Uros (Titikaka Lake, Peru): evolution and population genetics. *Hum Immunol*, Vol. 74, (4), pp. 478-482

[12] Arnaiz-Villena, A. Vargas-Alarcon, G. Serrano-Vela, J. I. Reguera, R. Martinez-Laso, J. Silvera-Redondo, C. Granados, J. and Moscoso, J. (2007). HLA-E polymorphism in Amerindians from Mexico (Mazatecans), Colombia (Wayu) and Chile (Mapuches): evolution of MHC-E gene. *Tissue Antigens*, Vol. 69 Suppl 1, pp. 132-135

[13] Bahri, R. Hirsch, F. Josse, A. Rouas-Freiss, N. Bidere, N. Vasquez, A. Carosella, E. D. Charpentier, B. and Durrbach, A. (2006). Soluble HLA-G inhibits cell cycle progression in human alloreactive T lymphocytes. *J Immunol*, Vol. 176, (3), pp. 1331-1339

[14] Baricordi, O. R. Stignani, M. Melchiorri, L. and Rizzo, R. (2008). HLA-G and inflammatory diseases. *Inflamm Allergy Drug Targets*, Vol. 7, (2), pp. 67-74

[15] Bland, F. A. Lemberg, M. K. McMichael, A. J. Martoglio, B. and Braud, V. M. (2003). Requirement of the proteasome for the trimming of signal peptide-derived epitopes presented by the nonclassical major histocompatibility complex class I molecule HLA-E. *J Biol Chem*, Vol. 278, (36), pp. 33747-33752

[16] Borrego, F. Kabat, J. Kim, D. K. Lieto, L. Maasho, K. Pena, J. Solana, R. and Coligan, J. E. (2002). Structure and function of major histocompatibility complex (MHC) class I specific receptors expressed on human natural killer (NK) cells. *Mol Immunol*, Vol. 38, (9), pp. 637-660

[17] Boyle, L. H. Gillingham, A. K. Munro, S. and Trowsdale, J. (2006). Selective export of HLA-F by its cytoplasmic tail. *J Immunol*, Vol. 176, (11), pp. 6464-6472

[18] Boyson, J. E. Erskine, R. Whitman, M. C. Chiu, M. Lau, J. M. Koopman, L. A. Valter, M. M. Angelisova, P. Horejsi, V. and Strominger, J. L. (2002). Disulfide bond-mediated dimerization of HLA-G on the cell surface. *Proc Natl Acad Sci U S A*, Vol. 99, (25), pp. 16180-16185

[19] Braud, V. Jones, E. Y. and McMichael, A. (1997). The human major histocompatibility complex class Ib molecule HLA-E binds signal sequence-derived peptides with primary anchor residues at positions 2 and 9. *Eur J Immunol*, Vol. 27, (5), pp. 1164-1169

[20] Braud, V. M. Aldemir, H. Breart, B. and Ferlin, W. G. (2003). Expression of CD94-NKG2A inhibitory receptor is restricted to a subset of CD8+ T cells. *Trends Immunol*, Vol. 24, (4), pp. 162-164

[21] Braud, V. M. Allan, D. S. O'Callaghan, C. A. Soderstrom, K. D'Andrea, A. Ogg, G. S. Lazetic, S. Young, N. T. Bell, J. I. Phillips, J. H. Lanier, L. L. and McMichael, A. J. (1998). HLA-E binds to natural killer cell receptors CD94/NKG2A, B and C. *Nature*, Vol. 391, (6669), pp. 795-799

[22] Braud, V. M. Allan, D. S. Wilson, D. and McMichael, A. J. (1998). TAP- and tapasin-dependent HLA-E surface expression correlates with the binding of an MHC class I leader peptide. *Curr Biol*, Vol. 8, (1), pp. 1-10

[23] Carosella, E. D. Favier, B. Rouas-Freiss, N. Moreau, P. and Lemaoult, J. (2008). Beyond the increasing complexity of the immunomodulatory HLA-G molecule. *Blood*, Vol. 111, (10), pp. 4862-4870

[24] Carosella, E. D.Horuzsko, A. (2007). HLA-G and cancer. *Semin Cancer Biol*, Vol. 17, (6), pp. 411-412

[25] Carosella, E. D. Moreau, P. Le Maoult, J. Le Discorde, M. Dausset, J. and Rouas-Freiss, N. (2003). HLA-G molecules: from maternal-fetal tolerance to tissue acceptance. *Adv Immunol*, Vol. 81, pp. 199-252

[26] Carvalho dos Santos, L. Tureck, L. V. Wowk, P. F. Mattar, S. B. Gelmini, G. F. Magalhaes, J. C. Bicalho Mda, G. and Roxo, V. M. (2013). HLA-E polymorphisms in an Afro-descendant Southern Brazilian population. *Hum Immunol*, Vol. 74, (2), pp. 199-202

[27] Castelli, E. C. Mendes-Junior, C. T. and Donadi, E. A. (2007). HLA-G alleles and HLA-G 14 bp polymorphisms in a Brazilian population. *Tissue Antigens*, Vol. 70, (1), pp. 62-68

[28] Castelli, E. C. Mendes-Junior, C. T. Veiga-Castelli, L. C. Roger, M. Moreau, P. and Donadi, E. A. (2011). A comprehensive study of polymorphic sites along the HLA-G gene: implication for gene regulation and evolution. *Mol Biol Evol*, Vol. 28, (11), pp. 3069-3086

[29] Castelli, E. C. Mendes-Junior, C. T. Viana de Camargo, J. L. and Donadi, E. A. (2008). HLA-G polymorphism and transitional cell carcinoma of the bladder in a Brazilian population. *Tissue Antigens*, Vol. 72, (2), pp. 149-157

[30] Castro, M. J. Morales, P. Rojo-Amigo, R. Martinez-Laso, J. Allende, L. Varela, P. Garcia-Berciano, M. Guillen-Perales, J. and Arnaiz-Villena, A. (2000). Homozygous HLA-G*0105N healthy individuals indicate that membrane-anchored HLA-G1 molecule is not necessary for survival. *Tissue Antigens*, Vol. 56, (3), pp. 232-239

[31] Caumartin, J. Favier, B. Daouya, M. Guillard, C. Moreau, P. Carosella, E. D. and LeMaoult, J. (2007). Trogocytosis-based generation of suppressive NK cells. *EMBO J*, Vol. 26, (5), pp. 1423-1433

[32] Cecati, M. Giannubilo, S. R. Emanuelli, M. Tranquilli, A. L. and Saccucci, F. (2011). HLA-G and pregnancy adverse outcomes. *Med Hypotheses*, Vol. 76, (6), pp. 782-784

[33] Chen, C. H. Liao, H. T. Chen, H. A. Liu, C. H. Liang, T. H. Wang, C. T. Tsai, C. Y. and Chou, C. T. (2010). Human leukocyte antigen-G in ankylosing spondylitis and the response after tumour necrosis factor-alpha blocker therapy. *Rheumatology (Oxford)*, Vol. 49, (2), pp. 264-270

[34] Christiansen, O. B. Kolte, A. M. Dahl, M. Larsen, E. C. Steffensen, R. Nielsen, H. S. and Hviid, T. V. (2012). Maternal homozygocity for a 14 base pair insertion in exon 8 of the HLA-G gene and carriage of HLA class II alleles restricting HY immunity predispose to unexplained secondary recurrent miscarriage and low birth weight in children born to these patients. *Hum Immunol*, Vol. 73, (7), pp. 699-705

[35] Chrul, S. Polakowska, E. Szadkowska, A. and Bodalski, J. (2006). Influence of interleukin IL-2 and IL-12 + IL-18 on surface expression of immunoglobulin-like receptors

KIR2DL1, KIR2DL2, and KIR3DL2 in natural killer cells. *Mediators Inflamm*, Vol. 2006, (4), pp. 46957

[36] Clements, C. S. Kjer-Nielsen, L. Kostenko, L. Hoare, H. L. Dunstone, M. A. Moses, E. Freed, K. Brooks, A. G. Rossjohn, J. and McCluskey, J. (2005). Crystal structure of HLA-G: a nonclassical MHC class I molecule expressed at the fetal-maternal interface. *Proc Natl Acad Sci U S A*, Vol. 102, (9), pp. 3360-3365

[37] Colonna, M. Navarro, F. Bellon, T. Llano, M. Garcia, P. Samaridis, J. Angman, L. Cella, M. and Lopez-Botet, M. (1997). A common inhibitory receptor for major histocompatibility complex class I molecules on human lymphoid and myelomonocytic cells. *J Exp Med*, Vol. 186, (11), pp. 1809-1818

[38] Colonna, M. Samaridis, J. Cella, M. Angman, L. Allen, R. L. O'Callaghan, C. A. Dunbar, R. Ogg, G. S. Cerundolo, V. and Rolink, A. (1998). Human myelomonocytic cells express an inhibitory receptor for classical and nonclassical MHC class I molecules. *J Immunol*, Vol. 160, (7), pp. 3096-3100

[39] Consiglio, C. R. Veit, T. D. Monticielo, O. A. Mucenic, T. Xavier, R. M. Brenol, J. C. and Chies, J. A. (2011). Association of the HLA-G gene +3142C>G polymorphism with systemic lupus erythematosus. *Tissue Antigens*, Vol. 77, (6), pp. 540-545

[40] Cordero, E. A. Veit, T. D. da Silva, M. A. Jacques, S. M. Silla, L. M. and Chies, J. A. (2009). HLA-G polymorphism influences the susceptibility to HCV infection in sickle cell disease patients. *Tissue Antigens*, Vol. 74, (4), pp. 308-313

[41] Curigliano, G. Criscitiello, C. Gelao, L. and Goldhirsch, A. (2013). Molecular Pathways: Human Leukocyte Antigen G (HLA-G). *Clin Cancer Res*, Vol. 19, (20), pp. 5564-5571

[42] Danzer, M. Polin, H. Proll, J. Haunschmid, R. Hofer, K. Stabentheiner, S. Hackl, C. Kasparu, H. Konig, J. Hauser, H. Binder, M. Weiss, R. Gabriel, C. and Krieger, O. (2009). Clinical significance of HLA-E*0103 homozygosity on survival after allogeneic hematopoietic stem-cell transplantation. *Transplantation*, Vol. 88, (4), pp. 528-532

[43] Dardano, A. Rizzo, R. Polini, A. Stignani, M. Tognini, S. Pasqualetti, G. Ursino, S. Colato, C. Ferdeghini, M. Baricordi, O. R. and Monzani, F. (2012). Soluble human leukocyte antigen-g and its insertion/deletion polymorphism in papillary thyroid carcinoma: novel potential biomarkers of disease? *J Clin Endocrinol Metab*, Vol. 97, (11), pp. 4080-4086

[44] de Kruijf, E. M. Sajet, A. van Nes, J. G. Natanov, R. Putter, H. Smit, V. T. Liefers, G. J. van den Elsen, P. J. van de Velde, C. J. and Kuppen, P. J. (2010). HLA-E and HLA-G expression in classical HLA class I-negative tumors is of prognostic value for clinical outcome of early breast cancer patients. *J Immunol*, Vol. 185, (12), pp. 7452-7459

[45] Derre, L. Corvaisier, M. Charreau, B. Moreau, A. Godefroy, E. Moreau-Aubry, A. Jotereau, F. and Gervois, N. (2006). Expression and release of HLA-E by melanoma

cells and melanocytes: potential impact on the response of cytotoxic effector cells. *J Immunol*, Vol. 177, (5), pp. 3100-3107

[46] Di Cristofaro, J. Buhler, S. Frassati, C. Basire, A. Galicher, V. Baier, C. Essautier, A. Regnier, A. Granier, T. Lepfoundzou, A. D. Chiaroni, J. and Picard, C. (2011). Linkage disequilibrium between HLA-G*0104 and HLA-E*0103 alleles in Tswa Pygmies. *Tissue Antigens*, Vol. 77, (3), pp. 193-200

[47] Diaz-Lagares, A. Alegre, E. LeMaoult, J. Carosella, E. D. and Gonzalez, A. (2009). Nitric oxide produces HLA-G nitration and induces metalloprotease-dependent shedding creating a tolerogenic milieu. *Immunology*, Vol. 126, (3), pp. 436-445

[48] Diehl, M. Munz, C. Keilholz, W. Stevanovic, S. Holmes, N. Loke, Y. W. and Rammensee, H. G. (1996). Nonclassical HLA-G molecules are classical peptide presenters. *Curr Biol*, Vol. 6, (3), pp. 305-314

[49] Donadi, E. A. Castelli, E. C. Arnaiz-Villena, A. Roger, M. Rey, D. and Moreau, P. (2011). Implications of the polymorphism of HLA-G on its function, regulation, evolution and disease association. *Cell Mol Life Sci*, Vol. 68, (3), pp. 369-395

[50] Dong, D. D. Yie, S. M. Li, K. Li, F. Xu, Y. Xu, G. Song, L. and Yang, H. (2012). Importance of HLA-G expression and tumor infiltrating lymphocytes in molecular subtypes of breast cancer. *Hum Immunol*, Vol. 73, (10), pp. 998-1004

[51] Dunn, G. P. Old, L. J. and Schreiber, R. D. (2004). The three Es of cancer immunoediting. *Annu Rev Immunol*, Vol. 22, pp. 329-360

[52] Fainardi, E. Rizzo, R. Melchiorri, L. Vaghi, L. Castellazzi, M. Marzola, A. Govoni, V. Paolino, E. Tola, M. R. Granieri, E. and Baricordi, O. R. (2003). Presence of detectable levels of soluble HLA-G molecules in CSF of relapsing-remitting multiple sclerosis: relationship with CSF soluble HLA-I and IL-10 concentrations and MRI findings. *J Neuroimmunol*, Vol. 142, (1-2), pp. 149-158

[53] Ferguson, R. Ramanakumar, A. V. Koushik, A. Coutlee, F. Franco, E. and Roger, M. (2012). Human leukocyte antigen G polymorphism is associated with an increased risk of invasive cancer of the uterine cervix. *Int J Cancer*, Vol. 131, (3), pp. E312-319

[54] Ferguson, R. Ramanakumar, A. V. Richardson, H. Tellier, P. P. Coutlee, F. Franco, E. L. and Roger, M. (2011). Human leukocyte antigen (HLA)-E and HLA-G polymorphisms in human papillomavirus infection susceptibility and persistence. *Hum Immunol*, Vol. 72, (4), pp. 337-341

[55] Furst, D. Bindja, J. Arnold, R. Herr, W. Schwerdtfeger, R. Muller, C. H. Recker, K. Schrezenmeier, H. and Mytilineos, J. (2012). HLA-E polymorphisms in hematopoietic stem cell transplantation. *Tissue Antigens*, Vol. 79, (4), pp. 287-290

[56] Garcia, A. Milet, J. Courtin, D. Sabbagh, A. Massaro, J. D. Castelli, E. C. Migot-Nabias, F. Favier, B. Rouas-Freiss, N. Donadi, E. A. and Moreau, P. (2013). Association

of HLA-G 3'UTR polymorphisms with response to malaria infection: a first insight. *Infect Genet Evol*, Vol. 16, pp. 263-269

[57] Geraghty, D. E. Koller, B. H. and Orr, H. T. (1987). A human major histocompatibility complex class I gene that encodes a protein with a shortened cytoplasmic segment. *Proc Natl Acad Sci U S A*, Vol. 84, (24), pp. 9145-9149

[58] Geraghty, D. E. Stockschleader, M. Ishitani, A. and Hansen, J. A. (1992). Polymorphism at the HLA-E locus predates most HLA-A and -B polymorphism. *Hum Immunol*, Vol. 33, (3), pp. 174-184

[59] Geraghty, D. E. Wei, X. H. Orr, H. T. and Koller, B. H. (1990). Human leukocyte antigen F (HLA-F). An expressed HLA gene composed of a class I coding sequence linked to a novel transcribed repetitive element. *J Exp Med*, Vol. 171, (1), pp. 1-18

[60] Ghandri, N. Gabbouj, S. Farhat, K. Bouaouina, N. Abdelaziz, H. Nouri, A. Chouchane, L. and Hassen, E. (2011). Association of HLA-G polymorphisms with nasopharyngeal carcinoma risk and clinical outcome. *Hum Immunol*, Vol. 72, (2), pp. 150-158

[61] Girdlestone, J. (1996). Transcriptional regulation of MHC class I genes. *Eur J Immunogenet*, Vol. 23, (5), pp. 395-413

[62] Gobin, S. J.van den Elsen, P. J. (2000). Transcriptional regulation of the MHC class Ib genes HLA-E, HLA-F, and HLA-G. *Hum Immunol*, Vol. 61, (11), pp. 1102-1107

[63] Gomez-Casado, E. Martinez-Laso, J. Vargas-Alarcon, G. Varela, P. Diaz-Campos, N. Alvarez, M. Alegre, R. and Arnaiz-Villena, A. (1997). Description of a new HLA-E (E*01031) allele and its frequency in the Spanish population. *Hum Immunol*, Vol. 54, (1), pp. 69-73

[64] Gonen-Gross, T. Achdout, H. Arnon, T. I. Gazit, R. Stern, N. Horejsi, V. Goldman-Wohl, D. Yagel, S. and Mandelboim, O. (2005). The CD85J/leukocyte inhibitory receptor-1 distinguishes between conformed and beta 2-microglobulin-free HLA-G molecules. *J Immunol*, Vol. 175, (8), pp. 4866-4874

[65] Gonen-Gross, T. Achdout, H. Gazit, R. Hanna, J. Mizrahi, S. Markel, G. Goldman-Wohl, D. Yagel, S. Horejsi, V. Levy, O. Baniyash, M. and Mandelboim, O. (2003). Complexes of HLA-G protein on the cell surface are important for leukocyte Ig-like receptor-1 function. *J Immunol*, Vol. 171, (3), pp. 1343-1351

[66] Gonzalez, A. Rebmann, V. LeMaoult, J. Horn, P. A. Carosella, E. D. and Alegre, E. (2012). The immunosuppressive molecule HLA-G and its clinical implications. *Crit Rev Clin Lab Sci*, Vol. 49, (3), pp. 63-84

[67] Gooden, M. Lampen, M. Jordanova, E. S. Leffers, N. Trimbos, J. B. van der Burg, S. H. Nijman, H. and van Hall, T. (2011). HLA-E expression by gynecological cancers restrains tumor-infiltrating CD8(+) T lymphocytes. *Proc Natl Acad Sci U S A*, Vol. 108, (26), pp. 10656-10661

[68] Goodridge, J. P. Burian, A. Lee, N. and Geraghty, D. E. (2010). HLA-F complex without peptide binds to MHC class I protein in the open conformer form. *J Immunol*, Vol. 184, (11), pp. 6199-6208

[69] Goodridge, J. P. Burian, A. Lee, N. and Geraghty, D. E. (2013). HLA-F and MHC class I open conformers are ligands for NK cell Ig-like receptors. *J Immunol*, Vol. 191, (7), pp. 3553-3562

[70] Goodridge, J. P. Lee, N. Burian, A. Pyo, C. W. Tykodi, S. S. Warren, E. H. Yee, C. Riddell, S. R. and Geraghty, D. E. (2013). HLA-F and MHC-I open conformers cooperate in a MHC-I antigen cross-presentation pathway. *J Immunol*, Vol. 191, (4), pp. 1567-1577

[71] Goodridge, J. P. Witt, C. S. Christiansen, F. T. and Warren, H. S. (2003). KIR2DL4 (CD158d) genotype influences expression and function in NK cells. *J Immunol*, Vol. 171, (4), pp. 1768-1774

[72] Grimsley, C. Kawasaki, A. Gassner, C. Sageshima, N. Nose, Y. Hatake, K. Geraghty, D. E. and Ishitani, A. (2002). Definitive high resolution typing of HLA-E allelic polymorphisms: Identifying potential errors in existing allele data. *Tissue Antigens*, Vol. 60, (3), pp. 206-212

[73] Grimsley, C.Ober, C. (1997). Population genetic studies of HLA-E: evidence for selection. *Hum Immunol*, Vol. 52, (1), pp. 33-40

[74] Gros, F. Cabillic, F. Toutirais, O. Maux, A. L. Sebti, Y. and Amiot, L. (2008). Soluble HLA-G molecules impair natural killer/dendritic cell crosstalk via inhibition of dendritic cells. *Eur J Immunol*, Vol. 38, (3), pp. 742-749

[75] Guzman-Fulgencio, M. Berenguer, J. Rallon, N. Fernandez-Rodriguez, A. Miralles, P. Soriano, V. Jimenez-Sousa, M. A. Cosin, J. Medrano, J. Garcia-Alvarez, M. Lopez, J. C. Benito, J. M. and Resino, S. (2013). HLA-E variants are associated with sustained virological response in HIV/hepatitis C virus-coinfected patients on hepatitis C virus therapy. *AIDS*, Vol. 27, (8), pp. 1231-1238

[76] Hassen, E. Ghedira, R. Ghandri, N. Farhat, K. Gabbouj, S. Bouaouina, N. Abdelaziz, H. Nouri, A. and Chouchane, L. (2011). Lack of association between human leukocyte antigen-E alleles and nasopharyngeal carcinoma in Tunisians. *DNA Cell Biol*, Vol. 30, (8), pp. 603-609

[77] He, X. Xu, L. Liu, Y. and Zeng, Y. (2004). Identification of a novel HLA-F allele - HLA-F*010102. *Tissue Antigens*, Vol. 63, (2), pp. 181-183

[78] Heinzel, A. S. Grotzke, J. E. Lines, R. A. Lewinsohn, D. A. McNabb, A. L. Streblow, D. N. Braud, V. M. Grieser, H. J. Belisle, J. T. and Lewinsohn, D. M. (2002). HLA-E-dependent presentation of Mtb-derived antigen to human CD8+ T cells. *J Exp Med*, Vol. 196, (11), pp. 1473-1481

[79] Hirankarn, N. Kimkong, I. and Mutirangura, A. (2004). HLA-E polymorphism in patients with nasopharyngeal carcinoma. *Tissue Antigens*, Vol. 64, (5), pp. 588-592

[80] Hoare, H. L. Sullivan, L. C. Pietra, G. Clements, C. S. Lee, E. J. Ely, L. K. Beddoe, T. Falco, M. Kjer-Nielsen, L. Reid, H. H. McCluskey, J. Moretta, L. Rossjohn, J. and Brooks, A. G. (2006). Structural basis for a major histocompatibility complex class Ib-restricted T cell response. *Nat Immunol*, Vol. 7, (3), pp. 256-264

[81] Hodgkinson, A. D. Millward, B. A. and Demaine, A. G. (2000). The HLA-E locus is associated with age at onset and susceptibility to type 1 diabetes mellitus. *Hum Immunol*, Vol. 61, (3), pp. 290-295

[82] Hofstetter, A. R. Sullivan, L. C. Lukacher, A. E. and Brooks, A. G. (2011). Diverse roles of non-diverse molecules: MHC class Ib molecules in host defense and control of autoimmunity. *Curr Opin Immunol*, Vol. 23, (1), pp. 104-110

[83] Hosseini, E. Schwarer, A. P. Jalali, A. and Ghasemzadeh, M. (2013). The impact of HLA-E polymorphisms on relapse following allogeneic hematopoietic stem cell transplantation. *Leuk Res*, Vol. 37, (5), pp. 516-519

[84] Howcroft, T.Singer, D. (2003). Expression of nonclassical MHC class Ib genes: comparison of regulatory elements. *Immunol Res*, Vol. 27, (1), pp. 1-30

[85] http://www.ebi.ac.uk/ipd/imgt/hla. (Ocober 2013). version 3.12.0.

[86] Hviid, T. V. (2006). HLA-G in human reproduction: aspects of genetics, function and pregnancy complications. *Hum Reprod Update*, Vol. 12, (3), pp. 209-232

[87] Hviid, T. V. Hylenius, S. Hoegh, A. M. Kruse, C. and Christiansen, O. B. (2002). HLA-G polymorphisms in couples with recurrent spontaneous abortions. *Tissue Antigens*, Vol. 60, (2), pp. 122-132

[88] Iodice, L. Sarnataro, S. and Bonatti, S. (2001). The carboxyl-terminal valine is required for transport of glycoprotein CD8 alpha from the endoplasmic reticulum to the intermediate compartment. *J Biol Chem*, Vol. 276, (31), pp. 28920-28926

[89] Ishitani, A. Kishida, M. Sageshima, N. Yashiki, S. Sonoda, S. Hayami, M. Smith, A. G. and Hatake, K. (1999). Re-examination of HLA-G polymorphism in African Americans. *Immunogenetics*, Vol. 49, (9), pp. 808-811

[90] Ishitani, A. Sageshima, N. and Hatake, K. (2006). The involvement of HLA-E and -F in pregnancy. *J Reprod Immunol*, Vol. 69, (2), pp. 101-113

[91] Ishitani, A. Sageshima, N. Lee, N. Dorofeeva, N. Hatake, K. Marquardt, H. and Geraghty, D. E. (2003). Protein expression and peptide binding suggest unique and interacting functional roles for HLA-E, F, and G in maternal-placental immune recognition. *J Immunol*, Vol. 171, (3), pp. 1376-1384

[92] Iwaszko, M.Bogunia-Kubik, K. (2011). Clinical significance of the HLA-E and CD94/NKG2 interaction. *Arch Immunol Ther Exp (Warsz)*, Vol. 59, (5), pp. 353-367

[93] Iwaszko, M.Bogunia-Kubik, K. (2011). [The role of HLA-E polymorphism in immunological response]. *Postepy Hig Med Dosw (Online)*, Vol. 65, pp. 616-626

[94] Jassem, R. M. Shani, W. S. Loisel, D. A. Sharief, M. Billstrand, C. and Ober, C. (2012). HLA-G polymorphisms and soluble HLA-G protein levels in women with recurrent pregnancy loss from Basrah province in Iraq. *Hum Immunol*, Vol. 73, (8), pp. 811-817

[95] Jin, Z. K. Xu, C. X. Tian, P. X. Xue, W. J. Ding, X. M. Zheng, J. Ding, C. G. Ge, G. Q. Mao, T. C. and Lin, Y. (2012). Impact of HLA-G 14-bp polymorphism on acute rejection and cytomegalovirus infection in kidney transplant recipients from northwestern China. *Transpl Immunol*, Vol. 27, (2-3), pp. 69-74

[96] Jones, D. C. Kosmoliaptsis, V. Apps, R. Lapaque, N. Smith, I. Kono, A. Chang, C. Boyle, L. H. Taylor, C. J. Trowsdale, J. and Allen, R. L. (2011). HLA class I allelic sequence and conformation regulate leukocyte Ig-like receptor binding. *J Immunol*, Vol. 186, (5), pp. 2990-2997

[97] Joosten, S. A. van Meijgaarden, K. E. van Weeren, P. C. Kazi, F. Geluk, A. Savage, N. D. Drijfhout, J. W. Flower, D. R. Hanekom, W. A. Klein, M. R. and Ottenhoff, T. H. (2010). Mycobacterium tuberculosis peptides presented by HLA-E molecules are targets for human CD8 T-cells with cytotoxic as well as regulatory activity. *PLoS Pathog*, Vol. 6, (2), pp. e1000782

[98] Kaiser, B. K. Barahmand-Pour, F. Paulsene, W. Medley, S. Geraghty, D. E. and Strong, R. K. (2005). Interactions between NKG2x immunoreceptors and HLA-E ligands display overlapping affinities and thermodynamics. *J Immunol*, Vol. 174, (5), pp. 2878-2884

[99] Kaiser, B. K. Pizarro, J. C. Kerns, J. and Strong, R. K. (2008). Structural basis for NKG2A/CD94 recognition of HLA-E. *Proc Natl Acad Sci U S A*, Vol. 105, (18), pp. 6696-6701

[100] Karhukorpi, J. Ikaheimo, I. Silvennoinen-Kassinen, S. and Tiilikainen, A. (1996). HLA-G polymorphism and allelic association with HLA-A in a Finnish population. *Eur J Immunogenet*, Vol. 23, (2), pp. 153-155

[101] Kikuchi-Maki, A. Yusa, S. Catina, T. L. and Campbell, K. S. (2003). KIR2DL4 is an IL-2-regulated NK cell receptor that exhibits limited expression in humans but triggers strong IFN-gamma production. *J Immunol*, Vol. 171, (7), pp. 3415-3425

[102] Kim, H. S. Garcia, J. Exley, M. Johnson, K. W. Balk, S. P. and Blumberg, R. S. (1999). Biochemical characterization of CD1d expression in the absence of beta2-microglobulin. *J Biol Chem*, Vol. 274, (14), pp. 9289-9295

[103] Kim, J. J. Hong, S. J. Hong, Y. M. Kim, S. Kang, M. J. Kim, K. J. Seo, E. J. Yoo, H. W. Cheong, H. S. Shin, H. D. Park, I. S. and Lee, J. K. (2008). Genetic variants in the HLA-G region are associated with Kawasaki disease. *Hum Immunol*, Vol. 69, (12), pp. 867-871

[104] Kim, S. K. Chung, J. H. Kim, D. H. Yun, D. H. Hong, S. J. and Lee, K. H. (2012). Lack of association between promoter polymorphisms of HLA-G gene and rheumatoid arthritis in Korean population. *Rheumatol Int*, Vol. 32, (2), pp. 509-512

[105] Kimkong, I. Mutirangura, A. and Pimtanothai, N. (2003). Distribution of human leukocyte antigens-E alleles in Thailand. *J Med Assoc Thai*, Vol. 86 Suppl 2, pp. S230-236

[106] Kotze, D. Kruger, T. F. Lombrd, C. Padayachee, T. Keskintepe, L. and Sher, G. (2013). The effect of the biochemical marker soluble human leukocyte antigen G on pregnancy outcome in assisted reproductive technology-a multicenter study. *Fertil Steril*, Vol., pp.

[107] Kovats, S. Main, E. K. Librach, C. Stubblebine, M. Fisher, S. J. and DeMars, R. (1990). A class I antigen, HLA-G, expressed in human trophoblasts. *Science*, Vol. 248, (4952), pp. 220-223

[108] Kren, L. Slaby, O. Muckova, K. Lzicarova, E. Sova, M. Vybihal, V. Svoboda, T. Fadrus, P. Lakomy, R. Vanhara, P. Krenova, Z. Sterba, J. Smrcka, M. and Michalek, J. (2011). Expression of immune-modulatory molecules HLA-G and HLA-E by tumor cells in glioblastomas: an unexpected prognostic significance? *Neuropathology*, Vol. 31, (2), pp. 129-134

[109] Lajoie, J. Hargrove, J. Zijenah, L. S. Humphrey, J. H. Ward, B. J. and Roger, M. (2006). Genetic variants in nonclassical major histocompatibility complex class I human leukocyte antigen (HLA)-E and HLA-G molecules are associated with susceptibility to heterosexual acquisition of HIV-1. *J Infect Dis*, Vol. 193, (2), pp. 298-301

[110] Lajoie, J. Jeanneau, A. Faucher, M. C. Moreau, P. and Roger, M. (2008). Characterisation of five novel HLA-G alleles with coding DNA base changes. *Tissue Antigens*, Vol. 72, (5), pp. 502-504

[111] Lauterbach, N. Voorter, C. E. and Tilanus, M. G. (2012). Molecular typing of HLA-E. *Methods Mol Biol*, Vol. 882, pp. 143-158

[112] Lawton, A. P. Prigozy, T. I. Brossay, L. Pei, B. Khurana, A. Martin, D. Zhu, T. Spate, K. Ozga, M. Honing, S. Bakke, O. and Kronenberg, M. (2005). The mouse CD1d cytoplasmic tail mediates CD1d trafficking and antigen presentation by adaptor protein 3-dependent and -independent mechanisms. *J Immunol*, Vol. 174, (6), pp. 3179-3186

[113] Le Bouteiller, P. (1994). HLA class I chromosomal region, genes, and products: facts and questions. *Crit Rev Immunol*, Vol. 14, (2), pp. 89-129

[114] Le Bouteiller, P. (1997). HLA-G: on the track of immunological functions. *Eur J Immunogenet*, Vol. 24, (5), pp. 397-408

[115] Le Rond, S. Le Maoult, J. Creput, C. Menier, C. Deschamps, M. Le Friec, G. Amiot, L. Durrbach, A. Dausset, J. Carosella, E. D. and Rouas-Freiss, N. (2004). Alloreactive CD4+ and CD8+ T cells express the immunotolerant HLA-G molecule in mixed lym-

phocyte reactions: in vivo implications in transplanted patients. *Eur J Immunol*, Vol. 34, (3), pp. 649-660

[116] Lee, N.Geraghty, D. E. (2003). HLA-F surface expression on B cell and monocyte cell lines is partially independent from tapasin and completely independent from TAP. *J Immunol*, Vol. 171, (10), pp. 5264-5271

[117] Lee, N. Goodlett, D. R. Ishitani, A. Marquardt, H. and Geraghty, D. E. (1998). HLA-E surface expression depends on binding of TAP-dependent peptides derived from certain HLA class I signal sequences. *J Immunol*, Vol. 160, (10), pp. 4951-4960

[118] Lee, N. Ishitani, A. and Geraghty, D. E. (2010). HLA-F is a surface marker on activated lymphocytes. *Eur J Immunol*, Vol., pp.

[119] Lee, N. Ishitani, A. and Geraghty, D. E. (2010). HLA-F is a surface marker on activated lymphocytes. *Eur J Immunol*, Vol. 40, (8), pp. 2308-2318

[120] Lee, N. Llano, M. Carretero, M. Ishitani, A. Navarro, F. Lopez-Botet, M. and Geraghty, D. E. (1998). HLA-E is a major ligand for the natural killer inhibitory receptor CD94/NKG2A. *Proc Natl Acad Sci U S A*, Vol. 95, (9), pp. 5199-5204

[121] LeMaoult, J. Krawice-Radanne, I. Dausset, J. and Carosella, E. D. (2004). HLA-G1-expressing antigen-presenting cells induce immunosuppressive CD4+ T cells. *Proc Natl Acad Sci U S A*, Vol. 101, (18), pp. 7064-7069

[122] LeMaoult, J. Zafaranloo, K. Le Danff, C. and Carosella, E. D. (2005). HLA-G up-regulates ILT2, ILT3, ILT4, and KIR2DL4 in antigen presenting cells, NK cells, and T cells. *FASEB J*, Vol. 19, (6), pp. 662-664

[123] Lemberg, M. K. Bland, F. A. Weihofen, A. Braud, V. M. and Martoglio, B. (2001). Intramembrane proteolysis of signal peptides: an essential step in the generation of HLA-E epitopes. *J Immunol*, Vol. 167, (11), pp. 6441-6446

[124] Lenfant, F. Pizzato, N. Liang, S. Davrinche, C. Le Bouteiller, P. and Horuzsko, A. (2003). Induction of HLA-G-restricted human cytomegalovirus pp65 (UL83)-specific cytotoxic T lymphocytes in HLA-G transgenic mice. *J Gen Virol*, Vol. 84, (Pt 2), pp. 307-317

[125] Levy, E. M. Sycz, G. Arriaga, J. M. Barrio, M. M. von Euw, E. M. Morales, S. B. Gonzalez, M. Mordoh, J. and Bianchini, M. (2009). Cetuximab-mediated cellular cytotoxicity is inhibited by HLA-E membrane expression in colon cancer cells. *Innate Immun*, Vol. 15, (2), pp. 91-100

[126] Li, C. Toth, I. Schulze Zur Wiesch, J. Pereyra, F. Rychert, J. Rosenberg, E. S. van Lunzen, J. Lichterfeld, M. and Yu, X. G. (2013). Functional characterization of HLA-G(+) regulatory T cells in HIV-1 infection. *PLoS Pathog*, Vol. 9, (1), pp. e1003140

[127] Li, J. Goldstein, I. Glickman-Nir, E. Jiang, H. and Chess, L. (2001). Induction of TCR Vbeta-specific CD8+ CTLs by TCR Vbeta-derived peptides bound to HLA-E. *J Immunol*, Vol. 167, (7), pp. 3800-3808

[128] Li, X. J. Zhang, X. Lin, A. Ruan, Y. Y. and Yan, W. H. (2012). Human leukocyte antigen-G (HLA-G) expression in cervical cancer lesions is associated with disease progression. *Hum Immunol*, Vol. 73, (9), pp. 946-949

[129] Liang, S. Ristich, V. Arase, H. Dausset, J. Carosella, E. D. and Horuzsko, A. (2008). Modulation of dendritic cell differentiation by HLA-G and ILT4 requires the IL-6--STAT3 signaling pathway. *Proc Natl Acad Sci U S A*, Vol. 105, (24), pp. 8357-8362

[130] Lin, A. Yan, W. H. Dai, M. Z. Chen, X. J. Li, B. L. Chen, B. G. and Fan, L. A. (2006). Maternal human leukocyte antigen-G polymorphism is not associated with pre-eclampsia in a Chinese Han population. *Tissue Antigens*, Vol. 68, (4), pp. 311-316

[131] Lin, A. Zhang, X. Ruan, Y. Y. Wang, Q. Zhou, W. J. and Yan, W. H. (2011). HLA-F expression is a prognostic factor in patients with non-small-cell lung cancer. *Lung Cancer*, Vol. 74, (3), pp. 504-509

[132] Little, A. M.Parham, P. (1999). Polymorphism and evolution of HLA class I and II genes and molecules. *Rev Immunogenet*, Vol. 1, (1), pp. 105-123

[133] Liu, X. X. Pan, F. H. and Tian, W. (2012). Characterization of HLA-E polymorphism in four distinct populations in Mainland China. *Tissue Antigens*, Vol. 80, (1), pp. 26-35

[134] Llano, M. Lee, N. Navarro, F. Garcia, P. Albar, J. P. Geraghty, D. E. and Lopez-Botet, M. (1998). HLA-E-bound peptides influence recognition by inhibitory and triggering CD94/NKG2 receptors: preferential response to an HLA-G-derived nonamer. *Eur J Immunol*, Vol. 28, (9), pp. 2854-2863

[135] Lopez-Botet, M.Bellon, T. (1999). Natural killer cell activation and inhibition by receptors for MHC class I. *Curr Opin Immunol*, Vol. 11, (3), pp. 301-307

[136] Loustau, M. Wiendl, H. Ferrone, S. and Carosella, E. D. (2013). HLA-G 2012 conference: the 15-year milestone update. *Tissue Antigens*, Vol. 81, (3), pp. 127-136

[137] Luo, M. Czarnecki, C. Ramdahin, S. Embree, J. and Plummer, F. A. (2013). HLA-G and mother-child perinatal HIV transmission. *Hum Immunol*, Vol. 74, (4), pp. 459-463

[138] Mallet, V. Blaschitz, A. Crisa, L. Schmitt, C. Fournel, S. King, A. Loke, Y. W. Dohr, G. and Le Bouteiller, P. (1999). HLA-G in the human thymus: a subpopulation of medullary epithelial but not CD83(+) dendritic cells expresses HLA-G as a membrane-bound and soluble protein. *Int Immunol*, Vol. 11, (6), pp. 889-898

[139] Malmberg, K. J. Levitsky, V. Norell, H. de Matos, C. T. Carlsten, M. Schedvins, K. Rabbani, H. Moretta, A. Soderstrom, K. Levitskaya, J. and Kiessling, R. (2002). IFN-gamma protects short-term ovarian carcinoma cell lines from CTL lysis via a CD94/NKG2A-dependent mechanism. *J Clin Invest*, Vol. 110, (10), pp. 1515-1523

[140] Marin, R. Ruiz-Cabello, F. Pedrinaci, S. Mendez, R. Jimenez, P. Geraghty, D. E. and Garrido, F. (2003). Analysis of HLA-E expression in human tumors. *Immunogenetics*, Vol. 54, (11), pp. 767-775

[141] Marsh, S. G. Albert, E. D. Bodmer, W. F. Bontrop, R. E. Dupont, B. Erlich, H. A. Fernandez-Vina, M. Geraghty, D. E. Holdsworth, R. Hurley, C. K. Lau, M. Lee, K. W. Mach, B. Maiers, M. Mayr, W. R. Muller, C. R. Parham, P. Petersdorf, E. W. Sasazuki, T. Strominger, J. L. Svejgaard, A. Terasaki, P. I. Tiercy, J. M. and Trowsdale, J. (2010). Nomenclature for factors of the HLA system, 2010. *Tissue Antigens*, Vol. 75, (4), pp. 291-455

[142] Martinetti, M. Pacati, I. Cuccia, M. Badulli, C. Pasi, A. Salvaneschi, L. Minola, E. De Silvestri, A. Iannone, A. M. and Maccabruni, A. (2006). Hierarchy of baby-linked immunogenetic risk factors in the vertical transmission of hepatitis C virus. *Int J Immunopathol Pharmacol*, Vol. 19, (2), pp. 369-378

[143] Matte, C. Lacaille, J. Zijenah, L. Ward, B. and Roger, M. (2000). HLA-G and HLA-E polymorphisms in an indigenous African population. The ZVITAMBO Study Group. *Hum Immunol*, Vol. 61, (11), pp. 1150-1156

[144] Matte, C. Lacaille, J. Zijenah, L. Ward, B. and Roger, M. (2002). HLA-G exhibits low level of polymorphism in indigenous East Africans. *Hum Immunol*, Vol. 63, (6), pp. 495-501

[145] Matte, C. Lajoie, J. Lacaille, J. Zijenah, L. S. Ward, B. J. and Roger, M. (2004). Functionally active HLA-G polymorphisms are associated with the risk of heterosexual HIV-1 infection in African women. *AIDS*, Vol. 18, (3), pp. 427-431

[146] Mazzarino, P. Pietra, G. Vacca, P. Falco, M. Colau, D. Coulie, P. Moretta, L. and Mingari, M. C. (2005). Identification of effector-memory CMV-specific T lymphocytes that kill CMV-infected target cells in an HLA-E-restricted fashion. *Eur J Immunol*, Vol. 35, (11), pp. 3240-3247

[147] Metcalfe, S. Roger, M. Faucher, M. C. Coutlee, F. Franco, E. L. and Brassard, P. (2013). The association between human leukocyte antigen (HLA)-G polymorphisms and human papillomavirus (HPV) infection in Inuit women of northern Quebec. *Hum Immunol*, Vol., pp.

[148] Metcalfe, S. Roger, M. Faucher, M. C. Coutlee, F. Franco, E. L. and Brassard, P. (2013). The frequency of HLA alleles in a population of Inuit women of northern Quebec. *Int J Circumpolar Health*, Vol. 72, pp.

[149] Michaelsson, J. Teixeira de Matos, C. Achour, A. Lanier, L. L. Karre, K. and Soderstrom, K. (2002). A signal peptide derived from hsp60 binds HLA-E and interferes with CD94/NKG2A recognition. *J Exp Med*, Vol. 196, (11), pp. 1403-1414

[150] Mittelbronn, M. Simon, P. Loffler, C. Capper, D. Bunz, B. Harter, P. Schlaszus, H. Schleich, A. Tabatabai, G. Goeppert, B. Meyermann, R. Weller, M. and Wischhusen, J. (2007). Elevated HLA-E levels in human glioblastomas but not in grade I to III astro-

cytomas correlate with infiltrating CD8+ cells. *J Neuroimmunol*, Vol. 189, (1-2), pp. 50-58

[151] Mizuki, N. Ota, M. Katsuyama, Y. Yabuki, K. Ando, H. Goto, K. Nakamura, S. Bahram, S. Ohno, S. and Inoko, H. (1999). Association analysis between the MIC-A and HLA-B alleles in Japanese patients with Behcet's disease. *Arthritis Rheum*, Vol. 42, (9), pp. 1961-1966

[152] Morales, P. Corell, A. Martinez-Laso, J. Martin-Villa, J. M. Varela, P. Paz-Artal, E. Allende, L. M. and Arnaiz-Villena, A. (1993). Three new HLA-G alleles and their linkage disequilibria with HLA-A. *Immunogenetics*, Vol. 38, (5), pp. 323-331

[153] Morales, P. J. Pace, J. L. Platt, J. S. Phillips, T. A. Morgan, K. Fazleabas, A. T. and Hunt, J. S. (2003). Placental cell expression of HLA-G2 isoforms is limited to the invasive trophoblast phenotype. *J Immunol*, Vol. 171, (11), pp. 6215-6224

[154] Morandi, F. Venturi, C. Rizzo, R. Castellazzi, M. Baldi, E. Caniatti, M. L. Tola, M. R. Granieri, E. Fainardi, E. Uccelli, A. and Pistoia, V. (2013). Intrathecal soluble HLA-E correlates with disease activity in patients with multiple sclerosis and may cooperate with soluble HLA-G in the resolution of neuroinflammation. *J Neuroimmune Pharmacol*, Vol. 8, (4), pp. 944-955

[155] Moreau, P. Contu, L. Alba, F. Lai, S. Simoes, R. Orru, S. Carcassi, C. Roger, M. Rabreau, M. and Carosella, E. D. (2008). HLA-G gene polymorphism in human placentas: possible association of G*0106 allele with preeclampsia and miscarriage. *Biol Reprod*, Vol. 79, (3), pp. 459-467

[156] Mosaad, Y. M. Abdel-Dayem, Y. El-Deek, B. S. and El-Sherbini, S. M. (2011). Association between HLA-E *0101 homozygosity and recurrent miscarriage in Egyptian women. *Scand J Immunol*, Vol. 74, (2), pp. 205-209

[157] Moscoso, J. Serrano-Vela, J. I. and Arnaiz-Villena, A. (2007). MHC-F polymorphism and evolution. *Tissue Antigens*, Vol. 69 Suppl 1, pp. 136-139

[158] Nardi Fda, S. Slowik, R. Wowk, P. F. da Silva, J. S. Gelmini, G. F. Michelon, T. F. Neumann, J. and Bicalho Mda, G. (2012). Analysis of HLA-G polymorphisms in couples with implantation failure. *Am J Reprod Immunol*, Vol. 68, (6), pp. 507-514

[159] Nattermann, J. Nischalke, H. D. Hofmeister, V. Ahlenstiel, G. Zimmermann, H. Leifeld, L. Weiss, E. H. Sauerbruch, T. and Spengler, U. (2005). The HLA-A2 restricted T cell epitope HCV core 35-44 stabilizes HLA-E expression and inhibits cytolysis mediated by natural killer cells. *Am J Pathol*, Vol. 166, (2), pp. 443-453

[160] Nattermann, J. Nischalke, H. D. Hofmeister, V. Kupfer, B. Ahlenstiel, G. Feldmann, G. Rockstroh, J. Weiss, E. H. Sauerbruch, T. and Spengler, U. (2005). HIV-1 infection leads to increased HLA-E expression resulting in impaired function of natural killer cells. *Antivir Ther*, Vol. 10, (1), pp. 95-107

[161] Nufer, O. Guldbrandsen, S. Degen, M. Kappeler, F. Paccaud, J. P. Tani, K. and Hauri, H. P. (2002). Role of cytoplasmic C-terminal amino acids of membrane proteins in ER export. *J Cell Sci*, Vol. 115, (Pt 3), pp. 619-628

[162] Ober, C. (1998). HLA and pregnancy: the paradox of the fetal allograft. *Am J Hum Genet*, Vol. 62, (1), pp. 1-5

[163] Ober, C. Rosinsky, B. Grimsley, C. van der Ven, K. Robertson, A. and Runge, A. (1996). Population genetic studies of HLA-G: allele frequencies and linkage disequilibrium with HLA-A1. *J Reprod Immunol*, Vol. 32, (2), pp. 111-123

[164] Ohya, K. Kondo, K. and Mizuno, S. (1990). Polymorphism in the human class I MHC locus HLA-E in Japanese. *Immunogenetics*, Vol. 32, (3), pp. 205-209

[165] Oliveira, C. C. van Veelen, P. A. Querido, B. de Ru, A. Sluijter, M. Laban, S. Drijfhout, J. W. van der Burg, S. H. Offringa, R. and van Hall, T. (2010). The nonpolymorphic MHC Qa-1b mediates CD8+ T cell surveillance of antigen-processing defects. *J Exp Med*, Vol. 207, (1), pp. 207-221

[166] Onno, M. Pangault, C. Le Friec, G. Guilloux, V. Andre, P. and Fauchet, R. (2000). Modulation of HLA-G antigens expression by human cytomegalovirus: specific induction in activated macrophages harboring human cytomegalovirus infection. *J Immunol*, Vol. 164, (12), pp. 6426-6434

[167] Paladini, F. Belfiore, F. Cocco, E. Carcassi, C. Cauli, A. Vacca, A. Fiorillo, M. T. Mathieu, A. Cascino, I. and Sorrentino, R. (2009). HLA-E gene polymorphism associates with ankylosing spondylitis in Sardinia. *Arthritis Res Ther*, Vol. 11, (6), pp. R171

[168] Pan, F. H. Liu, X. X. and Tian, W. (2013). Characterization of HLA-F polymorphism in four distinct populations in Mainland China. *Int J Immunogenet*, Vol. 40, (5), pp. 369-376

[169] Paquay, M. M. Schellekens, J. and Tilanus, M. G. (2009). A high-throughput Taqman approach for the discrimination of HLA-E alleles. *Tissue Antigens*, Vol. 74, (6), pp. 514-519

[170] Parham, P. Norman, P. J. Abi-Rached, L. and Guethlein, L. A. (2012). Human-specific evolution of killer cell immunoglobulin-like receptor recognition of major histocompatibility complex class I molecules. *Philos Trans R Soc Lond B Biol Sci*, Vol. 367, (1590), pp. 800-811

[171] Park, G. M. Lee, S. Park, B. Kim, E. Shin, J. Cho, K. and Ahn, K. (2004). Soluble HLA-G generated by proteolytic shedding inhibits NK-mediated cell lysis. *Biochem Biophys Res Commun*, Vol. 313, (3), pp. 606-611

[172] Park, K. S. Park, J. S. Nam, J. H. Bang, D. Sohn, S. and Lee, E. S. (2007). HLA-E*0101 and HLA-G*010101 reduce the risk of Behcet's disease. *Tissue Antigens*, Vol. 69, (2), pp. 139-144

[173] Park, Y. Kim, Y. S. Kwon, O. J. and Kim, H. S. (2012). Allele frequencies of human leukocyte antigen-G in a Korean population. *Int J Immunogenet*, Vol. 39, (1), pp. 39-45

[174] Peaper, D. R.Cresswell, P. (2008). Regulation of MHC class I assembly and peptide binding. *Annu Rev Cell Dev Biol*, Vol. 24, pp. 343-368

[175] Petrie, E. J. Clements, C. S. Lin, J. Sullivan, L. C. Johnson, D. Huyton, T. Heroux, A. Hoare, H. L. Beddoe, T. Reid, H. H. Wilce, M. C. Brooks, A. G. and Rossjohn, J. (2008). CD94-NKG2A recognition of human leukocyte antigen (HLA)-E bound to an HLA class I leader sequence. *J Exp Med*, Vol. 205, (3), pp. 725-735

[176] Pfeiffer, K. A. Fimmers, R. Engels, G. van der Ven, H. and van der Ven, K. (2001). The HLA-G genotype is potentially associated with idiopathic recurrent spontaneous abortion. *Mol Hum Reprod*, Vol. 7, (4), pp. 373-378

[177] Pietra, G. Romagnani, C. Moretta, L. and Mingari, M. C. (2009). HLA-E and HLA-E-bound peptides: recognition by subsets of NK and T cells. *Curr Pharm Des*, Vol. 15, (28), pp. 3336-3344

[178] Pirri, A. Contieri, F. C. Benvenutti, R. and Bicalho Mda, G. (2009). A study of HLA-G polymorphism and linkage disequilibrium in renal transplant patients and their donors. *Transpl Immunol*, Vol. 20, (3), pp. 143-149

[179] Prigione, I. Penco, F. Martini, A. Gattorno, M. Pistoia, V. and Morandi, F. (2011). HLA-G and HLA-E in patients with juvenile idiopathic arthritis. *Rheumatology (Oxford)*, Vol. 50, (5), pp. 966-972

[180] Pyo, C. W. Williams, L. M. Moore, Y. Hyodo, H. Li, S. S. Zhao, L. P. Sageshima, N. Ishitani, A. and Geraghty, D. E. (2006). HLA-E, HLA-F, and HLA-G polymorphism: genomic sequence defines haplotype structure and variation spanning the nonclassical class I genes. *Immunogenetics*, Vol. 58, (4), pp. 241-251

[181] Rahimi, R. Hosseini, A. Z. and Yari, F. (2010). The polymorphism of human leucocyte antigen-G gene in a healthy population of Iran. *Int J Immunogenet*, Vol. 37, (4), pp. 269-272

[182] Rajagopalan, S.Long, E. O. (1999). A human histocompatibility leukocyte antigen (HLA)-G-specific receptor expressed on all natural killer cells. *J Exp Med*, Vol. 189, (7), pp. 1093-1100

[183] Ren, E. C.Chan, S. H. (1996). Human leucocyte antigens and nasopharyngeal carcinoma. *Clin Sci (Lond)*, Vol. 91, (3), pp. 256-258

[184] Riteau, B. Rouas-Freiss, N. Menier, C. Paul, P. Dausset, J. and Carosella, E. D. (2001). HLA-G2, -G3, and -G4 isoforms expressed as nonmature cell surface glycoproteins inhibit NK and antigen-specific CTL cytolysis. *J Immunol*, Vol. 166, (8), pp. 5018-5026

[185] Rizzo, R. Bortolotti, D. Fredj, N. B. Rotola, A. Cura, F. Castellazzi, M. Tamborino, C. Seraceni, S. Baldi, E. Melchiorri, L. Tola, M. R. Granieri, E. Baricordi, O. R. and Fainardi, E. (2012). Role of HLA-G 14bp deletion/insertion and +3142C>G polymor-

phisms in the production of sHLA-G molecules in relapsing-remitting multiple sclerosis. *Hum Immunol*, Vol. 73, (11), pp. 1140-1146

[186] Rizzo, R. Farina, I. Bortolotti, D. Galuppi, E. Rotola, A. Melchiorri, L. Ciancio, G. Di Luca, D. and Govoni, M. (2013). HLA-G may predict the disease course in patients with early rheumatoid arthritis. *Hum Immunol*, Vol. 74, (4), pp. 425-432

[187] Rizzo, R. Hviid, T. V. Govoni, M. Padovan, M. Rubini, M. Melchiorri, L. Stignani, M. Carturan, S. Grappa, M. T. Fotinidi, M. Ferretti, S. Voss, A. Laustrup, H. Junker, P. Trotta, F. and Baricordi, O. R. (2008). HLA-G genotype and HLA-G expression in systemic lupus erythematosus: HLA-G as a putative susceptibility gene in systemic lupus erythematosus. *Tissue Antigens*, Vol. 71, (6), pp. 520-529

[188] Robinson, J. Halliwell, J. A. McWilliam, H. Lopez, R. Parham, P. and Marsh, S. G. (2013). The IMGT/HLA database. *Nucleic Acids Res*, Vol. 41, (Database issue), pp. D1222-1227

[189] Rodgers, J. R.Cook, R. G. (2005). MHC class Ib molecules bridge innate and acquired immunity. *Nat Rev Immunol*, Vol. 5, (6), pp. 459-471

[190] Roger, J. Faucher, M. C. and Roger, M. (2012). Identification of a new HLA-G allele, HLA-G*01:18, in a Canadian Caucasian individual. *Tissue Antigens*, Vol. 80, (5), pp. 472-473

[191] Romero, V. Larsen, C. E. Duke-Cohan, J. S. Fox, E. A. Romero, T. Clavijo, O. P. Fici, D. A. Husain, Z. Almeciga, I. Alford, D. R. Awdeh, Z. L. Zuniga, J. El-Dahdah, L. Alper, C. A. and Yunis, E. J. (2007). Genetic fixity in the human major histocompatibility complex and block size diversity in the class I region including HLA-E. *BMC Genet*, Vol. 8, pp. 14

[192] Rouas-Freiss, N. Marchal, R. E. Kirszenbaum, M. Dausset, J. and Carosella, E. D. (1997). The alpha1 domain of HLA-G1 and HLA-G2 inhibits cytotoxicity induced by natural killer cells: is HLA-G the public ligand for natural killer cell inhibitory receptors? *Proc Natl Acad Sci U S A*, Vol. 94, (10), pp. 5249-5254

[193] Salerno-Goncalves, R. Fernandez-Vina, M. Lewinsohn, D. M. and Sztein, M. B. (2004). Identification of a human HLA-E-restricted CD8+ T cell subset in volunteers immunized with Salmonella enterica serovar Typhi strain Ty21a typhoid vaccine. *J Immunol*, Vol. 173, (9), pp. 5852-5862

[194] Schulte, D. Vogel, M. Langhans, B. Kramer, B. Korner, C. Nischalke, H. D. Steinberg, V. Michalk, M. Berg, T. Rockstroh, J. K. Sauerbruch, T. Spengler, U. and Nattermann, J. (2009). The HLA-E(R)/HLA-E(R) genotype affects the natural course of hepatitis C virus (HCV) infection and is associated with HLA-E-restricted recognition of an HCV-derived peptide by interferon-gamma-secreting human CD8(+) T cells. *J Infect Dis*, Vol. 200, (9), pp. 1397-1401

[195] Selmani, Z. Naji, A. Zidi, I. Favier, B. Gaiffe, E. Obert, L. Borg, C. Saas, P. Tiberghien, P. Rouas-Freiss, N. Carosella, E. D. and Deschaseaux, F. (2008). Human leukocyte an-

tigen-G5 secretion by human mesenchymal stem cells is required to suppress T lymphocyte and natural killer function and to induce CD4+CD25highFOXP3+ regulatory T cells. *Stem Cells*, Vol. 26, (1), pp. 212-222

[196] Selvakumar, A. Steffens, U. and Dupont, B. (1996). NK cell receptor gene of the KIR family with two IG domains but highest homology to KIR receptors with three IG domains. *Tissue Antigens*, Vol. 48, (4 Pt 1), pp. 285-294

[197] Shawar, S. M. Vyas, J. M. Rodgers, J. R. and Rich, R. R. (1994). Antigen presentation by major histocompatibility complex class I-B molecules. *Annu Rev Immunol*, Vol. 12, pp. 839-880

[198] Shiroishi, M. Kuroki, K. Ose, T. Rasubala, L. Shiratori, I. Arase, H. Tsumoto, K. Kumagai, I. Kohda, D. and Maenaka, K. (2006). Efficient leukocyte Ig-like receptor signaling and crystal structure of disulfide-linked HLA-G dimer. *J Biol Chem*, Vol. 281, (15), pp. 10439-10447

[199] Shiroishi, M. Kuroki, K. Rasubala, L. Tsumoto, K. Kumagai, I. Kurimoto, E. Kato, K. Kohda, D. and Maenaka, K. (2006). Structural basis for recognition of the nonclassical MHC molecule HLA-G by the leukocyte Ig-like receptor B2 (LILRB2/LIR2/ILT4/CD85d). *Proc Natl Acad Sci U S A*, Vol. 103, (44), pp. 16412-16417

[200] Silva, I. D. Muniz, Y. C. Sousa, M. C. Silva, K. R. Castelli, E. C. Filho, J. C. Osta, A. P. Lima, M. I. and Simoes, R. T. (2013). HLA-G 3'UTR polymorphisms in high grade and invasive cervico-vaginal cancer. *Hum Immunol*, Vol. 74, (4), pp. 452-458

[201] Simoes, R. T. Goncalves, M. A. Castelli, E. C. Junior, C. M. Bettini, J. S. Discorde, M. L. Duarte, G. Quintana, S. M. Simoes, A. L. Moreau, P. Carosella, E. D. Soares, E. G. and Donadi, E. A. (2009). HLA-G polymorphisms in women with squamous intraepithelial lesions harboring human papillomavirus. *Mod Pathol*, Vol. 22, (8), pp. 1075-1082

[202] Singer, D. S.Maguire, J. E. (1990). Regulation of the expression of class I MHC genes. *Crit Rev Immunol*, Vol. 10, (3), pp. 235-257

[203] Sipak-Szmigiel, O. Cybulski, C. Lubinski, J. and Ronin-Walknowska, E. (2008). HLA-G polymorphism in a Polish population and reproductive failure. *Tissue Antigens*, Vol. 71, (1), pp. 67-71

[204] Sipak-Szmigiel, O. Cybulski, C. Wokolorczyk, D. Lubinski, J. Kurzawa, R. Baczkowski, T. Radwan, M. Radwan, P. and Ronin-Walknowska, E. (2009). HLA-G polymorphism and in vitro fertilization failure in a Polish population. *Tissue Antigens*, Vol. 73, (4), pp. 348-352

[205] Song, G. G. Choi, S. J. Ji, J. D. and Lee, Y. H. (2013). Genome-wide pathway analysis of a genome-wide association study on multiple sclerosis. *Mol Biol Rep*, Vol. 40, (3), pp. 2557-2564

[206] Strong, R. K. Holmes, M. A. Li, P. Braun, L. Lee, N. and Geraghty, D. E. (2003). HLA-E allelic variants. Correlating differential expression, peptide affinities, crystal structures, and thermal stabilities. *J Biol Chem*, Vol. 278, (7), pp. 5082-5090

[207] Suarez, M. B. Morales, P. Castro, M. J. Fernandez, V. Varela, P. Alvarez, M. Martinez-Laso, J. and Arnaiz-Villena, A. (1997). A new HLA-G allele (HLA-G*0105N) and its distribution in the Spanish population. *Immunogenetics*, Vol. 45, (6), pp. 464-465

[208] Sullivan, L. C. Clements, C. S. Rossjohn, J. and Brooks, A. G. (2008). The major histocompatibility complex class Ib molecule HLA-E at the interface between innate and adaptive immunity. *Tissue Antigens*, Vol. 72, (5), pp. 415-424

[209] Tamouza, R. Busson, M. Rocha, V. Fortier, C. Haddad, Y. Brun, M. Boukouaci, W. Bleux, H. Socie, G. Krishnamoorthy, R. Toubert, A. Gluckman, E. and Charron, D. (2006). Homozygous status for HLA-E*0103 confers protection from acute graft-versus-host disease and transplant-related mortality in HLA-matched sibling hematopoietic stem cell transplantation. *Transplantation*, Vol. 82, (11), pp. 1436-1440

[210] Tan, C. Y. Ho, J. F. Chong, Y. S. Loganath, A. Chan, Y. H. Ravichandran, J. Lee, C. G. and Chong, S. S. (2008). Paternal contribution of HLA-G*0106 significantly increases risk for pre-eclampsia in multigravid pregnancies. *Mol Hum Reprod*, Vol. 14, (5), pp. 317-324

[211] Terrazzano, G. Sica, M. Gianfrani, C. Mazzarella, G. Maurano, F. De Giulio, B. de Saint-Mezard, S. Zanzi, D. Maiuri, L. Londei, M. Jabri, B. Troncone, R. Auricchio, S. Zappacosta, S. and Carbone, E. (2007). Gliadin regulates the NK-dendritic cell cross-talk by HLA-E surface stabilization. *J Immunol*, Vol. 179, (1), pp. 372-381

[212] Todd, J. A. (1995). Genetic analysis of type 1 diabetes using whole genome approaches. *Proc Natl Acad Sci U S A*, Vol. 92, (19), pp. 8560-8565

[213] Tomasec, P. Braud, V. M. Rickards, C. Powell, M. B. McSharry, B. P. Gadola, S. Cerundolo, V. Borysiewicz, L. K. McMichael, A. J. and Wilkinson, G. W. (2000). Surface expression of HLA-E, an inhibitor of natural killer cells, enhanced by human cytomegalovirus gpUL40. *Science*, Vol. 287, (5455), pp. 1031

[214] Townsend, A.Bodmer, H. (1989). Antigen recognition by class I-restricted T lymphocytes. *Annu Rev Immunol*, Vol. 7, pp. 601-624

[215] Tripathi, P. Naik, S. and Agrawal, S. (2006). HLA-E and immunobiology of pregnancy. *Tissue Antigens*, Vol. 67, (3), pp. 207-213

[216] Tse, K. P. Su, W. H. Chang, K. P. Tsang, N. M. Yu, C. J. Tang, P. See, L. C. Hsueh, C. Yang, M. L. Hao, S. P. Li, H. Y. Wang, M. H. Liao, L. P. Chen, L. C. Lin, S. R. Jorgensen, T. J. Chang, Y. S. and Shugart, Y. Y. (2009). Genome-wide association study reveals multiple nasopharyngeal carcinoma-associated loci within the HLA region at chromosome 6p21.3. *Am J Hum Genet*, Vol. 85, (2), pp. 194-203

[217] Uchigiri, C. Mizuno, S. Wada, K. Tsutsumi, M. Kato, T. Kamiya, T. and Ozawa, K. (1997). An identification of the HLA-F null allele in Japanese. *Immunogenetics*, Vol. 45, (6), pp. 466-467

[218] Ulbrecht, M. Modrow, S. Srivastava, R. Peterson, P. A. and Weiss, E. H. (1998). Interaction of HLA-E with peptides and the peptide transporter in vitro: implications for its function in antigen presentation. *J Immunol*, Vol. 160, (9), pp. 4375-4385

[219] van der Ven, K. Skrablin, S. Engels, G. and Krebs, D. (1998). HLA-G polymorphisms and allele frequencies in Caucasians. *Hum Immunol*, Vol. 59, (5), pp. 302-312

[220] van der Ven, K. Skrablin, S. Ober, C. and Krebs, D. (1998). HLA-G polymorphisms: ethnic differences and implications for potential molecule function. *Am J Reprod Immunol*, Vol. 40, (3), pp. 145-157

[221] van Hall, T. Oliveira, C. C. Joosten, S. A. and Ottenhoff, T. H. (2010). The other Janus face of Qa-1 and HLA-E: diverse peptide repertoires in times of stress. *Microbes Infect*, Vol. 12, (12-13), pp. 910-918

[222] Veiga-Castelli, L. C. Castelli, E. C. Beauchemin, K. Donadi, E. A. and Roger, M. (2012). A novel HLA-E allele, E*01:03:05, identified in two Brazilian individuals. *Tissue Antigens*, Vol. 80, (2), pp. 200-201

[223] Veiga-Castelli, L. C. Castelli, E. C. Mendes, C. T., Jr. da Silva, W. A., Jr. Faucher, M. C. Beauchemin, K. Roger, M. Moreau, P. and Donadi, E. A. (2012). Non-classical HLA-E gene variability in Brazilians: a nearly invariable locus surrounded by the most variable genes in the human genome. *Tissue Antigens*, Vol. 79, (1), pp. 15-24

[224] Wainwright, S. D. Biro, P. A. and Holmes, C. H. (2000). HLA-F is a predominantly empty, intracellular, TAP-associated MHC class Ib protein with a restricted expression pattern. *J Immunol*, Vol. 164, (1), pp. 319-328

[225] Wang, X. Jiang, W. and Zhang, D. (2013). Association of 14-bp insertion/deletion polymorphism of HLA-G gene with unexplained recurrent spontaneous abortion: a meta-analysis. *Tissue Antigens*, Vol. 81, (2), pp. 108-115

[226] Wang, X. Li, B. Wang, J. Lei, J. Liu, C. Ma, Y. and Zhao, H. (2012). Evidence that miR-133a causes recurrent spontaneous abortion by reducing HLA-G expression. *Reprod Biomed Online*, Vol. 25, (4), pp. 415-424

[227] Warner, C. M. Tyas, D. A. Goldstein, C. Comiskey, M. Cohen, J. and Brenner, C. A. (2002). Genotyping: the HLA system and embryo development. *Reprod Biomed Online*, Vol. 4, (2), pp. 133-139

[228] Wei, X. H.Orr, H. T. (1990). Differential expression of HLA-E, HLA-F, and HLA-G transcripts in human tissue. *Hum Immunol*, Vol. 29, (2), pp. 131-142

[229] Wiendl, H. Feger, U. Mittelbronn, M. Jack, C. Schreiner, B. Stadelmann, C. Antel, J. Brueck, W. Meyermann, R. Bar-Or, A. Kieseier, B. C. and Weller, M. (2005). Expres-

sion of the immune-tolerogenic major histocompatibility molecule HLA-G in multiple sclerosis: implications for CNS immunity. *Brain*, Vol. 128, (Pt 11), pp. 2689-2704

[230] Wischhusen, J. Friese, M. A. Mittelbronn, M. Meyermann, R. and Weller, M. (2005). HLA-E protects glioma cells from NKG2D-mediated immune responses in vitro: implications for immune escape in vivo. *J Neuropathol Exp Neurol*, Vol. 64, (6), pp. 523-528

[231] Wisniewski, A. Bilinska, M. Klimczak, A. Wagner, M. Majorczyk, E. Nowak, I. Pokryszko-Dragan, A. and Kusnierczyk, P. (2010). Association of the HLA-G gene polymorphism with multiple sclerosis in a Polish population. *Int J Immunogenet*, Vol. 37, (4), pp. 307-311

[232] Wooden, S. L. Kalb, S. R. Cotter, R. J. and Soloski, M. J. (2005). Cutting edge: HLA-E binds a peptide derived from the ATP-binding cassette transporter multidrug resistance-associated protein 7 and inhibits NK cell-mediated lysis. *J Immunol*, Vol. 175, (3), pp. 1383-1387

[233] Yan, W. H. Fan, L. A. Yang, J. Q. Xu, L. D. Ge, Y. and Yao, F. J. (2006). HLA-G polymorphism in a Chinese Han population with recurrent spontaneous abortion. *Int J Immunogenet*, Vol. 33, (1), pp. 55-58

[234] Yusa, S. Catina, T. L. and Campbell, K. S. (2002). SHP-1- and phosphotyrosine-independent inhibitory signaling by a killer cell Ig-like receptor cytoplasmic domain in human NK cells. *J Immunol*, Vol. 168, (10), pp. 5047-5057

[235] Zeng, L. Sullivan, L. C. Vivian, J. P. Walpole, N. G. Harpur, C. M. Rossjohn, J. Clements, C. S. and Brooks, A. G. (2012). A structural basis for antigen presentation by the MHC class Ib molecule, Qa-1b. *J Immunol*, Vol. 188, (1), pp. 302-310

[236] Zhang, J. B. Wang, Z. Y. Chen, J. Wu, X. D. Zhou, B. and Yie, S. M. (2013). The expression of human leukocyte antigen G (HLA-G) is associated with sacroiliitis stages of ankylosing spondylitis. *Immunol Lett*, Vol. 152, (2), pp. 121-125

[237] Zhang, X. Lin, A. Zhang, J. G. Bao, W. G. Xu, D. P. Ruan, Y. Y. and Yan, W. H. (2013). Alteration of HLA-F and HLA I antigen expression in the tumor is associated with survival in patients with esophageal squamous cell carcinoma. *Int J Cancer*, Vol. 132, (1), pp. 82-89

[238] Zhao, L. Fan, L. Yang, J. Yao, F. and Xu, L. (2001). [Analysis on HLA-E polymorphism in Shanghai Han population]. *Zhonghua Yi Xue Yi Chuan Xue Za Zhi*, Vol. 18, (6), pp. 444-447

[239] Zhen, Z. J. Ling, J. Y. Cai, Y. Luo, W. B. and He, Y. J. (2013). Impact of HLA-E gene polymorphism on HLA-E expression in tumor cells and prognosis in patients with stage III colorectal cancer. *Med Oncol*, Vol. 30, (1), pp. 482

http://dx.doi.org/10.5772/57507

[240] Zheng, X. Q. Zhu, F. Shi, W. W. Lin, A. and Yan, W. H. (2009). The HLA-G 14 bp insertion/deletion polymorphism is a putative susceptible factor for active human cytomegalovirus infection in children. *Tissue Antigens,* Vol. 74, (4), pp. 317-321

[241] Zidi, I. Guillard, C. Marcou, C. Krawice-Radanne, I. Sangrouber, D. Rouas-Freiss, N. Carosella, E. D. and Moreau, P. (2006). Increase in HLA-G1 proteolytic shedding by tumor cells: a regulatory pathway controlled by NF-kappaB inducers. *Cell Mol Life Sci,* Vol. 63, (22), pp. 2669-2681

Chapter 4

Human Leucocyte Antigen Matching Strategy

Yuying Sun and Yongzhi Xi

Additional information is available at the end of the chapter

http://dx.doi.org/10.5772/57500

1. Introduction

The HLA system includes a complex array of genes located on chromosome number 6 and their molecular products that are involved in immune regulation and cellular differentiation. Human leukocyte antigen (HLA) molecules are expressed on almost all nucleated cells, and they are the major molecules that initiate graft rejection. There are three classical loci at HLA class I: HLA-A, -B, and -Cw, and five loci at class II: HLA-DR, -DQ, -DP, -DM, and -DO. HLA loci are the most genetically variable gene loci in human. Two hundred and twenty four loci of HLA complex have been identified so far. Among these, 128 are functional loci that encode proteins, and 39.8% of HLA genes are related to the immune system, particularly those belong to class II loci. Almost all these genes display immune-related functions. Approximately 100 HLA genes loci have been cloned and named and at least 18 of them have alleles. Since these loci have various amounts of alleles and each allele encodes a corresponding HLA antigen, the HLA complex has the most abundant genetic polymorphism in the human immune system.

Systemic investigations of the alleles in HLA loci began in 1987. There were just over 10 identified alleles at that time. The allele numbers in HLA-I and HLA-II loci were increased to 100 and 50 respectively in 1989. The allele number of HLA-I and HLA-II reached 1028 in 2000. As of July 2013, the total allele number of HLA loci has reached 9719. HLA-A, HLA-B and HLA-C loci have 2365, 3015 and 1848 alleles respectively. DRA site has 7 and DRB site has 1456 alleles. DQA1 and DQB1 sites have 51 and 416 alleles respectively; DPB1 sites have 37 and 190 alleles, respectively (Fig 1). Theoretically, it is very difficult to find an unrelated donor with a perfectly matched HLA genotype (at the allele level) in the general population.

The polymorphism of HLA makes it difficult to find a match between unrelated donor and recipient in the allo-transplantation. Currently, the most commonly used HLA typing in organ transplantations around the world is based on HLA-A, B, C and DR genes. There are up to 8600 alleles in these genes corresponding to more than 100 specific antigens. With the increasing number of patients who need hematopoietic stem cell transplantation, the lack of appropriate donors has become a significant challenge. Therefore, there is an urgent need to develop novel scientific, practical, and feasible HLA typing methods in the field of organ and hematopoietic stem cell transplantation.

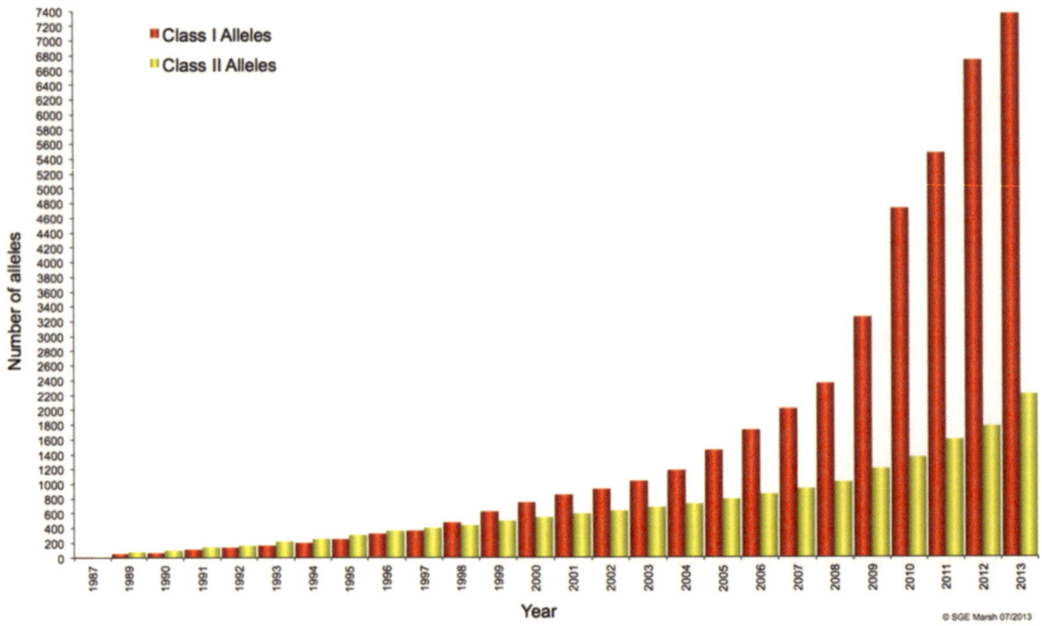

Figure 1. Increasing number of HLA alleles from 1987 to July 2013

2. The influence of HLA compatibility on organ and hematopoietic stem cell transplantation

The influence of HLA compatibility on organ transplant survival was analyzed in more than 150,000 recipients transplanted from 1987 to 1997 at transplant centers participating in the Collaborative Transplant Study. A statistically highly significant effect of HLA matching on graft and patient survival rates was found in the analysis of kidney transplants ($P < 0.0001$). Ten years after transplantation, the graft survival rate of first cadaver kidney transplants with a complete mismatch (6 HLA-A+B+DR mismatches) was 17% lower than that of grafts with no mismatch. During the first post-transplant year, the class II HLA-DR locus had a stronger impact than the class I HLA-A and HLA-B loci. During subsequent years, however, the influence on graft survival of the three loci was found to be equivalent and additive. For optimal graft outcome, compatibility at all three HLA loci is, therefore, desirable. The excellent correlation of HLA matching observed in recipients of cadaver kidneys with very short ischemic preservation (0-6 hours) or recipients of kidneys from living unrelated donors contradicts reports that short ischemia can eliminate the influence of matching.

Although HLA has a significant effect on graft outcome regardless of the state of presensitization, the matching effect is potentiated in patients with highly reactive preformed lymphocytotoxic antibodies. Among first cadaver transplant recipients with an antibody reactivity against > 50% of the test panel, the difference in graft survival at 5 years between patients with 0 or 6 mismatches reached 30%. A collaborative project, in which molecular DNA typing methods were employed, showed that the correction of serological HLA typing errors by more accurate DNA typing results in a significantly improved HLA matching effect. Moreover, matching for the class II locus HLA-DP, a locus that can be typed reliably only by DNA methods, showed a significant effect in cadaver kidney retransplants, especially in the presence of preformed lymphocytotoxic antibodies. The analysis of heart transplants showed a highly significant impact of HLA compatibility on graft outcome ($P < 0.0001$). This result is of particular interest because donor hearts are not allocated according to the HLA match. A biasing influence of donor organ allocation (i.e. a preferential allocation of good matches to good risk recipients) can, therefore, be excluded. In liver transplantation, neither matching for HLA class I nor HLA class II could be shown to influence transplant outcome.

The first successful human bone marrow transplantation between identical twins in 1957 has provided a new approach for the treatment of leukemia and other hematologic malignancies. After the successful hematopoietic stem cell transplantation between unrelated donor and recipient with matched HLA, a bone marrow donor registry was established in 1988 (National Marrow Donor Program, NMDP) in the USA. Later on, a public cord blood bank was established. According to the World Marrow Donor Association (WMDA), as of July 2012, the association has 68 bone marrow banks in 49 countries and regions. It also has 46 cord blood banks in 30 countries and regions. The registered bone marrow and umbilical cord blood donors have exceeded 20 million. Meanwhile, the technology of HLA typing has been transformed from simple serotyping to more accurate genotyping. Although there are hundreds of reports regarding the effect of HLA matching degree on the efficacy of hematopoietic stem cell transplantation, these results are not consistent due to the differences in sample size, disease type and stage, and HLA typing. In addition, the interpretation of HLA genotyping results and their biological significance is becoming increasingly complicated. It is challenging for the clinicians outside of the HLA field to select an unrelated donor with the best-matched HLA. To meet this challenge, WMDA, NMDP of the USA and European Federation of Immunogenetics (EFI) have provided guidelines for HLA typing.

3. The history of HLA typing strategy evolution

The technology for HLA typing has evolved from the serological level to the cellular level, to the molecular level. Serotyping was the mainstream method for HLA type and has played a critical role in organ transplantations before 1990s. However, most HLA antisera are polyclonal and often have cross-reactions, making it difficult to distinguish antigens with subtle structural differences, and leading to misidentifications. Furthermore, many factors, such as a prolonged transportation time of the blood sample and excessive amount of immature cells, may affect the result of serotyping and cellular typing.

The development of polymerase chain reaction (PCR) and its application in biomedical sciences has made the HLA typing at the DNA level possible. Therefore, using molecular methods to type HLA at the DNA level has gradually replaced serotyping and cellular typing. Commonly used DNA based HLA typing methods include PCR based sequence specific primers (PCR-SSP), and PCR based restriction fragment length polymorphism (PCR-RFLP), single-strand conformation polymorphism (PCR-SSCP), sequence-specific oligonucleotide (PCR-SSO) and single nucleotide polymorphism (PCR-SNP).

In recent years, there have been emerged many advanced techniques applied into HLA typing, such as microarray, reference strand mediated conformation (RSCA), Pyrosequencing^{TM}, flow cytometry and DNA sequencing. In the early 1990s, new permissible mismatching strategies based on HLA epitope and/or similarity between donor-recipient pairs were also established and employed in clinical application.

4. Serological typing and cellular typing

4.1. Serological typing

4.1.1. Principle of microlymphocyto toxicity test technology

As early as 1956, Gorer et al. created a complement-dependent cytotoxicity assay for detecting alloantibodies in mice. In 1964, at the University of California, Los Angeles (UCLA), the Terasaki group introduced the microlymphocytotoxicity testing technique (microcytotoxicity assay) to human leukocyte antigen (HLA) typing studies after making several improvements and scaling down the procedures of HLA serological testing. Because the method was simple, reliable, and precise, yielding reproducible results, it was widely adopted for serological study of HLA and became an international standard technology recognized by the United States National Institute of Health (NIH). HLA cytotoxic antibodies are IgG and IgM isotypes. In the presence of complements, these antibodies are capable of binding with their corresponding antigens on the surface of lymphocytes and inducing holes on the membrane. There is no such effect if the lymphocytes do not carry the corresponding antigens. The principle for this reaction is shown in Figure 2. Dead lymphocytes with damaged membrane can be observed in a number of ways, the simplest of which staining with eosin or trypan blue. Dead cells are stained and appear expanded due to incorporation of the dye; live cells are not stained. Generally, the extent of the antigen-antibody reaction is determined on the basis of the percentage of dead cells. NIH criteria are shown in Table 1.

Subsequently, an improved one-step method was developed in which antibodies, lymphocytes, and complement are successively added and then stained and fixed. Results were observed under a microscope. An operational diagram is shown in Figure 3.

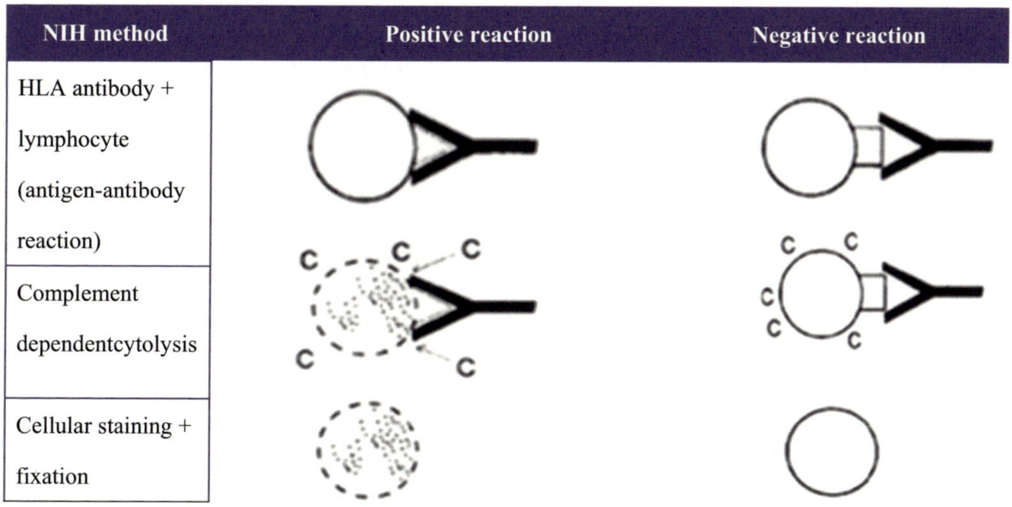

Figure 2. Microlymphocytotoxicity test principle diagram

Score	Mortality rate	Definition
1	0-10	Negative
2	11-20	Negative
4	21-50	Weak positive
6	51-80	positive
8	81-100	Strong positive
0		Not determinable

Table 1. NIH scoring criteria

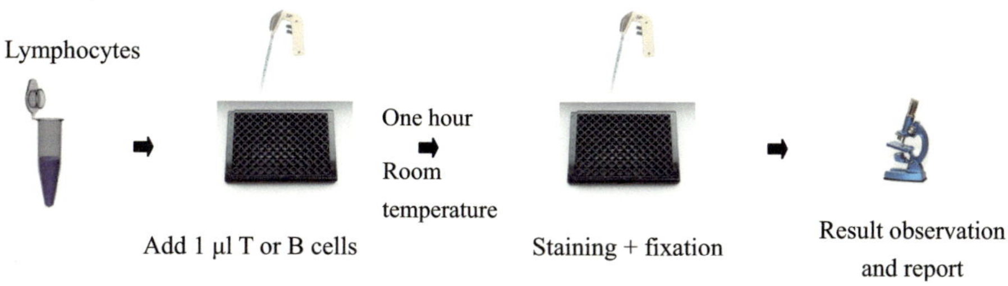

Figure 3. Schematic diagram of the one-step microlymphocytotoxicity test

4.1.2. Technique for HLA monoclonal antibody typing

Microlymphocytotoxicity tests have significantly promoted HLA research in basic and clinical applications since their introduction into serotyping. Some claim that serological typing techniques are the basis of HLA research because they are such important tools. In modern research, serological typing methods are still the main methods in HLA-I antigen typing. However, as advancing HLA research has placed increasing demands on typing techniques, shortcomings of serotyping methods have been identified, and these have been difficult to overcome. (1) The standard antiserum in serological methods is mainly from human serum or placenta. Because the rate of positive HLA antibody in sera is generally low, in particular, for some rare antibodies, it can only be obtained through collection and screening of a large number of serum samples. The technology for screening antisera is complex, difficult, and resource and labor intensive. (2) There are significant numbers of strong cross-reactions that can occur between serological tests; it is difficult to distinguish the sample antigen from the subtype antigen. (3) A high variability between serum batches significantly affects the quality of HLA typing reagents. (4) Serological match plates must be transported and preserved at low temperatures (−80°C), constraints that are inconvenient for clinical applications.

In order to solve such problems in serological typing, Terasaki et al. in the late 1980s began to develop HLA monoclonal antibodies to replace the standard antiserum. Formal production of HLA monoclonal antibody matching reagents plates began in 1992, and its availability has significantly improved the quality of HLA matching reagents. A comparison of the main technical indicators of monoclonal antibody match plates with serological match plate is shown in Table 2.

Main indexes	Serum plate	Monoclonal antibody plate
Identification of antigen determinants	specific and non-specific	specific
Specific	univalent and polyvalent	univalent
Titer	low (<1:8)	high (>20000)
Dosage	limited	almost unlimited
Anti-complement activity	may exist	non
Quality	stable	un-stable
Transportation	Dry ice low temperature	room temperature
Storage	-80°C	-20°C

Table 2. Comparison of key indicators of HLA monoclonal antibody typing plates with serological typing plates

4.2. Cellular typing

4.2.1. Homozygous typing cell

A homozygous typing cell (HTC) is homozygous for the A antigen, A/A. In the assay, HTCs are used as stimulator cells. Cells to be examined contain an unknown antigen, X/X, and are responding cells. In the reaction, a one way mixture lymphocyte culture (MLC) consists of

HTC (A/A) stimulator cells and the responder cells (X/X) being examined. An MLC reaction indicates that the responder cells could recognize the stimulator cells's A antigens, and that the responder cells being examined do not have A antigens. Absence of the MLC reaction indicates that the cells being examined have A antigens. The examined cells could be either A heterozygous (A/X) or A homozygous (A/A). In a repeated test, cells can be determined to have the same antigen only when the cells are examined with a negative HTC cell reaction. This procedure is also known as negative typing. This technique is rarely used because of the difficulty in identifying HTC individuals by this method.

4.2.2. Primed lymphocyte typing technique

In 1975 SheChy and others established a primed lymphocyte typing method (PLT) based on characteristics of a secondary response. It can specifically identify primed cells and it is also known as positive typing. In the initial MLC of responding cells A and stimulation cells B, after 9–12 days of culture, responding cells A proliferated into lymphoblastoid cells, after which they reverted to small lymphocytes. These inactive small lymphocytes were actually sensitized memory cells, also known as primed lymphocytes (PLs). When PLs and former stimulator cells were tested in a second MLC, there were very high responses within 20–24 hours. The stimulator cells are called primed cells (priming) in this process. According to this principle, experimental results of PLT depend on both priming and responding cells. Therefore, when conducting PLT, PL grouped cells must be carefully selected. More than one type of PL should be used in the identification of a PLT antigen. Preparation and sources of pretreatment cells are complex and difficult, so this method is rarely used.

4.2.3. Mixed lymphocyte culture

In 1964, Bain and Bach et al. found that lymphocytes from two unrelated individuals could stimulate each other in a mixed culture in a suitable in vitro environment. A lymphocyte could be activated and converted into a mother cell, resulting in the proliferation. After further research, other groups confirmed that mixed lymphocyte culture (MLC) is a good in vitro model for studying the cellular immune response, especially transplantation immunity. MLC technology was once widely used in organ transplantation and hematopoietic stem cell transplant matching. Because the technology is complex, has long testing cycles, involves radioactive elements, and has other drawbacks, it is gradually being replaced by the more convenient and higher-resolution genotyping methods. I will not go into the details of that method.

5. PCR based typing strategies

The technology for HLA typing has evolved from the serological level to the cellular level, to the molecular level. Serotyping was the mainstream method for HLA type and has played a critical role in organ transplantations before 1990s. However, most HLA antisera are polyclonal and often have cross-reactions, making it difficult to distinguish antigens with subtle structural differences, and leading to misidentifications. Furthermore, many factors, such as a prolonged transportation time of the blood sample and excessive amount of immature cells, may affect the result of serotyping and cellular typing. These are the limitations of traditional HLA typing methods. The development of polymerase chain reaction (PCR) and its application in biomedical sciences have made the HLA typing the DNA level possible. Therefore, using molecular methods to type HLA at the DNA level has been gradually replacing serotyping and cellular typing. Commonly used DNA based HLA typing methods include PCR with sequence specific primers (PCR-SSP), and PCR detection of restriction fragment length polymorphism (PCR-RFLP), single-strand conformation polymorphism (PCR-SSCP), sequence-specific oligonucleotide (PCR-SSO) and single nucleotide polymorphism (PCR-SNP).

5.1. PCR-SSP (PCR with sequence specific primers)

To identify point mutations in a DNA molecule, Newton invented the amplification refractory mutation system (ARMS) for in vitro DNA amplification. The technique requires an allele sequence specific 3′ primer for the PCR amplification. Otherwise the PCR reaction will not be effective. This is because the Taq DNA polymerase used in the PCR reaction has 5′ to 3′ polymerase activity and 5′ to 3′ exonuclease activity but 3′ to 5′ exonuclease activity. Therefore, the enzyme cannot repair the single mismatched nucleotide in the 3′ primer. In order to amplify the allele with a specific sequence, the primer with the corresponding sequence is designed. The conditions for PCR reaction are strictly controlled so that the amplification of the fragment with its sequence perfectly matching to the primer is much more effective than the sequence with one or more mismatched nucleotide. One mismatched nucleotide between the 3′ primer and the template is sufficient to prevent the amplification. The PCR product is further analyzed by electrophoresis to determine whether the amplicon corresponds to the anticipated primer-specific product. Since the DNA sequence of HLA class I and class II genes are known, PCR primers can be designed based on the specific sequence of each allele for PCR-SSP genotyping.

The encoding allele sequences of various HLA antigens can be amplified with sequence specific primers. By controlling the conditions of PCR reaction, a specific primer can only amplify its corresponding allele, not other alleles. Therefore, whether there is a PCR product can be used to determine the presence or absence of a specific allele. The specificity of PCR product can be further determined by agarose gel electrophoresis. Fig 4 shows the principle of PCR-SSP.

In the first step of PCR reaction, double-stranded DNA is denatured into single-stranded DNA. In the second step, specific primers anneal to the template DNA. In the third step, double stranded DNA is generated by TaqDNA polymerase by incorporating 4 types of dNTP into the newly synthesized DNA strand. After 30 cycles of amplification, the target gene is increased to 10^8 fold.

The main advantage of this method is that it is simple and fast, and the result is easy to interpret. The heterozygosity can be easily detected as well. Therefore, PCR-SSP is the currently most used method for HLA typing. There are several FDA approved high-resolution and low-resolution detection kits available for HLA class I and class II typing. Many clinical laboratories in China have been using this method for accurate pre-transplantation HLA typing. The

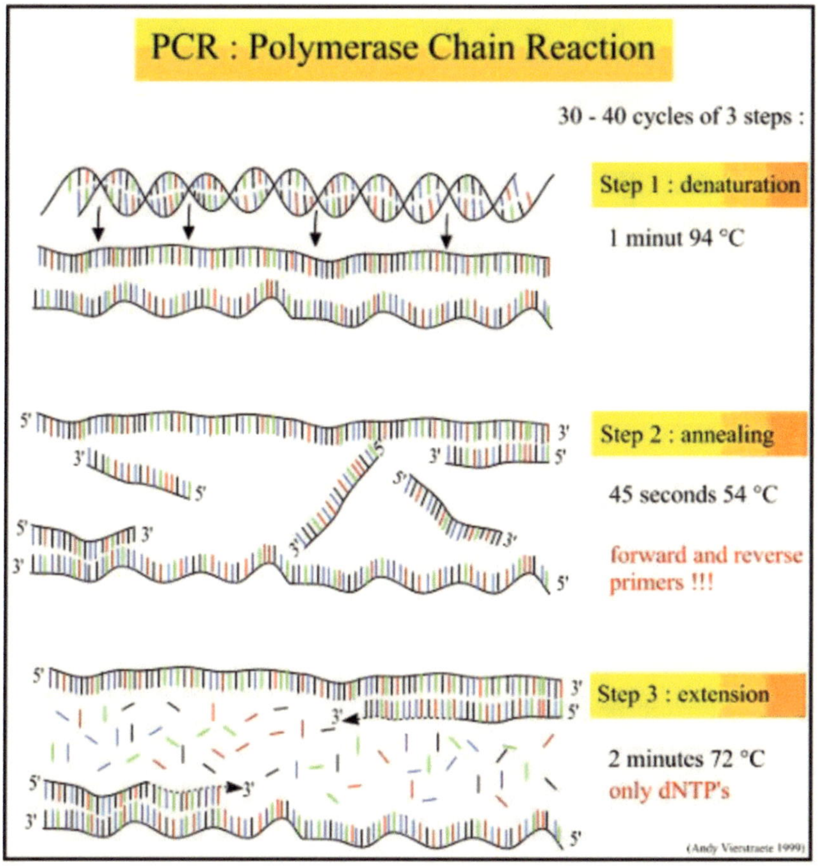

Figure 4. The diagram of PCR reaction

procedure of PCR-SSP is shown in Fig 5. One disadvantage of this method is that it requires multiple primers in order to amply all relevant alleles.

5.2. PCR-RFLP (restriction fragment length polymorphism)

Restriction endonucleases have unique recognition sites. Using computer software, restriction endonucleases that can recognize HLA sequence polymorphism are chosen to digest the PCR product. Because of sequence difference among the alleles, enzyme digestion will yield DNA fragments with unique patterns of length, which can be distinguished by electrophoresis.

Compared to serotyping, PCR-RFLP method is specific, simple and rapid and does not require probes. It can accurately detect single nucleotide difference and two linked polymorphic sites. The disadvantage of this method is that if the enzyme cannot completely digest the PCR product, the DNA fragments with similar lengths may be difficult to distinguish after electrophoresis. In addition, alleles need to have endonuclease recognition sites. Furthermore, PCR-RFLP cannot distinguish certain HLA heterozygosities. It requires multiple endonucleases for

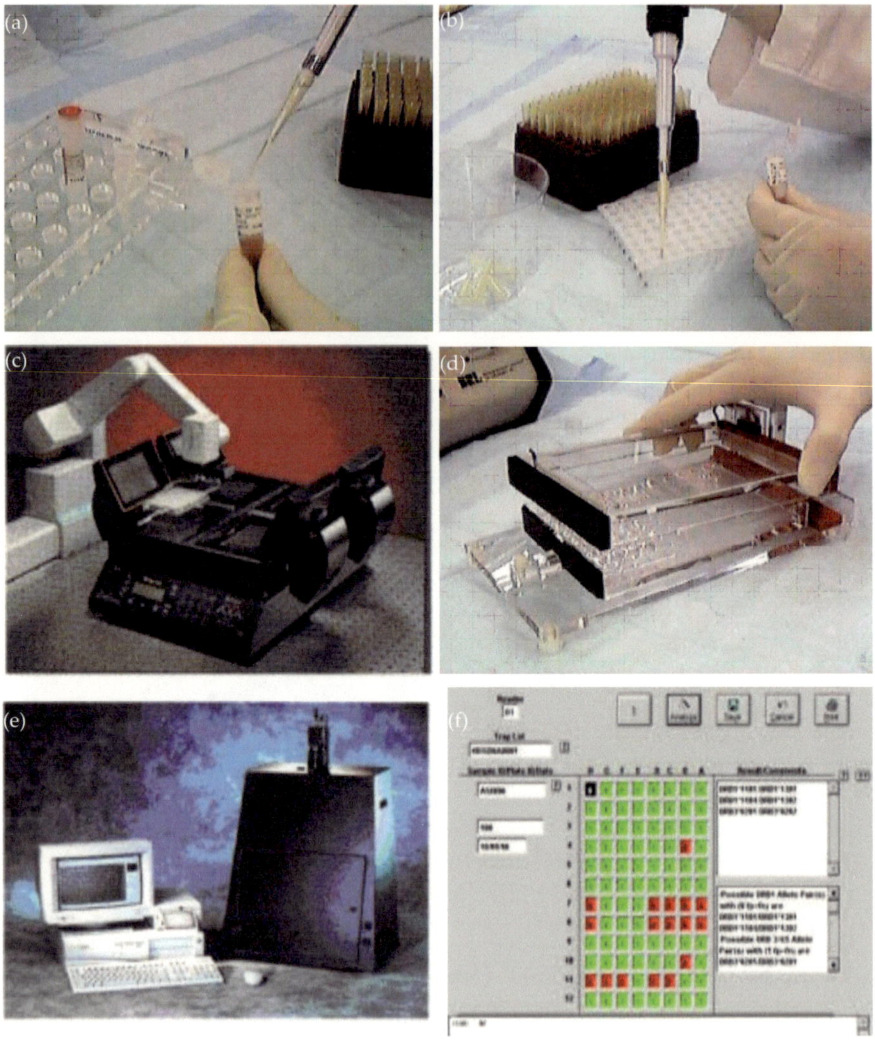

(a) DNA polymerase and DNA sample are added to the tube containing PCR reaction buffer and dNTP. (b) 10 μl of mixture of DNA and D-mix is added to the SSP kit. The negative control does not have this mixture. (c) PCR amplification, (d) electrophoresis (2-4 min) (e) Automatic gel imaging system, (f) Analysis of the result by software

Figure 5. The process of PCR-SSP

those alleles with high polymorphism such as HLA-DRB1, and may produce complicated restriction maps. For these reasons, this method is rarely used for HLA typing nowadays.

5.3. PCR-SSCP (single-strand conformation polymorphism)

Orita *et al* in Japan have found that single-stranded DNA fragment has complex spatial conformation. The three-dimensional structure is generated by the intramolecular interactions among the base pairs. Changing of one nucleotide will affect the spatial conformation of the

DNA strand, more or less. Single stranded DNA molecules have their unique size exclusion characters in polyacrylamide gels due to their molecular weights and three-dimensional structures. Therefore, they can be separated by non-denaturing polyacrylamide gel electrophoresis (PAGE). This method is sensitive enough to distinguish molecules with subtle structural differences, and is called single-stranded conformation polymorphism (SSCP). The authors later applied SSCP in the detection of mutations in PCR products and developed PCR-SSCP technique, which has further improved the sensitivity and simplicity for mutation detection.

This method is simple, rapid, sensitive, requiring no special equipment and suitable for clinical applications. However, this method can only detect mutations. The location and the type of the mutation need to be determined by sequencing. In addition, the conditions of electrophoresis need to be tightly controlled. Furthermore, point mutations in certain locations may have no effect or little effect on the DNA conformation. Therefore, different DNA molecules may not be able to separate by PAGE due to these reasons and other factors. Nevertheless, this method has a relatively high detection sensitivity compared with other methods. It can detect mutations in unknown locations in the DNA molecule. Takao has demonstrated that SSCP can detect 90% single nucleotide mutations in a DNA fragment smaller than 300bp. He believes that most of known single nucleotide mutations can be detected by this method. Mutant DNA molecules can be separated and purified by PAGE due to the different migration rates, and the mutation can be eventually identified by DNA sequencing.

In SSCP analysis, the separation of single stranded DNA by non-denaturing PAGE is not just based on their molecular weights and electric charges, but also on the retention force caused by their spatial conformations. Therefore, the migration rate of a DNA fragment does not reflect its molecular size. Since the wild type and mutant DNA molecules may migrate very closely and be difficult to be distinguished, it is generally required for DNA molecules to migrate for more than 16-18 cm in the gel. Mobility is calibrated using reference DNA as an internal control. Because of these reasons, this method cannot clearly determine the HLA genotype.

5.4. PCR-SSO (sequence specific oligonucleotide)

In PCR-SSO, specific probes are synthesized according to the sequence in the HLA polymorphic region. The target DNA fragment is amplified *in vitro* first. Then a specific probe will be hybridized to the PCR product under certain conditions based on base pair complementarity. The hybridized product can be detected by radioactive or non-radioactive signals. There are two types of SSO method, direct hybridization and reverse hybridization. In the direct hybridization, the PCR product is fixed on the membrane while in the reverse hybridization, the probe is fixed on membrane. Figure 6 is the diagram of PCR-SSO.

In 1986, Saiki *et al* were the first to report the analysis of DQA1 polymorphism using PCR and 4 ASO probes. Michelson has typed the DR loci by serotyping and PCR-SSO in 268 specimens. The success rate of serotyping is 91.0% while the success rate of PCR-SSO is 97.0%. Overall, PCR-SSO has a high success rate, a wide source of reagents, a high specificity and resolution. It can detect the difference of one nucleotide. In addition, PCR-SSO can be used for a large

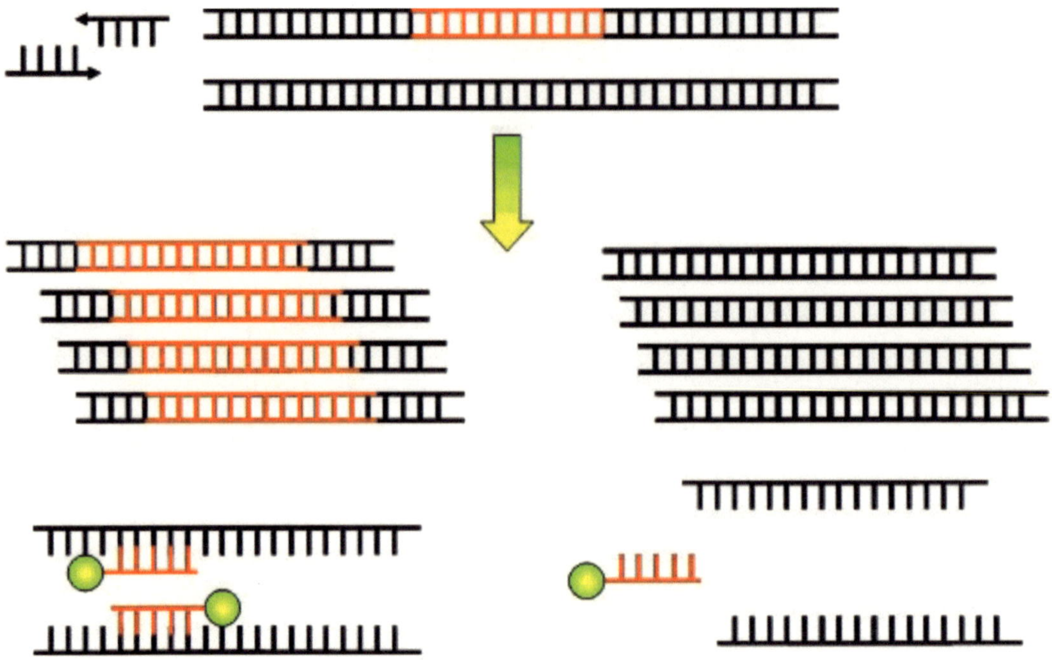

Figure 6. The diagram of PCR-SSO process

number of samples with accurate and reliable results. However, this method is time consuming. It often takes a few days and needs a large amount of probes. In addition, it is difficult to detect heterozygous alleles, particularly those of the complicated HLA-DRB1 genes.

Overall, PCR-SSO is an accurate HLA genotyping method, and can identify all known HLA alleles for accurate analysis of HLA polymorphism. HLA is a super gene family and new alleles are continuously been identified. SSO probes can only be designed based on the sequences of known alleles. Although PCR-SSO may discover new HLA polymorphism through its hybridization pattern, dot-hybridization often leads to false positives. In addition, when an allele is identified in the sample, it is difficult to determine whether the allele is homozygous or heterozygous. Therefore, the HLA allele frequency and haplotype frequency cannot be precisely determined by this method.

5.5. PCR-SNP (single nucleotide polymorphism)

Single nucleotide polymorphism (SNP) is the inheritable and stable biallelic single nucleotide difference. In the human genome, every 1000 base pairs have one to 10 SNPs. SNP may have some regulatory functions in gene expression and protein activity. High SNP density has been found in HLA class I genes with one SNP in every 400bp, setting the basis for high-throughput MHC-SNP analysis. Compared with other methods, SNP is less time consuming and with a low cost. Gou *et al* have developed a simple and effective oligonucleotide microarray to detect SNPs in the coding sequence of HLA-B locus. Based on the known polymorphism in the exon

2 and 3 of HLA-B genes, 137 specific probes were designed. In a double-blind experiment, these probes were used in the PCR-SNP analysis of 100 specimens from unrelated individuals. The result showed that this method could explicitly identify all SNPs in the HLA-B locus. Bu Ying *et al* have established a rapid, efficient and cost effective SNP detection method using a single tube.

In this method, 4 primers are used for the PCR amplification. Two primers are used to amplify the DNA fragment containing the SNP region, and the other two primers are SNP specific. The primer extension error is significantly reduced when 4 primers simultaneously carry out the PCR reaction, thereby the accuracy of SNP analysis is greatly improved. With the development of third-generation genetic markers, it is expected to find a series of single nucleotide polymorphisms in the HLA complex, and generate high-density SNP maps. In order to develop SNP technology into a simple and effective HLA typing method, production of high-density SNP maps in the HLA regions and development of HLA-SNP genotyping kits have been proposed in the 13th IHWC conference.

6. Reference-strand-mediated conformation analysis (RSCA)

Arguello *et al* invented the double-stranded conformation analysis (DSCA) technique in 1998 for the detection and analysis of gene mutations and complex polymorphic loci. Based on this technique, reference strand mediated conformation analysis (RSCA) has been developed. This is a major technical breakthrough in HLA typing. This technique combines sequencing and conformational analysis to overcome the limitations of the methods that just employ DNA sequencing or conformational analysis. The principle of RSCA is that fluorescent labeled reference strand is hybridized with the amplified product of a specific gene to form stable double stranded DNA with unique conformation. After non-denaturing polyacrylamide gel electrophoresis or capillary electrophoresis, HLA alleles can be detected by laser scanning and computer software based analysis. Figure 7 is the diagram of RSCA.

Compared with PCR-SSP, the most commonly used method of HLA genotyping, RSCA has the following advantages: (1) high resolution and sensitivity. RSCA is based on the differential migration rate of fluorescent-labeled double stranded DNA during the electrophoresis. Alleles with different sequences will produce DNA duplexes with different spatial structures after hybridization with their fluorescent labeled probes. Two alleles with one nucleotide difference will cause a change in the spatial structure of hybridized duplex, resulting in an altered migration rate in electrophoresis. Therefore, RSCA can distinguish the alleles with a single nucleotide difference. For example, HLA*0207 and A*0209 alleles only differ one nucleotide at the site 268 of exon 2 and 3. In this site, A*0207 has a G while A*0207 has an A. Likewise, HLA-A*0224 and A*0226 only differ one nucleotide. These alleles all can be distinguished by RSCA. (2) high reproducibility. In RSCA, each lane in the non-denature polyacrylamide gel has markers and each gel has a DNA ladder. Therefore, the alteration caused by different gels or lanes can be eliminated. (3) new allele or mutation identification. RSCA is based on the electrophoretic mobility difference caused by different spatial structure of the duplexes after

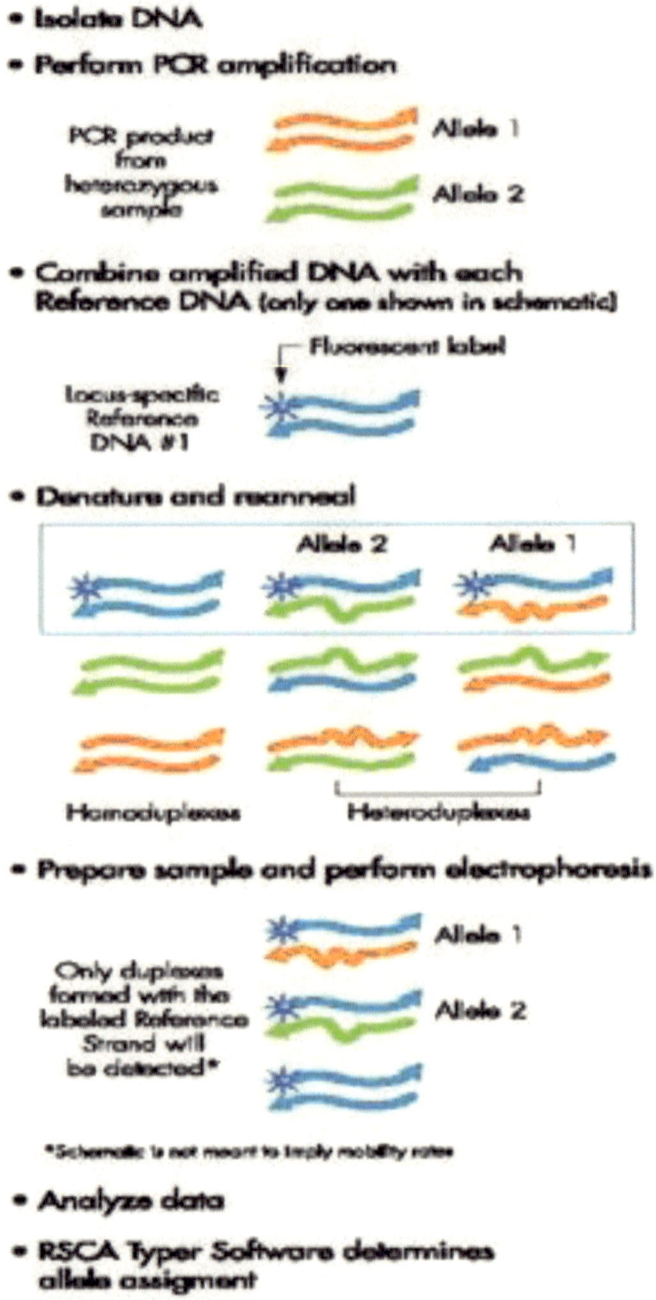

Figure 7. The diagram of RSCA

allele-FLR hybridization. New alleles or mutations will have electrophoretic mobility different from that of known alleles. (4) RSCA can be applied at a large scale with a low cost.

The disadvantages of RSCA are (1) time-consuming for a single sample; (2) requiring high quality samples; PCR-SSP requires 10-100ng/ml of DNA, which can be obtained with a regular DNA purification kit from patients even with a low amount of white blood cells. However, RSCA requires 50-100ng/ml of DNA. It may require an increased amount of blood sample for patients with low levels of white blood cell in order to obtain sufficient DNA; and (3) insufficient database.

7. Pyrosequencing™ — A high-resolution method for HLA typing

Pyrosequencing is a new HLA genotyping technology based on real time sequencing during DNA amplification. The reaction system contains 4 enzymes (DNA polymerase, ATP sulfurylase, luciferase and apyrase), substrate (APS: adenosine 5′ phosphosulfate), fluorescein (luciferin), primers and the single stranded DNA template. After one type of dNTP (dATP, dTTP, dCTP and dGTP) is added to the reaction system, it will be incorporated into the newly synthesized chain if it is complementary to the nucleotide on the template. Incorporation of dNTP will generate the same molar amount of pyrophosphate (PPi). ATP sulfurylase converts APS and PPi into ATP, which provides energy for luciferase to oxidate luciferin and emit light. The amount of light signal is proportional to the amount of ATP. The optical signal is detected by a CCD (charge couple device) camera and generates a peak in the pyrogram. The principle of Pyrosequencing is shown in Fig 8.

The height of each signal's peak is proportional to the number of incorporated nucleotide. Unincorporated dNTPs and excessive ATP are converted to dNDPs, which are further converted to dNMPs by apyrase. The optical signal is quenched and the system is regenerated for the next reaction. The next dNTP can be added to the system to start the next reaction after the unincorporated dNTPs and excessive ATP are removed. The reaction cycle continues until the complementary DNA strand is synthesized. Under the room temperature, it takes 3-4 seconds from polymerization to light detection. In this system, 1 pmol of DNA will generate 6×10^{11} pmol of ATP, which in turn yields 6×10^{9} pmol of photon with a wavelength of 560nm. The signal can be easily detected by a CCD camera. For the analysis of DNA with unknown sequence by Pyrosequencing, a cyclic nucleotide dispensation order (NDO) is used. dATP, dGTP, dTTP and dCTP are sequentially added to the reaction. After one nucleotide is incorporated, the other three will be degraded by the apyrase. For the DNA with known sequence, non-cyclic NDO can be used and will yield a predicted pyrogram. The sequence of the complementary DNA strand can be determined based on the NDO and peak value in the pyrogram.

Since nucleotides are differentially incorporated, Pyrosequencing can produce high-resolution results. Typing HLA-DRB1*04, 07 and DRB4* in the donor's DRB genes by Pyrosequencing not only yields the same result as using the SSOP typing kit, but also produces the result with a higher resolution. Compared with SSP, SSOP, direct or reverse hybridization, Pyrosequencing can be used to solve ambiguous allele combinations of HLA-DQ and HLA-A/B in a short time. The types of HLA-DQB1 and HLA-DRB alleles have been accurately determined by Pyrosequencing.

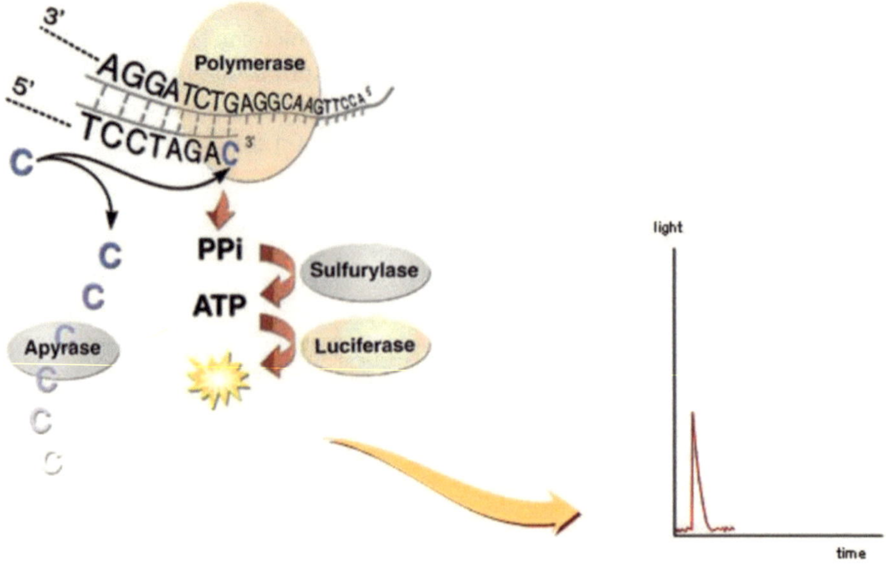

Figure 8. The principle of Pyrosequencing

An inherent problem with this technology is the de novo sequencing of polymorphic region in heterozygous DNA, although polymorphism can be detected in most cases. When the nucleotide in the polymorphic region is altered, synchronized extension can be achieved by the addition of the substituted nucleotides. If there is a deletion or insertion in the polymorphic region, and the deleted or inserted nucleotide is the same as the adjacent nucleotide on the template, the sequence after the polymorphic region will be synchronized. However, if the deleted or inserted nucleotide is different from the adjacent nucleotide on the template, the sequence reaction can be out of phase, making the subsequent sequence analysis difficult. Another issue with this technology is the difficulty in determining the number of incorporated nucleotides at the homopolymeric region. The light signal will become nonlinear after the incorporation of more than 5-6 identical nucleotides. Studies on the polymerization efficiency of the homopolymeric region have shown that it is possible to incorporate less than 10 identical nucleotides in the presence of apyrase. However, it needs specific software algorithm of signal integration to determine the precise number of incorporated nucleotides. For re-sequencing, the nucleotide is added twice to ensure complete polymerization in the homopolymeric region. Another limitation of this technology is the length of the sequencing.

8. Application of flow cytometry in HLA typing

Flow cytometry has failed to become a main method for HLA typing since it was applied to the field of immunology for the first time in 1977. This is mainly due to the large number of specific probes required for HLA typing. The flow analyzer LABScan100 that combines the flow cytometry and reverse SSO technology has a trend to replace three conventional methods, SSO, SSP and SBT (sequence-based typing, direct sequencing), in HLA typing.

On a suspension platform, multiple types of color-coded beads conjugated with SSO probes specifically bind to the single stranded DNA. Each type of bead has its unique spectral characteristics due to the different amount of fluorescent dye conjugated to the beads. When beads pass through a flow cytometer, the difference in the light scattering pattern from various angles can distinguish HLA genotypes.

Currently, LabType TM SSO is a relatively more mature technique compared with others in HLA typing. Its unique advantage is that thousands of molecules can be simultaneously analyzed in a matter of seconds. Therefore, this technique can be used for a large-scale analysis. Overall, this technique has following main advantages. (1) It has increased accuracy due to the automated detection system. (2) The workload and reagent consumption are reduced. One reaction tube can have 100 different SSO probes, thus greatly reducing the workload and reagent consumption. (3) It produces rapid and objective results. The ambiguous results can be avoided with Specialty Probe Technology TM (SP Technology). (4) Unlike regular flow cytometry that requires fresh samples, this technique can examine the sample at any time upon request or retrospectively. DNA samples can be analyzed right after extraction or stored at –20oC for more than 1 year without affecting the results. (5) The technique can analyze multiple HLA loci with low, medium and high resolutions. (6) It can be used in laboratories with large or small sample size. More than 100 probes can be put in one test tube for one sample or in a 96-well plate for 96 samples. The analysis of 96 samples takes less than 90 min after amplification. (7) The pollution to the environment and potential harm to the staff are reduced because electrophoresis is not required in this method.

9. Gene chip or DNA microarray

In gene chip or DNA microarray, large amount of probe molecules (usually $6x10^4$ molecules/cm^2) are attached to a solid surface. Labeled DNA samples are hybridized to the probes. The amount and sequence information of the target can be determined by the intensity of the hybridization signal. Gene chip or DNA microarray technology was first developed by Affymetrix in the USA, and has been improved significantly within a few years. The technology is based on the principle of reverse dot hybridization. Thousands of oligonucleotide probes representing different genes are spotted on a solid surface by a robot. These probes will bind to radioactive isotope or fluorescent dye labeled DNA or cDNA through complementary sequences. After autoradiography or fluorescence detection, signals are processed and analyzed by computer software. The intensity and distribution of hybridization signal reflect the expression level of the gene in the sample. The operation process of microarray is shown in Fig 9. Balazs *et al* spotted amplified DNA samples on silicon chips and compared the microarray results with PCR-SSO results in 768 specimens. It has been found that microarray has a high sensitivity and specificity. The consistent rate of genotyping results from microarray and PCR-SSO is 99.9%.

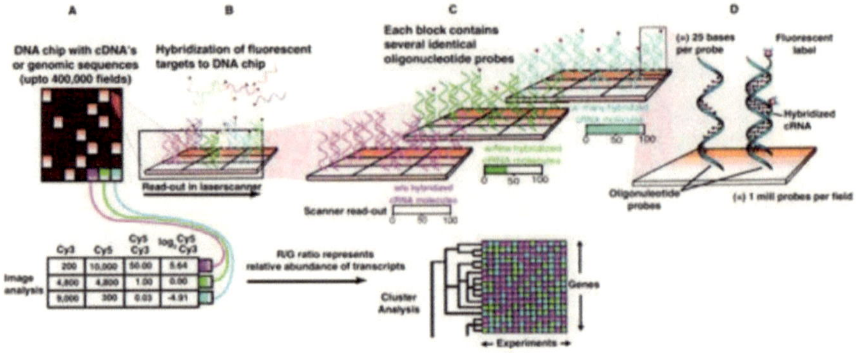

Figure 9. The procedure of gene chip/microarray analysis

Compared with existing genotyping methods, gene chip or microarray has the following advantages. (1) high intensity; The dot intensity on a chip can be higher than $6x10^4/cm^2$. Therefore, probes to thousands of HLA-A, B, C, DR, DQ and DP sequences can be spotted on a tiny chip of several square centimeters to obtain the information of individual HLA genes simultaneously. (2) high resolution; It can obtain information at the allele level. (3) simple operation; The results are generated by fluorescence scanning instead of gel electrophoresis, which greatly simplifies the procedure and shortens operation time. (4) high sensitivity; Signals are amplified twice with first PCR amplification of the template DNA and second amplification of fluorescence signal. Therefore, the sensitivity is greatly improved. (5) high accuracy; The intensity of the fluorescent signal generated by the perfect pairing of the probe and the sample is 5 to 35 times higher than the signal generated by the probe and the sample with one or two mismatched nucleotide. Accurate detection of fluorescent signal intensity is the basis of the detection specificity. Studies have shown that the consistency between microarray and Sanger sequencing in the detection of mutations and polymorphism is 99.9%. (6) high efficiency; The whole process is highly automatic, which saves manpower and time for data analysis. Genotyping of genes such as HLA-A, B, DR and DQ in multiple samples can be done with one PCR reaction and hybridization on one chip. (7) high level of standardization; Using a variety of multi-point synchronized hybridization and automated analysis, the human error is minimized to ensure the specificity and objectivity. (8) low cost. Since the chip fabrication and signal detection are all automatic, only small amount of probes and samples are required. One chip can be used for the analysis of samples from multiple individuals, which further reduces the cost. The biggest drawback of microarray analysis is its expensive equipment, which prevents it from becoming widely used. Only institutions with a large program can afford the equipment.

10. DNA sequencing technology

For the analysis of gene structure, sequencing is the most direct and accurate method. In this case, the DNA fragment is amplified by PCR and followed by sequencing. The basic process of this method is shown in Figure 10. Since the entire nucleotide sequence of the amplified fragment is obtained, this is the most reliable and through genotyping method. It can not only identify the sequence and genotype, but also lead to the discovery of new genotypes. Currently, the newly identified HLA alleles can only be verified by sequencing. It has been reported that if the HLA type cannot be determined by serotyping or the results from PCR-SSP and PCR-SSOP are inconsistent, sequence-based typing (SBT) often can yield accurate and reliable results with a high resolution. Hurley *et al* have typed HLA alleles by PCR-STB in 1775 bone marrow transplant patients and unrelated donors in NMDP, USA. The study has found that the degree of HLA allele mismatching between the recipient and donor of bone marrow transplantation is much higher than previously thought after examining the antigen matching results of HLA-A, HLA-B and HLA-DR.

The advantage of SBT over PCR-SSP and PCR-SSOP is its ability to analyze the entire gene sequence including the non-polymorphic region. SBT can be used not only for DNA sequencing but also for cDNA sequencing to determine gene expression. With increasing popularity of DNA sequencing technology, the PCR-SBT method has gained much attention for genotyping. PCR-SBT has advantages over other typing methods in terms of accuracy, efficiency and the degree of automation. Specialized software and solid phase sequencing kits with automatic loading are available for HLA typing. In addition, the cost of DNA sequencing has been greatly reduced. Therefore, PCR-SBT is an ideal method for HLA typing in researches. With the further decrease in the cost of automatic sequencing, this genotyping method will be widely used.

Currently, PCR-SBT is the gold standard of HLA typing. This method has several advantages. (1) It can accurately determine gene type in the exon 8 by a high-resolution sequencing, sufficient to meet the need in researches and clinics. (2) It can analyze more than 15,000 samples every month with high throughput detection. (3) Automated SOP and advanced data management system can reduce human error. (4) It has high quality assurance. Ten percent blind samples are used repeatedly as internal quality control and 100% accuracy is achieved for 10 consecutive times using UCLA external quality assurance samples. The results are confirmed by SSP. (5). It may lead to the discovery of new alleles. (6) HLA genotype can be updated by re-analyzing the sequence after the HLA database is updated.

11. HLA matchmaker

In organ transplantation, the degree of matching is generally determined by counting the number of mismatched HLA-A, B, DR antigens of the donor. It is well known that the zero-antigen mismatches have the highest success rates but why do so many mismatched transplants do so well? The answer to this question may be related to the fact that antibodies produced against HLA mismatches are significant risk factors for transplant failure. An important consideration is that HLA antigens have multiple epitopes that can be recognized by specific antibodies. The original description of the epitope repertoire was based on serological cross-reactivity between HLA antigens and antibody specificities against so-called

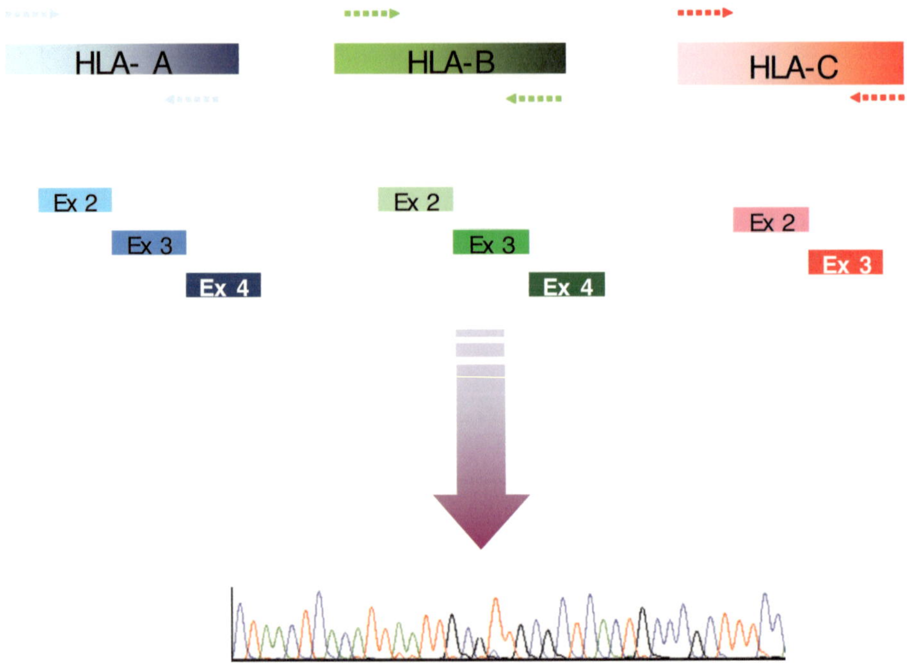

Figure 10. The diagram of DNA sequencing

private and public determinants. Elucidation of three-dimensional molecular structures and amino acid sequence differences between HLA antigens has made it possible to define the structural basis of HLA epitopes. The general concept is that HLA epitopes are determined by polymorphic amino acid residues on the molecular surface. Three-dimensional modeling of HLA antigens has revealed many clusters of polymorphic residues. In spite of this highly complex polymorphism it has become possible to determine HLA compatibility at the structural level.

HLA MATCHMAKER is a computer algorithm that assesses human leukocyte antigen (HLA) compatibility at a structural level by intralocus and interlocus comparisons of polymorphic amino acid sequences of HLA molecules. In its first version, each HLA antigen was seen as a chain of short, lineal sequences of polymorphic amino acids in an antibody-binding position (triplets); these triplets are considered the key elements of epitopes able to induce specific antibody production. The most recent version—Eplets HLA Matchmaker—introduces the concept of sequences of polymorphic amino acids in discontinuous positions that create on the surface of the HLA molecule conformational epitopes. The eplet version provides a broader repertoire of structural defined HLA epitopes and may provide a more accurate evaluation of the HLA compatibility.

HLA Matchmaker is based on the following principles. First, each HLA antigen is represented by different chains of epitopes structurally defined as potential immunogenic particles capable of inducing specific antibody production. Second, patients cannot produce antibodies against

http://dx.doi.org/10.5772/57500

epitopes present on their own HLA molecules. Initially, the program was developed to increase the chances of finding acceptable donors for hypersensitized patients. Subsequently, Duquesnoy et al demonstrated that it might also be useful in predicting the risk of graft loss according to the number of HLA-I mismatch triplets. This was proved in sensitized and nonsensitized patients.Háririan et al also showed that this triplet compatibility could give information about renal graft outcome in African-American patients. Nevertheless, Laux et al based on their own studies questioned the predictive role of triplet compatibility in graft survival. Other authors have also questioned the consistency of the epitopes in which this algorithm is based, pointing out that they might not be the unique epitopes inducing antibody formation. HLA Matchmaker has also been evaluated for clinical use in the selection of donors in pediatric renal desensitized receptors and HLA allosensitized thrombocytopenic patients. It has also been applied in unrelated bone marrow transplantation, lacking definitive proof of its benefit in patient survival.

12. HistoCheck

When there is no genotypically identical sibling and there are several alternative potential donors that all have a mismatch at an HLA class I or II locus, the allogenicity of mismatches may be estimated using the Sequence Similarity Matching concept described by our working group. In this concept the amino acid differences between HLA alleles are evaluated and rated with regard to position within the molecule (peptide binding, contact with the T-cell receptor) and with regard to functional similarity of amino acids within proteins. This procedure led to a dissimilarity score (allogenicity index) whereby high values represent high dissimilarity. When there are several mismatched donors, dissimilarity scores may be calculated for any of them, and the donor with the least may be preferred.

The importance of HLA-DPB1 matching for the outcome of allogeneic hematologic stem cell (HSC) transplantation is controversial. Previous findings identified HLA-DPB1 alleles as targets of cytoxic T cells mediating in vivo rejection of an HSC allograft. These HLA-DPB1 alleles encode T-Cell epitopes shared by a subset of HLA-DPB1 alleles that determine non-permissive mismatches for HSC transplantation. Retrospective evaluation of transplantations showed that the presence of non-permissive HLA-DPB1 mismatches was correlated with significantly increased hazards of acute grade II to IV graft-versus-host disease and transplantation-related mortality but not relapse as compared with the permissive group. Based on these findings, an algorithm for prediction of non-permissive HLA-DPB1 mismatches was developed (details in http://www.mh-hannover.de/institute/transfusion/histocheck/).

13. Conclusion

Currently, PCR-SSP genotyping is a commonly used method for HLA typing in clinical laboratories worldwide. Like SSP method, PCR-SSP method depends on specific primers for genotyping. Although the process is simple and rapid, high-resolution genotyping requires a large number of sequence specific primers, which leads to a high cost and prolonged operation time. Similarly, SSO technique is based on the sequence-specific oligonucleotide probes. High-resolution genotyping by SSO significantly increases the cost and complexity. Therefore, it is rarely used for HLA typing today. PCR-SNP is a simple and fast method with a high resolution. PCR-SNP is expected to become more popular in HLA typing as the technology continues to improve. Although RSCA and Pyrosequencing can achieve high-resolution results, their applications in HLA typing will be gradually eliminated as the technology of gene chip and sequencing continues to improve and the cost continues to decrease. HLA-chip genotyping is still largely dependent on the known sequence. It cannot identify new alleles with unknown sequence. At this moment, PCR-SBT technology has significant advantages over other HLA typing methods in terms of accuracy, efficiency and automation. There are specialized software and automatically loaded sequencing reagents for HLA typing by PCR-SBT. In addition, the operation cost has been greatly reduced. In conclusion, PCR-SBT technology with HLA-chip is the best method for HLA typing in research. With the reduction in the cost of automated nucleic acid sequencing, this genotyping method will be widely used in the field of basic research as well as in clinical transplantation.

Acknowledgements

Supported by grants from the State Key Development Program for Basic Research of China (No.2003CB515509 and 2009CB522401) and from National Natural Scientific Foundation of China(No.81070450 and 30470751) to Dr. X.-Y.Z.

Author details

Yuying Sun and Yongzhi Xi*

*Address all correspondence to: xiyz@yahoo.com

Department of Immunology and National Center for Biomedicine Analysis, Beijing Hospital Affiliated to Academy of Medical Sciences, Beijing, PRC

References

[1] Erlich HA, Opelz G, Hansen J: HLA DNA typing and transplantation. Immunity 2001, 14:347–356

[2] Methilinos J. HLA testing: the state of the art of genomic methods in 1996. Nephrol Dial Transplant 1996;11:2129-34.

[3] Opelz G, Methilinos J, Scherer S, et al. Survival of DNA-DR typed and matched cadaver kidney transplants. Lancet 1991;338:461-3.

[4] Otten HG, Tilanus MG, et al. Serology versus PCR-SSP in typing for HLA-DR and DQ: a practical evaluation. Tissue Antigens 1995;45:36-40.

[5] Bozon MV, Delgado JC, Selvakuman A, et al. Error rate for HLA-B antigen assignment by serology: implications for proficiency testing and utilization of DNA-based typing methods. Tissue Antigen 1997;50:387-94.

[6] Schrender GM, Hurley CK, March SG, et al. The HLA Dictionary: a summary of HLA-A, B, C DRB1 13, 14, 15, DQB1 alleles and their association with serologically defined HLA-A-B-C DR and DQ antigens. Tissue Antigens 1999;54:409-37.

[7] Opelz G, Wujciak T, Döhler B, Scherer S, Mytilineos J. HLA compatibility and organ transplant survival. Collaborative Transplant Study. Rev Immunogenet. 1999;1:334-42.

[8] Mahdi BM. A glow of HLA typing in organ transplantation. Clin Transl Med. 2013;2:6.

[9] Elsner HA, Blasczyk R. Sequence similarity matching: proposal of a structure-based rating system for bone marrow transplantation. Eur J Immunogenet 2002; 29: 229-236.

[10] Elsner HA, DeLuca D, Strub J,Blasczyk R. HistoCheck: rating of HLA class I and II mismatches by an internet-based software tool. Bone Marrow Transplant. 2004; 33: 165-169.

[11] Zino E, Frumento G, Marktel S, Sormani MP, Ficara F, Di Terlizzi S, Parodi AM, Sergeant R, Martinetti M, Bontadini A, Bonifazi F, Lisini D, Mazzi B, Rossini S, Servida P, Ciceri F, Bonini C, Lanino E, Bandini G, Locatelli F, Apperley J, Bacigalupo A, Ferrara GB, Bordignon C, Fleischhauer K. A T-cell epitope encoded by a subset of HLA-DPB1 alleles determines nonpermissive mismatches for hematologic stem cell transplantation. Blood. 2004 Feb 15; 103(4):1417-24.

[12] Crocchiolo R, Zino E, Vago L, Oneto R, Bruno B, Pollichieni S, Sacchi N, Sormani MP, Marcon J, Lamparelli T, Fanin R, Garbarino L, Miotti V, Bandini G, Bosi A, Ciceri F, Bacigalupo A, Fleischhauer K; Gruppo Italiano Trapianto di Midollo Osseo, Cellule Staminale Ematopoietiche (CSE) e Terapia Cellulare; Italian Bone Marrow Donor Registry. Nonpermissive HLA-DPB1 disparity is a significant independent risk factor for mortality after unrelated hematopoietic stem cell transplantation. Blood. 2009 Aug 13; 114(7):1437-44.

[13] Fleischhauer K, Locatelli F, Zecca M, Orofino MG, Giardini C, De Stefano P, Pession A, Iannone AM, Carcassi C, Zino E, La Nasa G. Graft rejection after unrelated donor hematopoietic stem cell transplantation for thalassemia is associated with nonper-

missive HLA-DPB1 disparity in host-versus-graft direction.Blood. 2006 Apr 1; 107(7): 2984-92.

[14] Zino E, Vago L, Di Terlizzi S, Mazzi B, Zito L, Sironi E, Rossini S, Bonini C, Ciceri F, Roncarolo MG, Bordignon C, Fleischhauer K. Frequency and targeted detection of HLA-DPB1 T cell epitope disparities relevant in unrelated hematopoietic stem cell transplantation. Biol Blood Marrow Transplant. 2007 Sep; 13(9):1031-40.

[15] Urlacher A, Dormoy A, Tongio MM. DP epitope mapping by using T-cell clones. Hum Immunol. 1992; 35:100-108.

[16] Cesbron A, Moreau P, Milpied N, Harousseau JL,Muller JY, Bignon JD. Crucial role of the third and fourth hypervariable regions of HLA-DPB1 allelic sequences in the mixed lymphocyte reaction. Hum Immunol. 1992; 33:202-207.

[17] Naruse TK, Nose Y, Kagiya M, et al. Cloned primed lymphocyte test cells recognize the fourth, fifth, and sixth hypervariable regions at amino acid positions 65-87 of the DPB1 molecule. Hum Immunol. 1995; 42:123-130.

[18] Brown JH, Jardetzky TS, Gorga JC, Stern LJ, Urban RG, Strominger JL, Wiley DC. Three-dimensional structure of the human class II histocompatibility antigen HLA-DR1. Nature 1993; 364: 33-9.

[19] Garboczi DN, Ghosh P, Utz U, Fan QR, Biddison WE, Wiley DC. Structure of the complex between human T-cell receptor, viral peptide and HLA-A2. Nature 1996; 384: 134-41.

[20] Hennecke J, Carfi A, Wiley DC. Structure of a covalently stabilized complex of a human alphabeta T-cell receptor, influenza HA peptide and MHC class II molecule, HLA-DR1. EMBO J 2000; 19: 5611-24.

[21] Risler JL, Delorme MO, Delacroix H, Henaut A. Amino acid substitutions in structurally related proteins. A pattern recognition approach. Determination of a new and efficient scoring matrix. J Mol Biol 1988; 204: 1019-29.

[22] Saper MA, Bjorkman, PJ, Wiley DC. Refined structure of the human histocompatibility antigen HLA-A2 at 2.6 Å resolution. J Mol Biol 1991; 219: 277-319.

[23] Sayle RA, Milner-White EJ. RASMOL: biomolecular graphics for all. Trends Biochem Sci. 1995; 20: 374.

[24] Stern LJ, Brown JH, Jardetzky TS, Gorga JC, Urban RG, Strominger JL, Wiley DC. Crystal structure of the human class II MHC protein HLA-DR1 complex with an influenza virus peptide. Nature 1994; 368: 215-21.

[25] Opelz G, Terasaki PI. International study of histocompatibility in renal transplantation. Transplantation. 1982, 33:87-95.

[26] Marsh SGE, Albert ED, Bodmer WF, et al. Nomenclature for factors of the HLA system, 2010. Tissue Antigens. 2010, 75:291-455.

[27] http://hla.alleles.org/

[28] Hansen JA, Petersdorf EW, Lin MT, Wang S, Chien JW, Storer B, Martin PJ. Genetics of allogeneic hematopoietic cell transplantation. Role of HLA matching, functional variation in immune response genes. Immunol Res. 2008, 41:56-78.

[29] Rubinstein P. HLA matching for bone marrow transplantation: How much is enough? N Engl J Med. 2001, 345: 1842-1844.

[30] Petersdorf EW, Hansen JA, Martin PJ, Woolfrey A, Malkki M, Gooley T, Storer B, Mickelson E, Smith A, Anasetti C. Major histocompatibility complex class I alleles and antigens in hematopoietic2cell transplantatio. N Engl J Med. 2001, 345:1794-1800.

[31] Petersdorf EW, Kollman C, Hurley CK, Dupont B, Nademanee A, Begovich AB, Weisdorf D, McGlave P. Effect of HLA class II gene disparity on clinical outcome in unrelated donor hematopoietic cell transplantation for chronic myeloid leukemia: the US national marrow donor program experience. Blood. 2001, 98:2922.

[32] McGlave PB, Shu XO, Wen W, Anasetti C, Nademanee A, Champlin R, Antin JH, Kernan NA, King R, Weisdorf DJ. Unrelated donor marrow transplantation for chronic myelogenous leukemia: 9 years' experience of the national marrow donor program. Blood. 2000, 95:2219-2225.

[33] Hadhoud A, Abdulaziz AM, Menawi LA, Shaheen FA, Abdulghaffar A, Abas FA, Al Mobrak MF. The relationship between HLA typing and HCV infection and outcome of renal transplantation in HCV positive patients. Exp Clin Transplant. 2003, 1:19-25.

[34] Erlich HA, Opelz G, Hansen J. HLA DNA typing and translation. Immunity, 2001, 14: 347- 356.

[35] Brown M, Wittwer C. Flow cytometry: principles and clinical application in hematology. Clin Chem. 2000, 46:1221-1229.

[36] Terasaki PI , Cho Y, Takemoto S et al. Twenty-year follow-up on the effect of HLA matching on kidney transplant survival and prediction of future twenty year survival. Transplant Proc. 1996, 28:1144-1145.

[37] Takemoto S, Terasaki PI. HLA compatibility can be predicted by matching only three residues with outward oriented sidechains.Transplant Proc. 1996, 28:1264-1266.

[38] Takemoto SK. HLA amino acid residue matching. Clin Transpl. 1996, 28:397-425.

[39] Takemoto SK, Terasaki PI, Gjertson DW,et al. Twelve years'experience with national sharing of HLA-matched cadaveric kidneys for transplantation. N Engl J Med. 2000,343: 1078-1084.

[40] Hata Y, Cecka JM, Takemoto S, et al. Effects of changes in the criteria for nationally shared kidney transplants for HLA-matched patients. Transplantation. 1998, 65: 208-212.

[41] Takemoto S, Cecka JM, Terasaki PI. Benefits of HLA-CREG matching for sensitized recipients as illustrated in kidney regraftes. Transplant Proc. 1997, 29:1417-1418.

[42] Orofino MG, Argiolu F, Sanna MA, Rosatelli MC, Tuveri T, Scalas MT, Badiali M, Cossu P, Puddu R, Lai ME, Cao A. Fetal HLA typing in beta thalassaemia: implications for haemopoietic stem-cell transplantation. Lancet. 2003, 362: 41-42.

[43] Karabon L, Polak M, Pacuszko T, Karabon L, Polak M, Pacuszko T. HLA typing for donor-recipient matching in unrelated donor hematopotetic stem cell transplantation.Transplant Proc. 2002, 34: 668-670.

[44] Torío A, Moya-Quiles MR, Muro M, Montes-Ares O, Ontañon J, Minguela A, Marin L, Alemany JM, Sánchez-Bueno F, Alvarez-López MR. Discrepancies in HLA-C typing in transplantation: comparison of PCR-SSP and serology results. Transplant Proc. 2002, 34: 419-420.

[45] Arrieta A, Maruri N, Rinon M, Riñón M, Fernández JR, Ortiz de Urbina J, García Masdevall MD. Confirmation of graft-versus-host disease by HLA typing after liver transplantation. Transplant Proc. 2002, 34: 278-279.

[46] Olerup O, Zetter H. HLA-DR typing by PCR amplification with sequence-specific primers (PCR-SSP) in 2 hours: an alternation to serological DR typing in clinical practice including donor-recipient matching in cadaveric transplantation. Tissue Antigens. 1992, 39: 225.

[47] Takemoto S, Terasaki PI. Refinement of permissible HLA mismatches. In: Terasaki PI, Cecka JM, eds. Clinical Transplants. Los Angeles: UCLA Tissue Typing Laboratory. 1994, 451.

[48] Stern LJ, Brown JH, Jardetzky TS, Gorga JC, Urban RG, Strominger JL, Wiley DC. Crystal structure of the human class II MHC protein HLA-DR1 complexed with an influenza virus peptide. Nature. 1994, 368:215-221.

[49] Smith PA, Brunmark A, Jackson MR, Potter TA. Peptide-independent recognition by alloreactive cytotoxic T lymphocytes (CTL). J Exp Med, 1997, 185: 1023-1033.

[50] Viret C, Wong FS, Janeway CA Jr. Designing and maintaining the mature TCR repertoire: the continuum of self-peptide: self-MHC complex recognition. Immunity. 1999, 10: 559.

[51] The MHC sequencing consortium: complete sequence and the gene map of a human major histocompatibility complex. Nature. 1999, 401:921.

[52] Jordan F, McWhinnie AJ, Turner S, Gavira N, Calvert AA, Cleaver SA, Holman RH, Goldman JM, Madrigal JA. Comparison of HLA-DRB1 typing by DNA-RFLP, PCR-SSO and PCR-SSP methods and their application in providing matched unrelated donors for bone marrow transplantation. Tissue Antigens. 1995, 45, 103-110.

[53] Zetterquist H, Bengtsson M, Backstrom G, Bäckström G, Egle-Jansson I, Ekdahl AM, Grunnet N, Gustafsson I, Knutsen I, Kuhle A, Rydberg L, Spurkland A, Steffensen R,

Storgärds M, Szojmer E, Söderholm G, Thuresson B, Turesson H, Olerup O. Report from the HLA class II typing by PCR-SSP Multicentre Study. Eur J Immunogenet. 1997, 24:191-199.

[54] Bryan CF, Harrell KM, Nelson PW, Pierce GE, Ross G, Shield CF 3rd, Warady BA, Aeder MI, Helling TS, Landreneau MD, Luger AM. HLA-DR and DQ typing by polymerase chain reaction using sequence-specific primer mixes reduces the incidence of phenotypic homozygosity (blanks) over serology. Transplantation. 1996, 62: 1819-1824.

[55] Suzuki Y, Orita M, Shiraishi M, Hayashi K, Sekiya T. Detection of ras gene mutations in human lung cancers by single-strand conformation polymorphism analysis of polymerase chain reaction products. Oncogene. 1990, 5:1037-1043.

[56] Hoshino S, Kimura A ,Fukuda Y, Dohi K, Sasazuki T. Polymerase chain reaction-single strand conformation polymorphism analysis of polymorphism in DPA1 and DPB1 genes :A simple ,economical and rapid method for histocompatibility testing. Hum Immunol. 1992, 33, 98-107.

[57] Pursall MC, Clay TM, Bidwell JL. Combined PCR-heteroduplex and PCR-SSCP analysis for matching of HLA-A, -B and -C allotypes in marrow transplantation. Eur J Immunogenet. 1996, 23: 41-53.

[58] Bradley BA, Bidwell JL. HLA-DQA1 and DQB1 genotyping by PCR-RFLP, heteroduplex and homoduplex analysis. Eur J Immunogenet, 1996. 23, 107-120.

[59] Saiki RK, Bugawan TL, Horn GT, ET AL. Analysis of enzymatically amplified beta-globin and HLA-DQ alpha DNA with allele-specific oligonucleotide probes. Nature. 1986, 324:163-166.

[60] Mickelson E, Smith A, McKinney S, Anderson G, Hansen JA. A comparative study of HLA-DRB1 typing by standard serology and hybridization of non-radioactive sequence-specific oligonucleotide probes to PCR-amplified DNA. Tissue Antigens. 1993, 41:86-93.

[61] Guo Z, Gatterman MS, Hood L, Hansen JA, Petersdorf EW. Oligonucleotide arrays for high-throughput SNPs detection in the MHC class I genes: HLA-B as a model system. Genome Res. 2002, 12:447-457.

[62] Consolandi C, Frosini A, Pera C,et al. Polymorphism analysis within the HLA-A locus by universal oligonucleotide array.Hum Mutat. 2004, 24:428-434.

[63] Li AX, Seul M, Cicciarelli J, et al. Multiplexed analysis of polymorphisms in the HLA gene complex using bead array chips.Tissue Antigens. 2004,63:518-528.

[64] Arguello JR, Little AM, Pay AL, et al. Mutation detection and typing of polymorphic loci through double-strand conformation analysis. Nature Genetics. 1998, 18:192-194.

[65] Arguello JR, Little AM, Bohan E, et al. A high resolution HLA class I and class II matching method for bone marrow donor selection. Bone Marrow Transplantation. 1998, 22:527-534.

[66] Lenz TL, Eizaguirre C, Becker S, Reusch TB. RSCA genotyping of MHC for high-throughput evolutionary studies in the model organism three-spined stickleback Gasterosteus aculeatus. BMC Evol Biol. 2009, 9:57.

[67] Sun Y, Zhao D, Jin L, Liu N, Liang F, Kong F, Xi Y. Human leukocyte antigens A and B Loci genotyping by reference strand-mediated conformation analysis in hematopoietic stem cell transplantation donor selection. Int J Hematol. 2007, 86:77-83.

[68] Shibata H, Yasunami M, Obuchi N, Takahashi M, Kobayashi Y, Numano F, Kimura A. Direct determination of single nucleotide polymorphism haplotype of NFKBIL1 promoter polymorphism by DNA conformation analysis and its application to association study of chronic inflammatory diseases. Hum Immunol. 2006, 67:363-73

[69] Kennedy LJ, Quarmby S, Fretwell N, Martin AJ, Jones PG, Jones CA, Ollier WE. High-resolution characterization of the canine DLA-DRB1 locus using reference strand-mediated conformational analysis. J Hered. 2005, 96:836-842.

[70] Ronaghi M, Elahi E. Pyrosequencing for microbial typing. J Chromatogr B. 2002, 782:67-72.

[71] Díaz S, Echeverría MG, It V, Posik DM, Rogberg-Muñoz A, Pena NL, Peral-García P, Vega-Pla JL, Giovambattista G. Development of an ELA-DRA gene typing method based on pyrosequencing technology. Tissue Antigens. 2008,72:464-468.

[72] Lank SM, Golbach BA, Creager HM, Wiseman RW, Keskin DB, Reinherz EL, Brusic V, O'Connor DH. Ultra-high resolution HLA genotyping and allele discovery by highly multiplexed cDNA amplicon pyrosequencing. BMC Genomics. 2012, 13(1): 378.

[73] Lank SM, Wiseman RW, Dudley DM, O'Connor DH. A novel single cDNA amplicon pyrosequencing method for high-throughput, cost-effective sequence-based HLA class I genotyping. Hum Immunol. 2010, 71:1011-1017.

[74] Gabriel C, Danzer M, Hackl C, Kopal G, Hufnagl P, Hofer K, Polin H, Stabentheiner S, Pröll J. Rapid high-throughput human leukocyte antigen typing by massively parallel pyrosequencing for high-resolution allele identification. Hum Immunol. 2009, 70: 960-964.

[75] Lu Y, Boehm J, Nichol L, Trucco M, Ringquist S. Multiplex HLA-typing by pyrosequencing. Methods Mol Biol. 2009, 496:89-114.

[76] Ringquist S, Styche A, Rudert WA, Trucco M. Pyrosequencing-based strategies for improved allele typing of human leukocyte antigen loci. Methods Mol Biol. 2007, 373:115-134.

[77] Loginova MA, Paramonov IV, Trofimova NP. Experience in using the LABType SSO reagent kits in the practice of a HLA typing laboratory. Klin Lab Diagn. 2011, 4:45-47.

[78] Testi M, Iannelli S, Testa G, Troiano M, Capelli S, Fruet F, Federici G, Bontadini A, Andreani M. Evaluation of DRB1 high resolution typing by a new SSO-based Luminex method. Mol Biol Rep. 2012, 39:13-16.

[79] Feng C, Putonti C, Zhang M, Eggers R, Mitra R, Hogan M, Jayaraman K, Fofanov Y. Ultraspecific probes for high throughput HLA typing. BMC Genomics. 2009, 10:85.

[80] Lee KR, Park E, Moon SH, Kim JM, Kwon OJ, Kim MH, Sohn YH, Ko SY, Oh HB. Development and clinical evaluation of a microarray for HLA-A and -DRB1 genotyping. Tissue Antigens. 2008, 72:568-577.

[81] Consolandi C. High-throughput multiplex HLA-typing by ligase detection reaction (LDR) and universal array (UA) approach. Methods Mol Biol. 2009, 496:115-127.

[82] Consolandi C, Frosini A, Pera C, Ferrara GB, Bordoni R, Castiglioni B, Rizzi E, Mezzelani A, Bernardi LR, De Bellis G, Battaglia C. Polymorphism analysis within the HLA-A locus by universal oligonucleotide array. Hum Mutat. 2004, 24:428-434.

[83] Pröll J, Danzer M, Stabentheiner S, Niklas N, Hackl C, Hofer K, Atzmüller S, Hufnagl P, Gülly C, Hauser H, Krieger O, Gabriel C. Sequence capture and next generation resequencing of the MHC region highlights potential transplantation determinants in HLA identical haematopoietic stem cell transplantation. DNA Res. 2011, 18:201-210.

[84] Noreen HJ, Trachtenberg E, Williams TM, Baxter-Lowe LA, Begovich AB, Petersdorf E, Selvakumar A, Stastny P, Hegland J, Hartzman RJ, Carston M, Gandham S, Kollman C, Nelson G, Spellman S, Setterholm M. A high degree of HLA disparity arises from limited allelie diversity: analysis of 1775 unrelated bone marrow transplant donor-recipient pairs. Hum mmunol. 2007, 68: 30-40

Chapter 5

In Phase HLA Genotyping by Next Generation Sequencing — A Comparison Between Two Massively Parallel Sequencing Bench-Top Systems, the Roche GS Junior and Ion Torrent PGM

Jerzy K. Kulski, Shingo Suzuki, Yuki Ozaki,
Shigeki Mitsunaga, Hidetoshi Inoko and
Takashi Shiina

Additional information is available at the end of the chapter

http://dx.doi.org/10.5772/57556

1. Introduction

Human Leukocyte Antigen (HLA) is the major histocompatibility complex in humans and it is critically involved in the rejection of hematopoietic stem cell or organ transplants [1-3] and in the pathogenesis of numerous autoimmune diseases [4]. Rejection and autoimmunity is believed to occur because the HLA presents aberrant histocompatibility antigen or public epitopes that play a key role in self-nonself recognition via various mechanisms including molecular mimicry and antibody mediated rejection [5-9]. The HLA genomic region on chromosome 6p21 encodes more than 200 genes including nine classical HLA genes, HLA-A, -B, -C in the class I region and HLA–DPA1, -DPB1, -DQA1, -DQB1, -DRA, -DRB1 in the class II region, that are the most polymorphic in the human genome contributing to over 7000 alleles and numerous HLA haplotypes implicated in disease resistance or susceptibility [10]. There are also a variety of non-classical HLA genes, such as HLA-DO and HLA-DM [11], HLA-E, -F, -G, MICA and MICB, which have received less attention in clinical medical research than the classical HLA genes [12,13].

The determination of the classical HLA alleles by DNA typing techniques over the past thirty years has assisted with the efficient and rapid HLA matching in transplantation therapy [2,14,15], research into autoimmunity and HLA related diseases [4,10], population diversity studies [16-18] and in forensic and paternity testing [19]. HLA gene alleles are also a target for pharmacogenomics research into drug hypersensitivity [20], such as the association of HLA-B*57:01 with hypersensitivity to the antiviral agent abacavir [21] and the association of HLA-B*15:02 with anticonvulsants in Asian populations [20].

Many variations of the conventional PCR typing method have been used for HLA DNA typing, such as incorporating restriction fragment polymorphisms [22], single strand conformation polymorphism [23], sequence specific oligonucleotides (SSOs) [24], sequence specific primers (SSPs) [25] and sequence based typing (SBT), like the Sanger method [26]. The HLA DNA typing methods mainly applied today are PCR-SSO, such as the Luminex commercial methodology [27,28], and SBT by the Sanger method employing capillary sequencing of cloned chain-termination reactions [26,29]. However, the current, conventional DNA typing methods cannot readily distinguish between polymorphisms on the same chromosome (*cis*) or different chromosomes (*trans*), thereby creating ambiguities that are difficult, time-consuming and expensive to resolve. Because we cannot assign a single HLA allele to a particular chromosome when using these conventional methods in routine HLA-typing, we have to predict the most probable HLA allele assignment based on the information of allele frequency of a population or by computation using complex statistical likelihoods. Therefore, in most cases, the HLA gene haplotype that is the cluster of SNPs within a gene sequence inherited from a single parent is a statistical prediction rather than a proper empirical determination [30].

The next generation sequencing (NGS) technologies, which are also referred to as second-generation sequence technologies, are new sequencing developments [31-33] that have followed on from the first generation sequencing technologies of the Sanger-Coulson sequencing method using chain-termination dideoxynucleotide sequencing of single-stranded DNA [34] and chemical cleavage of double-stranded DNA using the Maxam-Gilbert method [35]. Recent advances in technology and cost effectiveness of NGS point the way for its implementation and wider use in HLA research and diagnostic settings with the generation of haplotype (in-phase) sequencing and a massive level of parallelism producing millions of sequencing reads for analysis [36-43]. There are a variety of commercial NGS platforms currently available for HLA gene amplicon resequencing, such as those from Roche-454 (454 GS-FLX-Titanium, GS Junior), Applied Biosystems-Agencourt (3730XL, SOLiD 3), Illumina-Solexa (Genome Analyzer GAII, MiSeq, HiSeq models), Life Technologies (Ion Torrent Proton with different high density sequencing Chips), HeliScope (Helicos) and PacBio RS II (PacBio); including three small benchtop sequencers, the Roche Genome Sequencer (GS) Junior, Ion Personal Genome Machine (PGM) sequencer and the Illumina MiSeq, that are much cheaper than their larger counterparts and that provide faster turnover rates, but a more limited data throughput [31,44-46].

Recently, the performances of the three commercially available benchtop sequencers were compared against each other directly by different investigators comparing the sequencing of bacterial genomes [45-47]. There were large differences obtained from the three platforms in cost, sequence capacity and in performance outcomes of genome depth, stability of coverage and read lengths and quality, due in part to their different sequencing methods. The Roche GS Junior was of intermediate price with the lowest sequencing capacity of >6 Mb per run and a run time of 8 h, but the highest cost per run because of expensive reagents. Its sequencing is dependent on using the pyrosequencing technique, measuring the fluorescent light emitted when fluorophore-labeled dNTPs are added to sample DNA templates during the polymerase reaction [31,32]. The MiSeq was the most expensive instrument with the highest throughput at 1.5-2 Gb and a run time of 27 h. The running cost was 60 times cheaper than the Roche GS Junior. The MiSeq uses reversible terminator chemistry for sequencing in a cyclic method that involves fluorophore-labeled nucleotide incorporation, fluorescence imaging and cleavage [31,48]. The Ion PGM was the cheapest instrument with a throughput of 100 Mb using the 316 Chip, and 1 Gb using the 318 Chip, and a run time of 2-3 h. The running cost was 8 to 50 times cheaper than the Roche GS Junior depending on which Chip was purchased. The Ion PGM uses semi-conductor technology and ion-sensitive transistors to sequence DNA using only DNA polymerase and natural nucleotides in a sequencing-by-synthesis approach, with each polymerisation event resulting in pH and voltage changes identified by electronic sensors [33]. Therefore, the Ion PGM is the only "non-light" sequencer currently available in the market place.

Most pre-sequencing workflows for the benchtop sequencers and the other machines require DNA template fragmentation and library preparation where the fragments are labeled in vitro with oligonucleotide tags and adapters using commercial kits such as NimbleGen, Sure Select and other systems in order to be captured by beads or probes in preparation for clonal amplification of single stranded DNA fragments [31]. The labeling of DNA libraries with barcode sample tags, such as the multiplex identifier (MID) for Roche/454 sequencing, allows the libraries to be pooled to maximize the sequence output as a multiplex amplicon sequencing step for each sequencing run [49,50]. After construction of the template libraries, the DNA fragments are clonally amplified by emulsion PCR [51,52] or by solid phase PCR using primers attached to a solid surface [53] in order to generate sufficient single stranded DNA molecules and detectable signal for generating sequencing data [31]. Apart from selecting a suitable sequencing machine, NGS also provides challenges in analyzing and interpreting complex HLA genomic data from the millions of sequencing reads generated from the next-generation sequencers, which are different to those generated from traditional sequencers, and other HLA DNA typing methods and platforms.

We have described a new HLA DNA typing method, called Super high-resolution Single molecule - Sequence Based Typing (SS-SBT), that employs NGS and the Roche GS Junior [54] and the Ion PGM [55] massively parallel sequencing bench-top platforms (Figure 1). The SS-SBT method allows sequencing of the entire HLA gene region (promoter/enhancer, 5'UT, exons, introns, 3'UT) to detect new alleles and null alleles and solves the problem of phase ambiguity by using bioinformatics and computing for accurate phase alignments, after long-range PCR and sequencing clonally amplified single DNA molecules [42, 56].

This chapter updates our progress with the SS-SBT method [42] and describes some of the tasks required to identify the polymorphisms and other variants generated by NGS for SNP haplotyping from different classical HLA loci of individuals such as tissue donors and recipients in a relatively simple and economical way.

1.1. Aims of chapter

Here we describe and examine our latest modifications to the SS-SBT method for six-classical class I and class II HLA loci (HLA-A, -B, -C, -DPB1, -DQB1 and -DRB1) at a super-high resolution (formerly known as the 8-digit level of resolution) and three non classical class II HLA loci HLA-DRB3, -DRB4 and –DRB5 at high resolution using single DNA molecules to solve the ambiguity problem by undertaking:

1. Specific amplification of the entire gene sequence.
2. Comparisons between two different NGS platforms, the Roche GS Junior and Ion PGM.
3. Comparisons between different DNA typing software for in phase sequence analysis and validation of the huge amounts of NGS data.
4. Comparison of workflow differences in the construction of single gene and multiplex gene sequencing template libraries for 11 HLA class I and class II loci.
5. Application of the SS-SBT method including PCR multiplexing for the construction of template libraries for more efficient sequencing runs.

2. Materials and methods

2.1. HLA allele nomenclature and definition of super-high resolution

HLA genotyped alleles can be assigned at different levels of detail according to a recommended, standardized nomenclature [57]. Designations begin with HLA- as the prefix for an HLA gene and the locus name, followed by a separator * and then one or more two-digit numbers separated by colons (field separators) that specify the allele. The first two digits specify a group of alleles (first order, field one or a low resolution level). The third and fourth digits specify a non- synonymous allele (second order, field two or an intermediate resolution level). Digits five and six denote any synonymous mutations within the coding frame of the gene (third order, field three or a high resolution level). The seventh and eighth digits distinguish mutations outside the coding region (fourth order, field four or a super high resolution level). A ninth digit usually specifies an expression level or other non-genomic data and it is designated by a letter such as A ('Aberrant' expression), C (present in the 'Cytoplasm' but not on the cell surface), L ('Low' cell surface expression), N ('Null' alleles), Q ('Questionable' expression) or S (expressed as a soluble 'Secreted' molecule but is not present on the cell surface). Thus, a completely described allele may be up to 9 digits long. An example of an eight-digit or a super high resolution of an HLA-A allele that includes sequence variation within the introns or 5'/3' extremities of the gene is HLA-A*01:01:01:01.

2.2. DNA samples

One hundred genomic DNA samples were obtained from Japanese subjects for this study on PCR amplification and NGS of HLA genes. We obtained written consent from each individual and ethical approval from Tokai University School of Medicine where the research was performed. The DNA samples were isolated from the peripheral white blood cells using the QIAamp DNA Blood Mini Kit (QIAGEN, Germany). The HLA class I and class II gene alleles for nine samples (TU1 to TU8 and TU10) had been previously assigned to the field 2 allelic level of resolution (formerly known as 4-digit typing) [57] by the Luminex method [27,58] and LABType SSO kits (One Lambda, CA).

2.3. DNA extraction

Genomic DNA samples were isolated from the peripheral white blood cells using the QIAamp DNA Blood Mini Kit (Qiagen). The purity of the genomic DNA for each sample was determined by measuring the absorbance at 260 and 280 nm, with the A260/A280 values being in the range of 1.5-1.9, and the concentration of the DNA was adjusted to 10-20 ng/μl using PicoGreen assay (Life Technologies, CA).

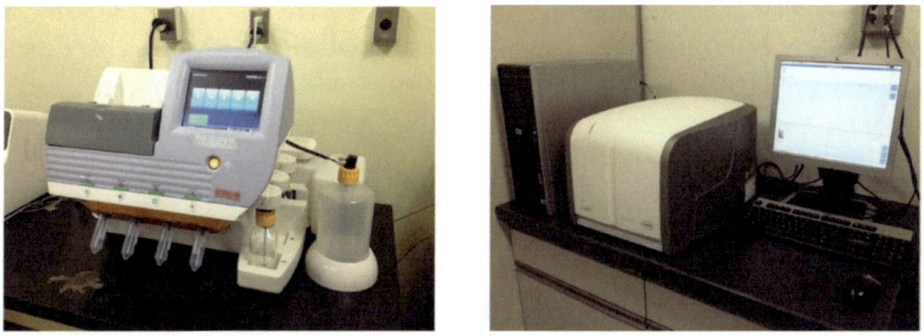

Ion Torrent PGM system **Roche 454 GS Junior**

Figure 1. The benchtop sequencers, Ion PGM from Ion Torrent and GS Junior from Roche/454

2.4. HLA DNA typing of genomic DNA samples by the Luminex method

The samples were typed at HLA-A, -B, -C, -DRB1, -DQB1 and -DPB1 using the Luminex method [27,28,58] and reagents supplied by the LABType SSO kits (One Lambda). An outline of the workflow for the Luminex method is shown in Figure 2.

2.5. HLA DNA typing of genomic DNA samples by SBT and the Sanger sequencing method

The DNA samples were typed at HLA-A, -B and -C (exons 2, 3 and 4) and -DRB1 (exon 2) using AlleleSEQR HLA-SBT Reagents (Abbott Laboratories, Abbott Park, IL). To confirm that the HLA alleles from both chromosomes were amplified with a 1:1 ratio and to validate newly discovered SNPs and indels, the nucleotide sequences of the PCR products were also directly sequenced by using the Sanger method and the ABI3130 genetic analyzer (Life Technologies, CA) in accordance with the protocol of the Big Dye terminator method (Life Technologies). The sequence-generated chromatogram data was analyzed by the Sequencher ver.4.10 DNA sequence assembly software (Gene Code Co., MI). Sequence data were also analyzed using the assign-atf software (Conexio Genomics, Australia, [59]). An outline of the workflow for the Sanger sequencing method is shown in Figure 2.

2.6. SS-SBT by NGS

We used two different benchtop NGS platforms (Figure 1); massively parallel pyrosequencing with the Roche GS Junior Bench Top system [54] and massively parallel semiconductor sequencing with the Ion Personal Genome Machine (PGM) system [55]. A general review of the NGS workflows used for the Roche 450 system is presented by Margulies et al. [51], Metzger [31] and Erlich [41] and for the Ions PGM/Torrents system by Rothberg et al. [33].

For SS-SBT, we used a five-step workflow for HLA DNA genotyping and haplotyping for both the Roche GS Junior Bench Top system and the Ions PGM (Figure 2). These steps were LR-PCR, amplicon library construction, template preparation by emulsion (em) PCR, NGS run and HLA DNA data analysis. The first and last steps were essentially the same for both platforms, whereas steps 2 to 4 were platform specific. Two different sequencing runs, a single gene-sequencing run (SGSR) or a multiplex gene sequencing run (MGSR) were performed for the different HLA gene loci. SGSR was performed for only a single gene locus per run, whereas MGSR was performed at the same time for all of the HLA gene loci, whereby all of the LR-PCR amplicons were pooled together to construct the template libraries required for the sequencing platforms.

2.6.1. Step 1: LR-PCR

Single LR-PCR

We developed and used LR-PCR primers for eleven HLA loci, A, B, C, DRB1, DRB3, DRB4, DRB5 (DRB3/4/5), DQA1, DQB1, DPA1 and DPB1 [42, 56]. For amplification of the HLA-DRB1, group-specific primers were employed to prevent concomitant amplification of DRB1-like genes, such as DRB3, DRB4, DRB5 and DRB pseudogenes including DRB2, DRB6, DRB8 and DRB9. Others have reported different LR-PCR primer sets for some of the same HLA genes [40,43].

Pooling the LR-PCR amplicons

Amplicons from all class I and class II loci for each individual were pooled in equal amounts to yield 2-3 μg per pool of a single sample.

2.6.2. Steps 2 to 4: Amplicon library construction, emPCR and NGS

Both NGS platforms require the preparation of a fragmented template library of the PCR products and further clonal amplification of the templates by emPCR for sequencing of singled stranded DNA and detection of base-called signals (Figure 2).

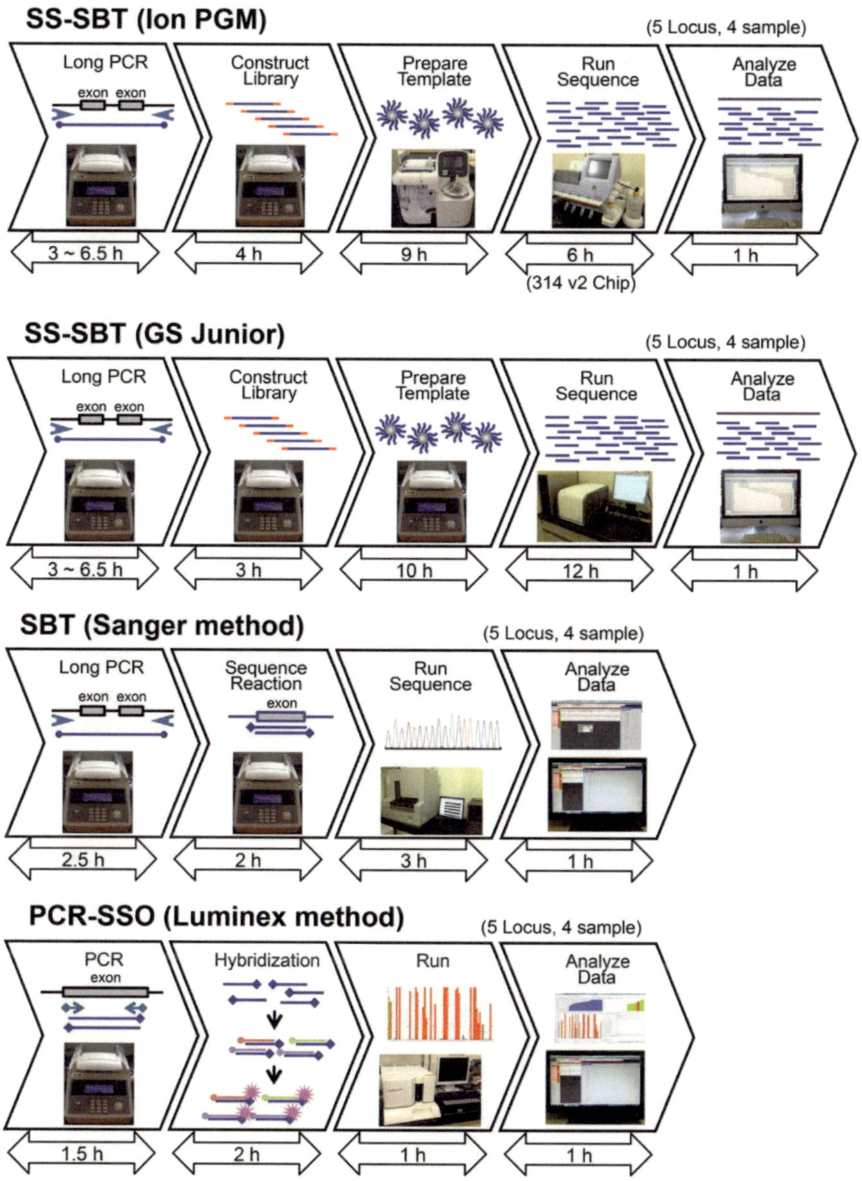

Figure 2. Workflow and time (hours) taken for each HLA genotyping step using the SS-SBT method by NGS with the Ion PGM or Roche GS Junior sequencers, by SBT using the Sanger sequencing method or by PCR-SSO using the Luminex method. The times are for typing five HLA loci using four DNA samples

2.6.2.1. Workflow for Roche GS Junior Bench Top system

Titanium libraries of single-stranded template DNA fragments were prepared for emPCR and sequencing using a GS FLX Titanium Rapid Library Preparation kit (cat no.

05608228001, 454 Life Sciences, Schweiz, CA) together with the GS Titanium Rapid Library MID Adaptors Kit (cat no. 05619211001, 454 Life Sciences) that permits the preparation of up to 12 individually MID labeled libraries per kit [60]. The workflow with the preparation kit involved fragmenting the LR-PCR amplicons by nebulization using disposable nebulisers, repairing fragment ends in a thermocycler reaction with T4 polymerase and Taq polymerase, adding adaptors such as the fusion A and B capture/sequence adapters and MID tags to the fragmented DNA by ligation with ligase and then linking the fragments of 100 bp or larger to the AMPure paramagnetic beads (Beckman Coulter Genomics, MA) with a selective binding buffer. Small fragments, primers and nucleotides were removed from the magnetic beads by washing them with 70% ethanol. Each single-strand DNA library was eluted from the beads with water or a Tris-acetate buffer, pH 8.

A MID adaptor was substituted for the adaptor provided in the GS FLX Titanium Rapid Library Preparation kit during the preparation of a library from a PCR DNA sample. The MID adaptor was ligated to each fragmented sequence of a library to provide a recognizable sequence tag at the beginning of each read. In this way, multiple libraries prepared with different MIDs can be sequenced together allowing the data analysis software to assign each read to the correct library and therefore a particular sample.

The libraries were quantified in 96-well format using the Fluoroskan Ascent CF Ver. 2.6 software (Thermo Fisher Scientific, DE) to detect the fluorescence in a PicoGreen assay (Life Technologies). The library size for each sample was measured by an Agilent 2100 Bioanalyzer using an Agilent High Sensitivity DNA Kit (Agilent Technologies, CA) and pooled with the other libraries at equimolar concentrations to create a multiplexed library.

The multiplexed libraries were clonally amplified by emPCR in order to produce hundreds of thousands or millions of copies of the same template sequence so that sufficient signal would be generated to be easily detected and recorded by the sequencing system. For preparation of emulsion beads, the single-stranded DNA fragmented libraries were added to the capture beads A and B, emulsified with oil and then amplified for at least 6 hours with an enzyme and reaction mix provided in the GS Junior Titanium emPCR Kit (Lib-L). An emulsion of PCR reagents in microreactors was prepared by adding beads A and B to the PCR reaction mix (1X amplification mix, Amplification Primers, 0.15U/ml Platinum Taq (Life Technologies), and emulsion oil and mixing vigorously using a Tissue Lyser (Qiagen, Germany).

The emulsion PCR of the library templates was carried out in an ABI 9700 (Life Technologies) thermocycler using the following cycling conditions: hotstart activation for 4 minutes at 94°C, 50 cycles of 94°C for 30 seconds, 58°C for 4.5 minutes, 68°C for 30 seconds. Sequencing primers were added to the mixture of beads and annealing buffer and annealed to the template using the following thermocycler conditions: 65°C for 5 minutes, and kept on ice for 2 minutes..

After emPCR, the emulsion was broken by isopropanol, the beads carrying the single-stranded DNA templates were enriched with primers A and B, counted, and 0.5 million beads deposited along with enzymes and buffer into a single loading port of a GS Junior Titanium PicoTiterPlate (PTP) (Cat. No 05 996 619 001, 454 Life Sciences, Carlsbad, CA) to obtain sequence reads by pyrosequencing using the Roche GS Junior system. Packing beads, sample beads and enzyme beads were applied to the PTP as per manufacturer instructions. The GS Junior Titanium PicoTiterPlate permits only a single sequencing run per PTP. During sequencing, nucleotides flowed across the PicoTiterPlate in a fixed order and a cooled CCD camera recorded the amount of light generated by the pyrosequencing reactions. The images from the CCD camera were then converted to sequence data by the instrument's software. Bi-directional sequencing for the fragments was achieved because the single strands captured by the A and B beads allow both forward and reverse reads to be identified.

After the DNA sequencing run by the Roche GS Junior Bench Top system, data analysis such as image processing, signal correction and base-calling, binning, trimming and mapping of the sequence reads and assignment of HLA alleles were carried out in accordance with our previous publication [42]. Image processing, signal correction and base-calling were performed by the GS Run Processor Ver. 2.5 (454 Life Sciences) with full processing for shotgun or filter analysis. Quality-filter sequence reads that were passed by the assembler software (single sff file) were binned on the basis of the MID labels into 10 separate sequence sff files using the sfffile software (454 Life Sciences). These files were further quality trimmed to remove poor sequence at the end of the reads with quality values (QVs) of less than 20.

2.6.2.2. *Workflow for Ion PGM system*

Barcoded-library DNAs were prepared from PCR amplicons with an Ion Xpress Plus Fragment Library Kit and Ion Xpress Barcode Adaptors 1-16 Kit according to the manufacture's protocol for 200 base-read sequencing (Life Technologies). One hundred nanograms of the HLA pooled amplicon products from four individuals were used for the preparation of each DNA library. Each DNA library was clonally amplified by eight cycles of PCR. The DNA size for each library was measured by an Agilent 2100 Expert Bioanalyzer using the Agilent High Sensitivity DNA Kit (Agilent Technologies) and the concentration of each library was measured with the Ion Library Quantitation Kit using the 7500 Real-Time PCR System (Life Technologies). Each barcoded-library was mixed at equimolar concentrations then diluted according to the manufacture's recommendation. emPCR was performed using the resulting multiplexed library with the Ion Xpress Template 200 Kit on an ABI 9700 (Life Technologies) with the following cycling parameters: primary denaturation 94°C/6 min, followed by 40 cycles for 94°C/30 s, 58°C/30 s and 72°C/90 s, and 10 cycles for 94°C/30 s and 68°C/6 min. After the emulsion was broken with 1-butanol, a magnetic-bead-based process according to the manufacture's recommendation enriched the beads carrying the single-stranded DNA templates. Sequencing was performed using the Ion Sequencing 200 Kit and Ion 316 chip with a flow number of 440 for 200 base-read [61].

Ion Torrent uses a pH change (release and detection of a proton) to detect the incorporation of a base into the growing DNA strand rather than a flash of light, as used in the 454 Sequencing System [33].

In the case of the Ion PGM DNA sequencing system, the raw data processing and base-calling, trimming and output of quality-filter reads that were binned on the basis of the Ion Xpress Barcodes into 10 separate sequence sff files were all performed by the Torrent Suite 1.5.1 (Life Technologies) with full processing for shotgun analysis. These files were further quality trimmed to remove poor sequence at the end of the reads with QVs of less than 10.

2.6.2.3. Sequencing parameters, variables and definitions

The NGS methodology generates a number of sequencing parameters, variables and errors that need to be defined and noted.

A sequencing read is a contiguous length of nucleotide bases that is generated using a sequencing machine. The full set of aligned reads (coverage) reveals the entire genomic sequence in the DNA sample selected for sequencing.

Both the NGS methods described here are designed to generate hundreds of thousands to millions of short (100 to 800 bp) contiguous reads of low to high quality. Intrinsic quality measures or filters are automatically built into the sequencing analysis software to recognize and measure or statistically predict quality values (QV or Q) and remove incorrect repetitive sequence, indels, low-quality sequence at the beginning and end of runs (end clipping) and recognize accurate consensus sequences [62,63].

Generally, the QVs or Q's are based on estimated Phred quality scores [64] so that a quality score of 10 represents a 1 in 10 probability of an incorrect base call or 90% base call accuracy, 20 represents a 1 in 100 probability of an incorrect base call or 99% base call accuracy, 30 represents a 1 in 1000 probability of an incorrect base call or 99.9% base call accuracy, 40 represents a 1 in 10000 probability of an incorrect base call or 99.99% base call accuracy, and so on.

QV scores are clearly valuable because they can reveal how much of the data from a given run is usable in a resequencing or assembly experiment. Sequencing data with lower quality scores can result in a significant portion of the reads being unusable, resulting in wasted time and expense. A QV of ≥ 20 is usually considered a satisfactory cut-off score for base calling accuracy. The QV and Q reads from the GS Junior and the Ion PGM are slightly different from each other and not directly comparable, with some studies showing the GS Junior overestimates the base-calling accuracy while the Ion PGM underestimates the base-call accuracy [45,65-67].

Read depth is the number of individual sequence reads that align to a particular nucleotide position [40]. The average read depth (coverage, redundancy or depth) is the number of average reads representing or covering a given nucleotide in the reconstructed sequence, often calculated as N x L/G where G is the original length of the genome sequence, N is the number of reads and L is the average read length. Thus, for a 1000 bp sequence G reconstructed from 10 reads N with and average length of 200 nucleotides per read L, there is a 2x coverage or redundancy. However, reads are not distributed evenly over an entire genome and many bases will be covered by fewer reads than the average coverage, while other bases will be covered by more reads than average [68].

Another important variable to consider, particularly for HLA typing with NGS is the allelic balance [40] or the ratio of the average depth [42], which is the relative number of reads originating from each of the two alleles of each locus. This variable is important to monitor in order to prevent allele drop-out. Allelic imbalance is usually not a sequencing problem, but most often is due to poor genomic PCR primer design where a set of primers favours the amplification of one haplotype over the other.

Sequence accuracy to estimate the quality of a sequencing run was estimated by including internal control DNA beads of known sequence with each run.

2.6.3. Step 5: DNA sequence data analysis and HLA assignments

The trimmed and MID or barcoded binned sequences were mapped as perfectly matched parameters using the GS Reference Mapper Ver. 2.5 (Life Technologies). Reference sequences used for mapping of the sequence reads were selected by nucleotide similarity searches with HLA allele sequences in the IMGT-HLA database using the BLAT program [69]. If a reference sequence covering the entire gene region was not available, we converted the sff files to ace files and constructed a new virtual sequence by *de novo* assembly using the sequencher Ver. 4.10 DNA sequence assembly software (Gene Code Co, Ann Arbor, MI), and used it as a reference sequence.

Three different automated NGS data processing systems, the Sequence Alignment Based Assigning Software (SEABASS) (an in house development of Tokai University, Isehara), Omixon Target (Omixon, [70]) and Assign MPS v1 (Conexio, [59]) were also assessed and compared for in phase sequence alignment of HLA genes and for allele assignment at the 8-digit level. The three programs were designed to provide software or a suite of software tools for analyzing targeted sequencing data from the next generation sequencing platforms, Roche 454, Ion Torrent and Illumina. The HLA edition of the Omixon Target can be obtained for use with MacOSX or Windows as a credit-based or annual based license fee. Conexio software for Windows can be purchased outright, whereas SEABASS is an in house development for Linux and is not available commercially at this time.

3. Results

3.1. HLA typing by Sanger SBT, the Luminex method or SS-SBT by NGS

Ten genomic samples (TU1-TU10) were genotyped at six HLA loci (HLA-A, -B, -C, -DRB1, -DQB1 and –DPB1) by three different typing methods, the Luminex, the Sanger SBT and the NGS SS-SBT method. At least one or more pairs of unresolved alleles were detected in the samples by the SBT and/or Luminex methods, whereas all the samples were easily resolved at least to the 4-digit level by the SS-SBT typing method (see the Tables and Supplementary Tables in the paper by Shiina et al [42]). Table 1 shows an example of the DNA typing results obtained for the HLA-C locus by the Luminex, SBT or SS-SBT methods as previously reported.

HLA-C typing by Luminex method				
DNA Sample ID	Allele 1	Allele 2	Number of ambiguities	
			Allele 1	Allele 2
TU1	C*01:02/07/11/+	C*03:03/11/12/+	18	17
TU2	C*01:02/07/11/+	C*03:04/06/09/+	18	23
TU3	C*03:03/04/06/+	C*07:02/10/13/+	40	29
TU4	C*03:03/04/06/+	C*14:03/10	41	2
TU5	C*03:02/04/05/+	C*07:02/10/13/+	40	29
TU6	C*03:03/04/06/+	C*14:03/10	41	2
TU7	C*01:02/07/11/+	C*07:02/32/38/+	17	25
TU8	C*08:03/06/14	**C*14:03**	3	0
TU9	C*08:01/08/20/+	C*15:02/03/10/+	7	5
TU10	C*07:02/10/19/+	C*15:02/03/07/+	27	7
HLA-C typing by SBT method				
	Allele 1	**Allele 2**	**Ambiguities (Allele 1 and Allele 2)**	
TU1	C*01:02/22/51	C*03:03/04/20/+	9	
TU2	C*01:02/22/31/+	C*03:04/28/64/+	8	
TU3	C*03:03/04/13/+	C*07:02/10/50/+	18	
TU4	C*03:03/04/20	C*14:03/10	4	
TU5	C*03:04/32/35/+	C*07:02/10/29/+	15	
TU6	C*03:03/04/20	C*14:03/10	4	
TU7	C*01:02/17/22	C*07:02/37/39/+	10	
TU8	**C*08:03:01**	**C*14:03**	0	
TU9	C*08:01/10/22	C*15:02/17	3	
TU10	C*07:02/19/39/+	C*15:02/03/07/+	8	
HLA-C typing by SS-SBT using Roche GS Junior				
	Allele 1	**Allele 2**	**Ambiguities**	
TU1	C*01:02:01	C*03:03:01	0	
TU2	C*01:02:01	C*03:04:01:02	0	
TU3	C*03:03:01	C*07:02:01:03	0	
TU4	C*03:03:01	C*14:03	0	
TU5	C*03:04:01:02	**C*07:02:01:(04)**	0	
TU6	C*03:03:01	C*14:03	0	
TU7	C*01:02:01	**C*07:02:01:(05)**	0	
TU8	C*08:03:01	C*14:03	0	
TU9	C*08:01:01	C*15:02:01	0	
TU10	C*07:02:01:01	C*15:02:01	0	

Table 1. Results of HLA DNA typing for the HLA-C locus by the Luminex, SBT or SS-SBT methods. The / is possible ambiguity, + is more than the possible ambiguities indicated by /, Parenthesis and bold letters indicate tentative allele names, not yet officially approved by the WHO Nomenclature Committee.

http://dx.doi.org/10.5772/57556

Figure 3 shows how the SS-SBT NGS typing method resolves the phase ambiguity at the HLA-DRB1 locus of a sample that the Luminex beads and other conventional typing methods were not able to resolve. Essentially, the Luminex bead method analyzed the mixture of the PCR products amplified from the paternal and maternal chromosomes and could not distinguish between HLA-DRB1*15:01/DRB1*04:05 on Sample "A" and HLA-DRB1*15:02/DRB1*04:10 on Sample "B", and therefore, resulting in ambiguity. On the other hand, in the SS-SBT method the sequenced PCR products were each amplified from a single DNA molecule (clonal amplification method by emulsion PCR), which helps to determine whether each polymorphism is paternal or maternal, thus resolving phase ambiguity. In the case shown in Figure 3, the sample was typed as DRB1*15:02/DRB1*04:10 on Sample "B".

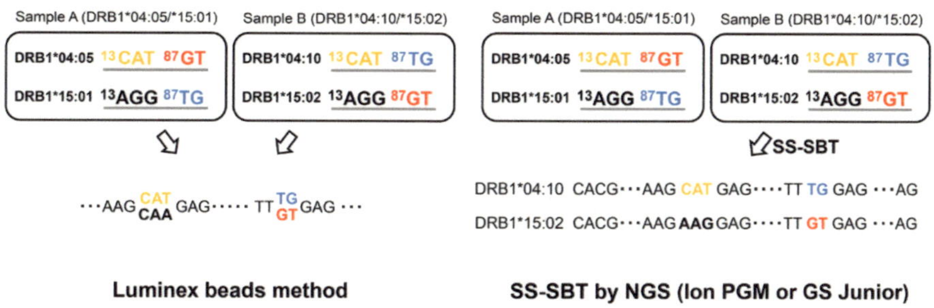

Figure 3. SS-SBT resolves phase ambiguity, which is an inherent problem of the Luminex beads method and other conventional methods

3.2. HLA typing by SS-SBT using two different NGS benchtop platforms

3.2.1. LR-PCR

3.2.1.1. Single LR-PCR

Long-range PCR (LR-PCR) was developed to amplify eleven HLA genes (HLA-A, -C, -B, -DRB1, -DQA1, -DQB1, -DPA1, -DPB1, -DRB3, -DRB4 and –DRB5) that are known to be highly polymorphic. PCR primers were designed to avoid annealing to any known polymorphic sites and to amplify regions spanning from the 5′ promoter to the 3′UTR region of the HLA genes in either a single amplification reaction or as two separately divided amplifications that could be easily merged when sequenced.

The PCR primer sets for the HLA-A, -B and -C genes were designed to amplify their sequences from the 5′-enhancer-promoter region to the 3′UTR with an amplicon size of about 5 kb. PCR primer sets were designed for HLA-DQA1, -DQB1, and -DPA1 to amplify sequences from the 5′- enhancer-promoter region to the 3′UTR with amplicon sizes of about 7 to 10 kb bases. Because the gene sizes for HLA-DRB1 and -DPB1 were too long to successfully amplify the whole gene in a single reaction, we divided the amplification of these genes into two parts. One PCR primer pair was designed to amplify the 5′-enhancer-promoter region to exon 2 and the other primer pair was designed to amplify exon 2 to the 3'UTR, resulting in amplicon sizes of about 6 to 11 kb and 5 to 7 kb, respectively (Figure 4). The DRB1 locus produced different amplicon sizes because of allelic differences in the length of its introns.

LR-PCR methods were also designed and tested to amplify HLA-DRB3, -DRB4 and -DRB5 (*DRB3/4/5)* from intron 1 to exon 6 (3'UTR) with the product size of 5.6 kb for *DRB3*, 5.1 kb for *DRB4* and 4.7 kb for *DRB5*. The *DRB3/4/5* specific primer sets successfully amplified the HLA-DRB3, -DRB4 and -DRB5 genes from 19 positive genomic DNA samples (TU1 to TU8, TU10 to TU17 and TU20 to TU22) with PCR products varying in size between 4.7 kb to 5.6 kb (Figure 4, [56]).

Although some LR-PCR methods are known to produce low frequency extra amplification of pseudogenes, as previously reported [43], our LR-PCR methods generally produced specific amplicons of targeted genes with little or no evidence of extra sequences (Figure 4). In addition, allelic imbalance for all the LR-PCR methods was minimal as judged by the sequencing results with allelic ratios ranging on average between 0.6 and 1.6 in heterozygous samples.

3.2.1.2. Pooling LR-PCR products for library construction

In order to expedite the number of samples and HLA loci required for NGS, the single LR-PCR products were pooled in equimolar amounts to produce a single multiplex (up to 13 PCR products) for the construction of a multiplexed, barcoded sample library. Figure 5 shows an example of an electrophoretogram of the pooled PCR amplicons from the HLA-A, -B, -C and -DRB1 genes.

3.2.2. Roche GS Junior NGS system

3.2.2.1. Library preparations using different gene loci and sample numbers

Initially, we applied an individual tagging per gene amplicon method for SGSR by preparing a tagged library for each of the ten individual samples with the aim of sequencing one HLA locus at a time [42]. Thus, ten libraries were constructed from each PCR amplicon of a particular HLA locus, with each library representing an HLA gene with ten tagged individual samples. The ten individual MID-labelled ssDNA libraries were then combined into a single tube for clonal emPCR and sequencing. In this way, we performed a single sequencing run for each HLA locus represented by ten MID labelled individuals, one locus at a time. For example, Run 1 was HLA-A with samples one to ten; Run 2 was HLA-B with samples one to ten, Run 3 was HLA-B with samples one to ten, and so on until we finished Run 13, our last run, Run 13, representing the 13th LR-PCR amplicon we had amplified from the 11 HLA gene loci that we had chosen to analyze.

Later, we changed from SGSR to an individual tagging and gene-pooling method for MGSR in order to markedly reduce the number of required sequencing runs. In this approach, we first pooled the PCR amplicons obtained from the eleven separate HLA genes (HLA-A, -B, -C, -DQA1, -DQB1, -DPA1, -DRB1 (part a and b), -DPB1 (part a and b), -DRB3, -DRB4

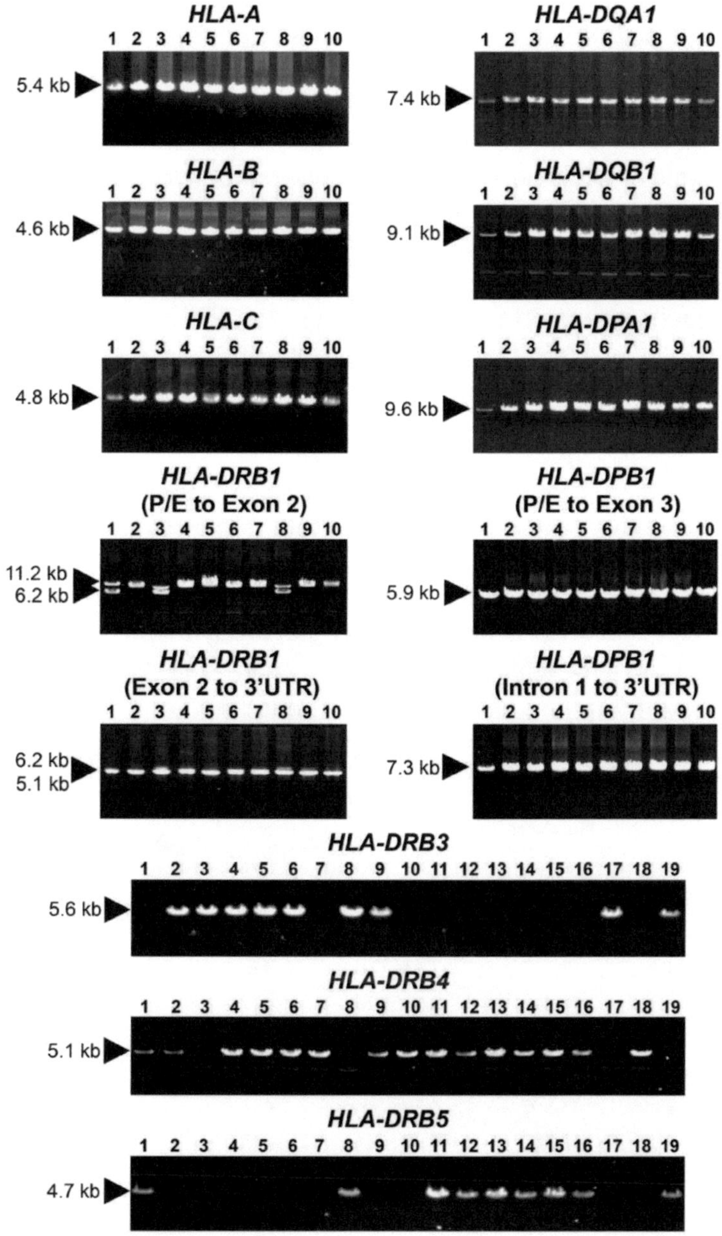

Figure 4. Agarose gel electrophoresis of LR-PCR products obtained from 10 to 19 unrelated genomic DNA samples using locus-specific primers for 11 HLA genes. The individual LR-PCR amplicons were used for SGSR or were combined into a single pooled mix for MGSR. Figure adapted from [42] and [56]

and -DRB5 of each individual at equimolar concentrations and then prepared the MID-labeled NGS libraries using the pooled amplicons from each individual. In this way, a single sequencing run was performed for all eleven HLA loci and for a multiple number of MID-labelled individuals or DNA samples. This was possible because the sequencing adapters specifically identified and grouped the gene loci, whereas the MID tags identified the individual samples. Figure 5 shows an electrophoretogram of pooled LR-PCR amplicons amplified from samples with known DR sub-types in parenthesis such that lane 1 is a heterozygous sample of DR6 and DR9, lane 2 is heterozygote of DR2 and DR6, lane 3 is a heterozygote of DR2 and DR4, lane 4 is a heterozygote of DR3 and DR8 and lane 5 is a heterozygote of DR1 and DR7. Consequently, the PCR product from the DRB1 gene varies in size depending on the DR sub-type and associated HLA-DRB1 allele so that it is 5.1 kb (orange) and 5.2 kb (blue) in lane 1, 5.2 kb (blue) and 5.6 kb (green) in lane 2, 5.6 kb (green) and 6.2 kb (purple) in lane 3, 5.2 kb (blue) in lane 4 and 5.1 kb (orange) and 5.2 kb (blue) in lane 5.

3.2.2.2. Sequencing multiplex libraries prepared for SGSR

Table 2 shows the number of draft sequences or reads (sequences passing a quality control criteria after base calling), generated by the Roche GS Junior Bench Top system for HLA-C in ten samples using multiplex libraries prepared for SGSR. The results for the sequence information about HLA-C were reported previously by Shiina et al [42] and Ozaki et al [56] as part of the data obtained in their NGS analysis of the eleven HLA loci.

DNA Sample ID	MID type	Draft Read Numbers	Draft Read Bases (bp)	Avg Read Length (bp)	Edited Reads (% of Draft Reads)	No. Mapping Bases (bp) post edit
TU1	MID1	7,873	3,213,949	408.2	5,075 (64.5%)	1,640,715
TU2	MID2	17,926	7,472,332	416.8	12,002 (67.0%)	4,003,792
TU3	MID3	8,211	3,326,703	405.2	5,553 (67.6%)	1,678,658
TU4	MID4	18,617	7,782,001	422.5	12,600 (67.7%)	4,223,267
TU5	MID5	12,432	5,185,865	417.1	8,318 (66.9%)	2,617,187
TU6	MID6	8,292	3,468,588	418.3	5,784 (69.8%)	1,982,456
TU7	MID7	10,900	4,503,252	413.1	7,042 (64.6%)	2,181,140
TU8	MID8	11,507	4,793,240	416.5	7,801 (67.8%)	2,554,949
TU9	MID9	12,082	4,995,156	413.4	8,101 (67.1%)	2,709,149
TU10	MID10	17,674	7,415,292	419.6	12,929 (73.2%)	3,968,608
Total		125,514	52,156,378	416.2	85,205 (67.9%)	27,559,921

Table 2. Sequence read information obtained by the Roche GS Junior for HLA-C.

Draft read numbers for eight genes, HLA-A, -C, -B, -DRB1, -DQA1, -DQB1, -DPA1 and -DPB1, were 1,015,526 sequence reads in total for 10 samples per locus with a range of reads between 49,048 in HLA-DQA1 and 153,610 sequence reads in exon 2 to 3'UTR of HLA-DRB1 [42]. These were high quality reads with QV ≥ 20 and an average QV of 30.4 ranging between 28.6 and 32.4. The draft read bases for eight genes, HLA-A, -C, -B, -DRB1, -DQA1, -DQB1, -DPA1, -

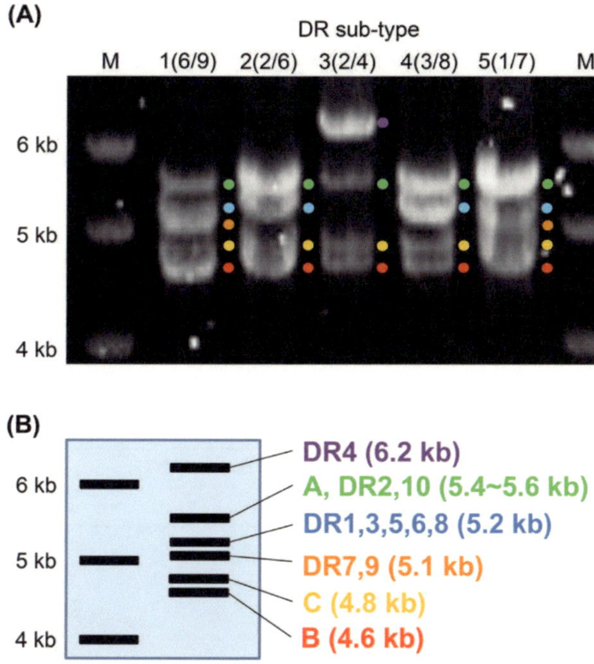

Figure 5. (A) Agarose gel electrophoresis of pooled LR-PCR amplicons of HLA-A (green), -B (red), -C (yellow) and -DRB1 (purple, green, blue and orange) used for MGRS. The lanes labeled M are bands of the 1 kb DNA size marker ladder. (B) Schematic of the expected PCR product band patterns and sizes seen in the PCR multiplex amplified from samples with different DR subtypes

DPB1, were 412,956,301 bp in total with a range between 18,077,833 bp in HLA-DQA1 and 65,384,530 bp in exon 2 to 3'UTR of HLA-DRB1 [42]. There was an overall average sequence length of 414.2 bp, ranging from 321.8 bp in intron 1 to 3'UTR of HLA-DPB1 to 441bp in HLA-DPA1. Of the draft reads, excluding error reads such as artificial insertion or deletion (indel) and nucleotide substitutions, 49.7%–75.4% matched perfectly with HLA allele sequences released from the IMGT-HLA database or our newly constructed virtual reference sequences. Therefore, the sequence reads had high quality and sufficient sequence volume for further HLA DNA genotyping and haplotyping analysis.

The HLA-DRB3, -DRB4 and -DRB5 (DRB3/4/5) gene loci were each sequenced separately by the Roche GS Junior Bench Top system using 19 samples and two separate multiplex libraries. After the sequencing run for each gene, a total of 147,269 sequence reads were provided for mapping and allele assignment of DRB3/4/5. The sequence reads were high quality reads (QV≥20) with an average QV of 30.9 ranging between 28.6 and 32.4. The draft read bases in total were 62.3 Mb in DRB3/4/5, with an overall average sequence length of 423.2 bp, ranging from 361 bp to 445.6 bp. This data suggested that the sequence reads had sufficient high quality and sequence volume for further HLA DNA genotyping and haplotyping analysis.

3.2.2.3. HLA SS-SBT DNA typing

HLA typing was applied to 10 genomic DNA samples (TU1-TU10) all of which gave more than one pair of unresolved alleles when defined by the SBT and/or Luminex methods (Table 1 and Table 3). In comparison, the pyrosequencing reads using Roche GS Junior system matched perfectly with the HLA allele sequences previously deposited in the IMGT-HLA database or against the virtual allele sequences constructed by *de novo* assembly as reference sequences. HLA allele sequences were determined at the 8-digit level in both phases in all samples of HLA-C (Table 1) and –DRB1 (Table 3) as well as HLA-A, -B, and -DQB1. Ambiguous alleles were resolved by in phase (haplotype) sequencing through the heterozygous positions thereby eliminating any doubt about possible alternative allele combinations (Figure 3). Cloning and Sanger sequencing validated the accuracy of the sequencing results by NGS (data not shown).

DNA sample ID	Sanger-SBT	
	Allele 1	**Allele 2**
TU1	DRB1*09:01/06	DRB1*15:01/02
TU2	DRB1*09:01/06	DRB1*14:05/44
TU3	DRB1*01:01/17/20	DRB1*14:05/44/100
TU4	DRB1*04:10/11	DRB1*14:01/32/54
TU5	DRB1*09:01:02	DRB1*13:02:01
TU6	DRB1*04:05/28/43/+	DRB1*13:02/36/65/+
TU7	DRB1*04:03/07/11/+	DRB1*08:03/10/29/+
TU8	DRB1*13:02/29/36	DRB1*16:02/05/10
TU9	DRB1*14:05:01	-
TU10	DRB1*09:01:02	DRB1*12:01/06/10/+
DNA sample ID	**PCR-SSOP**	
	Allele 1	**Allele 2**
TU1	DRB1*09:01/04/05	DRB1*15:01/13/16/+
TU2	DRB1*09:01/04/05/+	DRB1*14:05/23/43/+
TU3	DRB1*01:01/05/07/+	DRB1*14:05/23/45/+
TU4	DRB1*04:10	DRB1*14:01/26/54/+
TU5	DRB1*09:01/04/05	DRB1*13:02/96
TU6	DRB1*04:05/29/45/+	DRB1*13:02/73/96
TU7	DRB1*04:03/39/41/+	DRB1*08:03/23/27/+
TU8	DRB1*13:02/73/96	DRB1*16:02
TU9	DRB1*14:05/23/43/+	-
TU10	DRB1*09:01/04/05/+	DRB1*12:01/06/08/+
DNA sample ID	**SS-SBT**	
	Allele 1	**Allele 2**
TU1	DRB1*09:01:02:(01)	DRB1*15:01:01:01/02/03
TU2	DRB1*09:01:02:(02)	DRB1*14:05:01:(02)

TU3	DRB1*01:01:01	DRB1*14:05:01:(02)
TU4	DRB1*04:10:(03):(01)	DRB1*14:54:01:(02)
TU5	DRB1*09:01:02:(01)	DRB1*13:02:01:(02)
TU6	DRB1*04:05:01:(01)	DRB1*13:02:01:(02)
TU7	DRB1*04:03:01:(02)	DRB1*08:03:02:(02)
TU8	DRB1*13:02:01:(02)	DRB1*16:02:01:(02)
TU9	DRB1*14:05:01:(02)	-
TU10	DRB1*09:01:02:(01)	DRB1*12:01:01:(02)

Table 3. Results of HLA DNA typing for the HLA-DRB1 locus by the Sanger SBT, PCR-SSOP and NGS SS-SBT methods. The / is possible ambiguity, + is more than the possible ambiguities indicated by /, parenthesis and bold letters indicate tentative allele names, not yet officially approved by the WHO Nomenclature Committee. Blue background indicates HLA alleles with ambiguous allele.

An average sequencing depth was 387.9 in total, ranging between a depth of 53.5 in TU7 of HLA-DQB1 and 924.0 in TU4 of HLA-C. An example of the minimum and maximum depth and ratio of depth between two allele sequence reads for HLA-C in five DNA samples using the Roche GS Junior is shown in Table 4. The average depth ratio between haplotypes or alleles of HLA-A, -B, -C, -DRB1 (mix 2), -DQB1 ranged from 0.6 to 1.6, suggesting a satisfactory allelic balance was achieved with the PCR reactions. In comparison, the ratio of depth between two alleles in the HLA-DRB1 (mix 1) sequences was more variable exceeding a ratio delta of 1.0, which may be due to the marked difference in the sizes of PCR products among DRB1 groups (6-11 kb). However, this ratio of depth between two alleles did not affect sequence determination from the enhancer–promoter region to the exon 2 region of the DRB1 gene when the number of draft reads was increased.

			Depth			
Allele	**Sample ID**	**Read Num.**	**Min**	**Max**	**Ave**	**Ratio***
	TU1	4,766	87	628	339.9	0.9
	TU2	11,296	246	1,433	847.4	1.0
Allele 1	TU3	3,648	91	595	290.9	1.1
	TU4	12,232	245	1,446	924.0	1.1
	TU5	5,339	171	843	433.5	1.0
	TU1	4,876	106	634	371.1	0.9
	TU2	11,465	234	1,425	883.5	1.0
Allele 2	TU3	3,392	85	616	262.6	1.1
	TU4	12,103	230	1,447	870.6	1.1
	TU5	5,265	156	868	427.5	1.0

Table 4. Minimum and maximum depth and ratio of depth between two-allele sequence reads for HLA-C from five DNA samples using the Roche GS Junior. *Ratio is the average depth of allele 1/average depth of allele 2.

Overall, in this analysis, 21 HLA allele sequences were newly determined, 17 of them were newly identified alleles and four were alleles extended from 2-digit to 8-digit level sequences. Most of the newly identified SNPs and/or indels for 16 alleles were observed in the introns, whereas a synonymous SNP was identified in one allele of DRB1*04:10:(03):(01)) (parenthesis indicates tentative allele name, not yet officially approved by the WHO Nomenclature Committee). A comparison of the alleles detected for HLA-DRB1 by Sanger-SBT and SS-SBT in ten samples is shown in Table 3.

The HLA-DQA1, -DPA1 and -DPB1 alleles were assigned only at the 6-digit level of exon 2 with no novel alleles discovered in the 10 genomic DNA samples. This lower level assignment was likely due in part to low SNP densities preventing the haplotype genomic segments to be properly aligned and the phases separated from each other.

DRB3/4/5 sequences were identified to the field 4 level in both phases and validated by Sanger sequencing [56]. An average depth of DRB3/4/5 was 277 in total (107 in TU1 to 561.7 in TU11. The number of newly determined allele sequences at the field 4 level of resolution was two for DRB3 (DRB3*01:01:02:(02) and DRB3*02:02:01:(03)), three for DRB4 (DRB4*01:03:01:(04), DRB4*01:03:01:(05) and DRB4*01:03:01:(06)) and one for DRB5 (DRB5*01:01:01:(02)) (the allele names at field 4 are tentative as they have not yet been officially approved by the WHO Nomenclature Committee). Six allele sequences were extended from a field 2 or 3 level to a field 4 level with one for DRB3 (DRB3*03:01:01:(01)), one for DRB4 (DRB4*01:03:02:(01)) and two for DRB5 (DRB5*01:02:(01):(01) and DRB5*02:02:(01):(01)). Field 4 level haplotype structure of DRB1-DRB3/4/5 were also determined by SS-SBT and reported by [56].

3.2.2.4. Sequencing multiplex LR-PCR generated libraries prepared for MGSR

Using the libraries prepared from pooled LR-PCR for MGSRs (Figure 5), we sequenced 81 Japanese and Caucasian genomic samples by the Roche GS Junior instrument and assigned the aligned alleles across the entire gene regions of the eleven HLA gene loci without any ambiguities at least to the field 3 assignment level. Of the 164 alleles detected at the field 4 assignment level, 78 (47.6%) were newly detected alleles. We were unable to determine the allele sequences of HLA-DQA1, -DPA1 and -DPB1 at field 4 due to a lack of tag SNPs available to identify and separate the two phases within some of the noncoding regions. However, all the HLA exonic alleles were assigned without ambiguity at the field 3 level.

3.2.3. Sequence read information from the Ion PGM system

The amplicons amplified from eight HLA loci (A, B, C, DRB1, DQA1, DQB1, DPA1 and DPB1), representing a total of 60 kb of the entire gene regions (from the enhancer-promoter region to the 3'UT region), were prepared and pooled for the construction of barcoded DNA libraries from four DNA samples (TU1, TU3, TU5 and TU8) that had been previously sequenced by the Roche Junior system (Table 1). The four-barcoded samples were sequenced as a multiplex in a single run on an Ion 316™ chip. Figure 6 shows the workflow of the SS-SBT method performed by the Ion PGM™ sequencer that completed the processes from sample preparation to sequence analysis within three days. Previously, four days were needed for the manual sample preparation and library construction from the time of PCR amplification to HLA allele definition [42]. Now, with the use of automated procedures, such as the AB Library Builder™ system and Ion OneTouch™ system from Life Technologies, we have shortened the workflow significantly to just two to three days.

The number of reads, number of bases, and median read-length of each sample are shown in Table 5. A total of 522 Mb of sequence data was produced (about 600K to 720K reads per sample) with a range between 123.3 Mb for TU1 and 141.6 Mb for TU5, with an overall average read length of 197.3 bp. The median read length was about 214 bp, which was sufficient to resolve the phase ambiguity in all of the samples that were tested. Draft read numbers in total were 2,646,446 reads with a range of reads from 605,501 for TU1 to 721,499 reads for TU5 that were high quality reads with QV ≥ 10 at an average QV of 19.2 in the high quality reads.

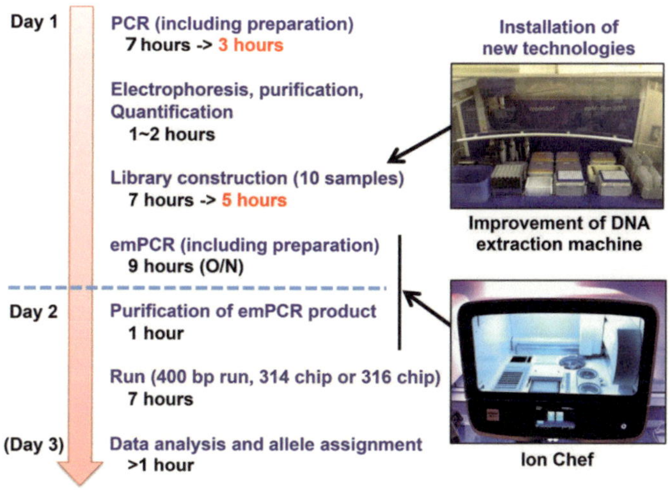

Figure 6. Improved workflow and time reduction to simplify the SS-SBT method using the Ion PGM

Sample ID	Number of Reads	Number of Bases (Mbp)	Median Read Length (bp)
TU01	605,501	123.3	220
TU03	644,314	127.2	214
TU05	721,499	141.6	214
TU08	675,132	130.2	214
Total	2,646,446	Total 522.2	Ave. 214

Table 5. Number of reads, number of bases, and median read length of each of four samples using the Ion PGM sequencer.

Alleles of HLA class I genes obtained from the typing method using Ion PGM™ are shown in Table 6. The 1,292,006 draft sequence reads (48.8% of the passed assembly reads) when compared with the reference sequences using the GS Reference Mapper (Ver. 2.5) matched consistently with the HLA alleles that were assigned by Roche GS Junior sequencing. The average depth between two-allele sequence reads spanned from 581 for *HLA-DRB1* in the TU1 sample to 2177 for *HLA-B* in the TU5 sample. The ratio between the average depth of allele 1 and average depth of allele 2 was 0.87 to 2.03. These typing results using the Ion PGM were consistent with the results obtained by Roche Junior system at an 8-digit level with no phase ambiguity. Also, for HLA class II genes, the Ion PGM typing results for HLA-DRB1, -DQA1, -DQB1, -DPA1 and -DPB1 by the SS-SBT methods was an exact match with the results obtained by Roche Junior system demonstrating that complete and correct HLA typing was carried out efficiently by both sequencing systems [42].

A comparison between the Ion PGM and the Roche GS Junior for the depth distribution obtained for HLA-B is shown in Figure 7.

The depth distribution of nucleotide calls across the HLA-B DNA sequence in different samples occurred with numerous peaks and valleys. For HLA-B the depth of nucleotide calls was lowest at a depth of 38 for allele 2 in sample TU01 where a string of polyG was sequenced in intron 7 by the Ion PGM sequencer. However, a depth of > 30 appears to be sufficient for accurate calls and a sequence run of more than 15 identical nucleotides seemed to be accurate enough both by the Roche Junior and Ion PGM sequencers in this study. Overall, the trend in the variation of depth distributions tended to be similar between the samples for both the Roche GS Junior and Ion PGM suggesting that read depth was probably more dependent on the gene sequence and grouping of nucleotides than other factors such as read length, fragmentation of PCR products for the library construction, fragment size selection, emPCR variability and efficiency of sequencing primer locations.

Locus	Sample ID	Allele 1		Allele 2	
		Allele name	Depth Ave.	Allele name	Depth Ave.
HLA-A	TU01	A*02:06:01:01	1281	A*11:01:01:01	1297
	TU03	A*24:02:01:01	1171	A*31:01:02:01	1194
	TU05	A*26:01:01:01	1922	A*31:01:02:01	1923
	TU08	A*24:02:01:01	1280	A*332:03:01:01	1267
HLA-B	TU01	B*40:02:01:01	1509	B*55:02:01(:02)*	1419
	TU03	B*02:06:01:01	1337	B*35:01:01:02	1330
	TU05	B*02:06:01:01	2167	B*35:01:01:02	2177
	TU08	B*02:06:01:01	1478	B*48:01:01:01	1428
HLA-C	TU01	C*02:06:01:01	1612	C*03:03:01:01	1576
	TU03	C*02:06:01:01	1328	C*07:02:01:03	1296
	TU05	C*02:06:01:01	1831	C*07:02:01:04	1808
	TU08	C*02:06:01:01	1661	C*14:03:01:01	1642

Table 6. Class I alleles for each sample identified by typing with Ion PGM.

3.3. HLA assignment software comparisons

We developed an in-house software system (SEABASS) for HLA sequence analysis, allele and in phase haplotyping and compared it to two commercial software systems, the Conexio Genomics genotyping software, Assign-MPS v1 [59], and the Omixon Target HLA Typing software program [70]. The user interface for the Assign-MPS v1 is shown in Figure 8 for (A) accurately genotyping the HLA-B*56:01:01(02) sequence and (B) not detecting DQB1*03:03:02 because of too many low quality sequence reads.

All three software systems imported and converted the.fna files (FASTA format sequence files for each read) generated by the GS Junior or the Ion PGM software into the appropriate files for HLA genotype assignments. All the software programs analysed the various sequence reads, sorted them according to genomic primer and MID tag or barcodes, compared the sequences to the IMGT/HLA sequence database and generated a consensus sequence with allele assignment taking into account the exonic and intronic sequence and phase relationship. The numbers of different reverse and forward reads for each amplicon were indicated, phased and automatically assigned a genotype only if the aligned sequences were perfectly matched with the alleles listed in the HLA sequence database (Figure 9). In cases where the aligned sequence reads were mismatched at one or more bases with the database, manual editing allowed for further investigation and assignment of a genotype.

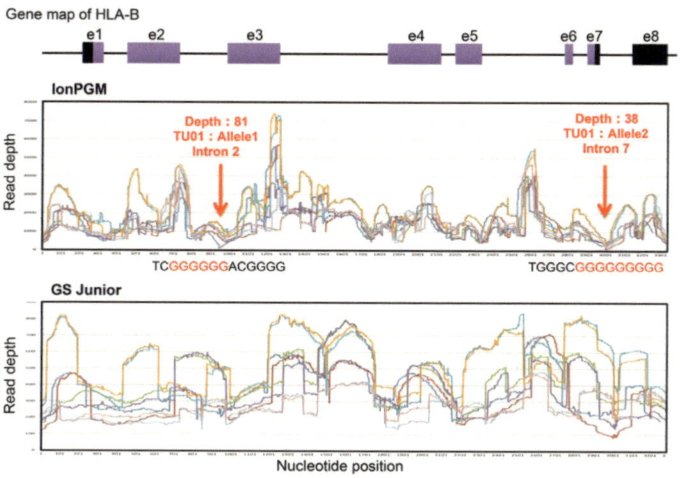

Figure 7. Distribution of depth of base calls for all samples at each nucleotide position of the HLA-B gene using Ion PGM and Roche GS Junior sequencers

A comparison of the three software systems for allele assignment in terms of platform, convenience, analysis speed, detection of new alleles, field 2 and field 4 level of typing assignment are shown in Table 7. All three software systems performed excellently for HLA typing at the field 2 level, but the SEABASS method was better than Assign and Omixon for HLA typing at the field 4 level. In addition, the SEABASS and Assign software could detect new alleles whereas the Omixon did not provide this possibility. However, Omixon was best for analysis speed and convenience of use. Overall, there was marginal difference in the efficiency, performance, analysis and outputs between the three output systems, although we favored our in house system over the commercially available Conexio Genomics software on a cost benefits basis.

	SEABASS	Omixon 1.6.0	Assign MPS
Platform	Linux	Mac/Windows	Windows
Convenience	*	***	*
Analysis speed	*	***	**
Detection of NEW allele	YES	NO	YES
Field 2 level typing	***	**	**
Field 4 level typing	***	*	*

Table 7. Comparison of allele assignment software systems

4. Discussion

Our NGS study focused on developing a suitable SS-BT method for in phase HLA genotyping for research and diagnostic laboratories using two of the commercially available low to medium throughput capacity NGS systems, the Roche GS Junior and the Ion PGM [42,56]. So far, in our best-case scenario, we were able to sequence 11 HLA loci for 5 individuals in a single sequencing run by Roche GS Junior or the Ion PGM. We have not used the full capacity of the Ion Torrents sequencing chip and, therefore, there is a potential to use a greater number of loci or individual samples (at least 57 samples) than we have already used for a single sequencing run. Moreover, both platforms provided high-resolution or super high resolution HLA typing without ambiguities, depending on the LR-PCR design to amplify the HLA gene loci.

High-throughput HLA genotyping methodologies were previously developed using massively parallel sequencing strategies, such as Roche/454 [36,37,40-42,56,71] and Illumina MiSeq sequencing [43,72]. Most of these high-throughput HLA-genotyping studies amplified a few individual exons (usually exons two, three and four) in an exon based strategy and sequenced in a multiplexed manner. LR-PCR was used by a few of the investigators to amplify large genomic regions of each gene including introns and all or most of the exons in a single PCR [40,42,43,56,72]. We also chose to combine LR-PCR with NGS because LR-PCR requires only one or two primer sets and eliminates the need to validate multiple sets of primers to amplify all alleles in the exon-based strategy. In addition, the error rates of the polymerase enzymes used in LR-PCR, because of error repair, are typically two- to six-fold lower than that of Taq polymerase that is used in conventional PCR [73]. We amplified and sequenced from the 5′ promoter to the 3′ UTR including exons 1-7 for HLA class I and class II genes in order to substantially improve the allele resolution for genotyping in comparison with the previous conventional genotyping methods, such as SSOP and SBT, with which allele calling of

http://dx.doi.org/10.5772/57556

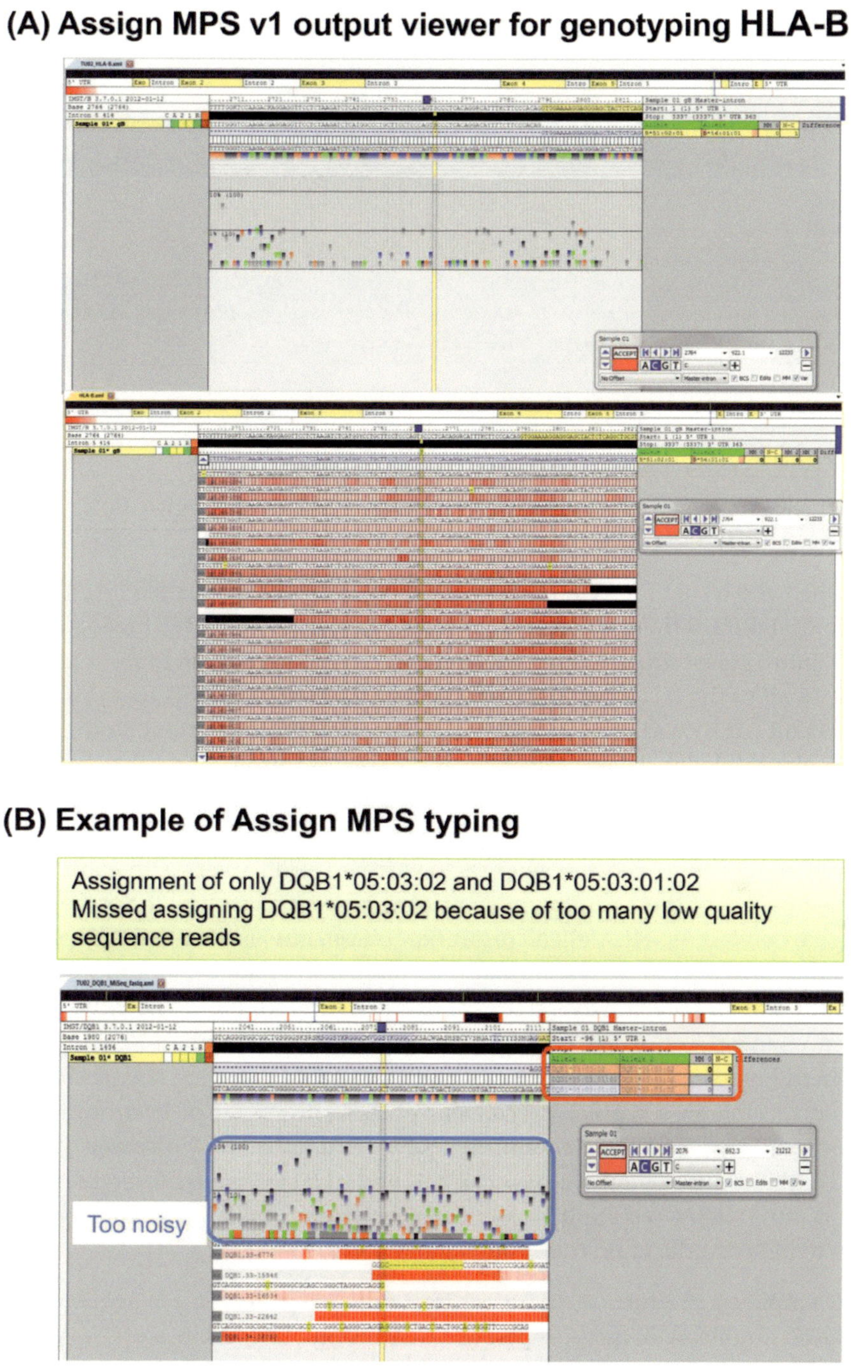

Figure 8. Assign-MPS v1 user interface (A) accurately genotyping the HLA-B*56:01:01(02) sequence, and (B) not detecting DQB1*03:03:02 because of too many low quality sequence reads

sequences was largely limited to exons 2 and 3 for HLA class I genes and exon 2 for HLA-DRB1.

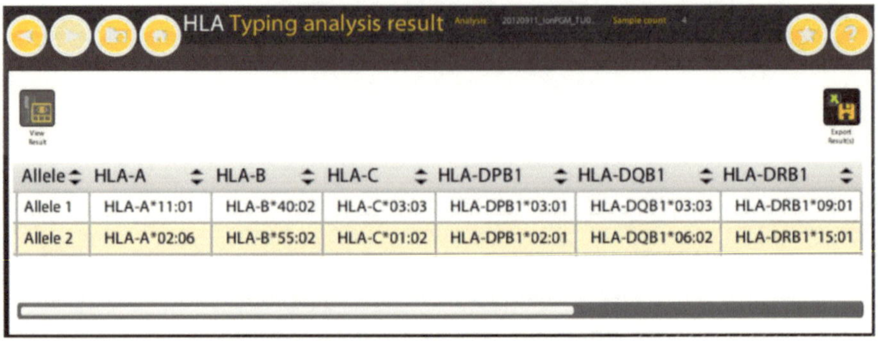

Figure 9. Omixon software system output viewer of HLA typing analysis results for HLA-A, -B, -C, -DPB1, -DQB1 and -DRB1 at the field 2 level of allele resolution

We developed and tested LR-PCR for the following 11 class I and class II HLA genes, HLA-A, -B. -C, -DRB1, -DRB3, -DRB4, -DRB5, -DQA1, -DQB1, -DPA1 and -DPB1 using 13 separate LR-PCRs. The entire gene sequence from the enhancer/promoter region to the 3'UTR-region was amplified for all of the HLA gene loci, except for HLA-DRB1, -DPB1 and -DRB3/4/5. PCR of HLA-DRB1 and -DPB1 was divided into two parts with enhancer/promoter to exon 2 and exon 2 to 3'UTR for HLA-DRB1, and enhancer/promoter to intron 2 and intron 1 to 3'UTR for DRB1*15:01:01:03 because of the large size of intron 1 (~ 8kb) and/or the complexity of nucleotide repeat (microsatellite) polymorphisms in intron 2 (Figure 7). The three DRB3/4/5 specific primer sets amplified the gene regions from intron 1 across to exon 6 and into the 3'UTR. The LR-PCR of these HLA genes revealed intronic as well as the exonic polymorphic sites, which extended the HLA allelic resolution phase, but also provided important phasing information to assist with the resolution of combination ambiguities and identifying previously unknown alleles outside the regions of exon 2 and 3. Although the IMGT/HLA database has sequences mostly of exons 2 and 3 [74,75], the promoter/enhancer, intron, and 3'UTR variants should not be ignored for more comprehensive HLA typing now and into the future. The genetic variants in a regulatory element such as promoter or even introns need to be extensively analyzed because autoimmune [76] and infectious diseases [77] have been associated with the differential expression levels of the HLA genes in different haplotypes [78]. In addition, null alleles resulting from intronic polymorphisms warrant investigation and resolution to better understand their functional effects [79-82].

After PCR amplicon production, there are four main steps leading to sequencing and HLA data analysis; amplicon library preparation, emulsion PCR, NGS and HLA data analysis (Figure 2). The preparation of the template library is an important step because the PCR amplicons are used either singly or pooled together into a multiplex and then labeled with sequence tags (indexes, barcodes or MIDs) during library construction to facilitate sample multiplexing prior to emulsion PCR and sequencing. The addition of different barcodes to different sample libraries enables the independent detection of sequences in a mixture of different samples. Computing software is used to accurately parse the tagged sample files during the analysis of sequencing data. However, a possible disadvantage of using too many multiple barcoding tags is to lose sequencing depth because when samples are pooled for multiplexing the amount of input DNA for each sample, due to the increased sample number, is reduced.

In previous studies, most investigators using either the Roche or Illumina systems pooled their PCR amplicons at equimolar concentrations for even gene distribution before constructing barcoded libraries [36,37,40,41,43,56,71,72]. The ligation of barcodes to the fragmented DNA templates during library construction allowed a varying number of different samples to be sequenced during a single sequencing run, depending on read lengths, the capacity of the sequencing platform and the number of pooled amplicons that were used. For example, Erlich et al. [71] reported sequencing a maximum of 760 samples per run after loading a multiplex of 95-96 barcoded samples into a single lane of an 8-region PicoTiter Plate using the 454 Genome Sequencer FLX instrument. Initially, we used only a single gene-sequencing run (SGSR) by sequencing a single PCR amplicon and up to ten barcoded samples per sequencing run with the Roche GS Junior and chose to use only up to four barcoded samples per sequencing run with the Ion PGM [42]. As described in this chapter, we now have changed from SGSR to a multiplex gene-sequencing run (MGSR), for which we pooled all 13 LR-PCR amplicons together into a single sample (Figure 5) prior to constructing libraries for five barcoded samples per sequencing run. This change, from SGSR to MGSR, reduced the number of sequencing runs from 13 to 1, thereby greatly reducing the workload, the cost per sample and the overall cost per individual. Currently, five barcoded samples using 13 LR-PCR amplicons in a single sample is close to Roche GS Junior's maximum sequencing capacity of 80 Mb of sequence reads per run (assuming an average 100-bp read length) without compromising depth of coverage and increasing sequencing or genotyping errors. A statistically adequate depth of sequence coverage is essential to prevent alignment errors and minimize genotyping errors. In comparison, the Ion PGM 318 sequencing chip has far greater sequencing capacity of 1000 Mb ((assuming an average 200 bp read length) and potentially we could use the Ion PGM for genotyping up to 57 barcoded samples using the 13 LR-PCR amplicons in a single sample, if necessary. Although the sample number per sequencing run is low for the Roche GS Junior compared to high capacity NGS platforms, often a small HLA typing laboratory for transplantation matching would require the typing results from only a small number of samples on a weekly basis. If sequencing is required for a very large number of samples, such as for association studies or population diversity studies, our workflow for the Roche Junior can be easily adapted to the larger capacity platforms such as the Roche 454 Genome Sequencer FLX instrument.

Apart from different sequencing capacities, the Roche Junior and Ion PGM use different sequencing principles and procedures. Roche uses a pyrosequencing fluorescence technology with a light output detected by camera scanning [31, 32], whereas the Ion PGM uses Ion Torrent semiconductor sequencing technology with simple sequencing flow chemistry and no light [33]. Ion PGM is the first commercial sequencing machine that does not require fluorescence and camera scanning, resulting in higher speed, lower cost, and smaller instrument size. Currently, it enables 200 bp reads in 3 hours and the sample preparation time is less than 13 hours for 8 samples in parallel. Because every new sequencing technology introduces unique errors and biases into the resulting DNA sequences, a proper understanding of the NGS specific characteristics that are used to identify and interpret reads is crucial in assessing the accuracy and applications for this new technology. Both manufacturers provide their own unique software to processes the raw acquisition data and produce read files that contain high quality consensus reads and draft assemblies. Roche has the GS analysis software and Ion Torrent has a web browser driving the Torrent Suite Software on computers attached to their respective sequencing instruments. For both platforms, we used the manufacturers software to preprocess the DNA sequencing raw data before transferring the edited data onto our HLA genotyping software. Therefore, we have not directly addressed what errors are introduced into the raw reads by the NGS apparatus. However, others have shown that the major sequencing errors with both sequencing instruments prior to pre-processing are largely related to high frequency indel polymorphisms, homopolymeric regions, replicate bias, and substitution errors that mostly increase in rate with distance from the read start [45,65-67]. In addition, the quality scores that are Phred-based can be only used to detect inserted and substituted bases for both the Roche and Ion Torrent platforms. While the Ion PGM quality scores underestimate the base accuracy, the Roche 454 quality scores tend to over estimate the base accuracy [45,65-67]. Although there are no key studies of raw error reads directly comparing the Roche GS Junior with Ion PGM outputs, a recent statistical study has concluded that the accuracy of the Ion PGM is poorer than that of light-based technologies [65]. On the other hand, direct comparisons of the Roche light-based technologies and Ion PGM of pre-edited sequencing data of bacteria has generally concluded that there is little difference in the accuracy of the sequencing data and that most errors arise with indel polymorphisms and homopolymeric regions [45-47]. Currently, we are conducting our NGS sequencing experiments with 100 DNA samples using the Roche Junior and 200 DNA samples with the Ion PGM, so, at this stage, we have not performed any accurate or meaningful statistical comparisons for the various sequencing variables produced by the two different platforms. In general, however, the indels and homopolymers are only a minor problem for SS-SBT HLA genotyping by NGS using either of the two platforms.

After pre-editing the sequences generated by the two NGS platforms using the manufacturers software, we transferred the edited data to HLA typing software. We compared a software program, called the Suzuki method, which was developed in-house, against two commercial programs, Omixon Target (Omixon) and Assign MPS (Conexio). These stand-alone software programs were assessed and compared for in phase sequence alignment of HLA genes and for allele assignment at different levels including the 8-digit level. Most genotype-calling algorithms select the HLA type candidates based on optimized alignment to cDNA references from the IMGT-HLA database due to the lack of genomic reference sequences. All three software programs consolidated and assessed the various sequence reads, sorted them according to genomic primer and barcodes, compared the sequences to the IMGT/HLA sequence database references and generated a consensus sequence with allele assignment taking into account the exonic and intronic sequence and phase relationship. The barcodes or

MID tags identified by the software were used to reveal the reads of the various samples. Scores for sequence measures and quality assurances were provided including sequence depth, allele depth and allelic balance. Reads were aligned to the various loci and regions based on 100% matching between the read sequence and the reference library. Finally, a consensus sequence was generated and allele assignment made taking into account exonic and intronic sequence as well as phase relationship. The numbers of different reverse and forward reads for each amplicon were indicated, phased and automatically assigned a genotype only if the aligned sequences were perfectly matched with the alleles of genomic references or constructed references. A mapping procedure was applied for each candidate allele to verify the accuracy of the HLA typing and to detect novel alleles. In cases of less than 100% match, even at 99%, mis-mapping can occur among the HLA loci. Also, at least an average 30-fold depth was necessary to identify genetic variants with high sensitivity and resolution. When sequencing read numbers were too few, then we could not make exact assignments. If aligned sequence reads were mismatched at one or more bases with the database, manual editing allowed for further investigation and assignment of a genotype. Overall, there was little difference in the efficiency, performance, analysis and outputs between the three software systems, although we favored our in house program over the commercially available software on a cost benefits basis. Because the IMGT/HLA sequence database has relatively few genomic sequences, at less than 6% of the database entries, a major task remains to continue building a suitable reference library for all the known polymorphic HLA genes.

Our main aim in using the NGS technology was to eliminate the ambiguities currently associated with the conventional HLA genotyping methods. So far, we found that the SS-SBT method is superior to other HLA DNA typing methods, especially to efficiently detect new HLA alleles and null alleles at the 8-digit level of DNA typing without ambiguity. Although, at most, only 100 Japanese and Caucasian genomic DNA samples were used in this study, we unequivocally defined the HLA-A, -B, -C, -DRB1 and -DQB1 loci to single HLA alleles at the 8-digit level without any ambiguity. In addition, 17 DRB allele sequences, seven in DRB1, three in DRB3, four in DRB4 and three in DRB5, were newly determined to the field 4 level of allele resolution without phase ambiguity by SS-SBT. However, achieving a complete depth of correct sequence information in most samples of DRB1 and in some samples of DRB3/4/5, such as TU20 in DRB3, was compromised by the presence of microsatellites in a limited number of intronic sites. Major sequence instabilities were encountered in our study with $T^{5\sim17}$ and $T^{2\sim27}$ mono-stretch sequences and $GT^{7\sim28}$ and $GA^{3\sim23}$ microsatellite repeats in intron 1 of DRB1, intron 5 of DRB1 and intron 2 of DRB1 and DRB3/4/5 alleles that were obtained in our study and from the IMGT-HLA database. These instabilities within the microsatellite repeats are probably compounded by PCR and sequencing errors [65], but could be solved by Sanger sequencing of PCR products using high fidelity DNA polymerase.

All the allele sequences, excluding DRB1*09:21, were perfectly matched to at least the previously reported field 1 or field 2 level of allele information [83]. Therefore, the newly designed primers and PCR conditions for HLA-A, -B, -C, -DRB1, -DQA1, -DQB1, -DPA1 and -DPB1 [42] and -DRB3/4/5 [56] are efficient for DNA typing by the SS-SBT method. Of the 164 alleles detected at the field 4 assignment level in 81 Japanese and Caucasian samples, 78 (47.6%) were newly detected alleles. Therefore, simply increasing the sample size in future analyses of HLA polymorphisms by the SS-SBT method could identify new non-synonymous substitutions along with indels that generate a null allele. A new allele DRB1*09:21 that we identified in only one sample so far, in comparison to the 129 DRB1*09:01 positive genomic DNA samples typed by SS-SBT in the Japanese population, suggests that the new allele has extremely low frequency in the Japanese.

We encountered problems with some microsatellite sequences, especially for DRB1*15:01:01:03 with the complexity of microsatellite polymorphisms in intron 2. In addition, the 8-digit level HLA alleles could not be assigned in HLA-DQA1, -DPA1 and -DPB1 because the SNP and indel densities to separate both of the phases were much lower than in the other HLA loci. Resolution was difficult for phase ambiguities in the conserved sequences at HLA loci, such as exon 3 in the HLA class II genes. Therefore, most HLA allele sequences are still unknown at the 8-digit level. In this respect, collection of the 8-digit level reference sequences using HLA homozygous DNA samples, haplotype extraction methods [84] or third generation sequencers such as one molecule real time DNA sequencer PacBio RS [85,86] (Pacific Biosciences, Menlo Park, CA) that provide a 3 kb read length on average are necessary for solving the current genotyping problems to improve the SS-SBT method.

The collection of HLA allele sequences at the 8-digit level and the development of HLA allele assignment programs are necessary to improve the SS-SBT method. The average depth of HLA-A, -B and -C was stable with a ratio of ~1:1. However, in comparison, the average depth of HLA-DRB1 for LR-PCR mix 2 and -DQB1 was less stable with ratios varying between 1:1 and 1: <2 [42]. Monitoring the depth ratio and potential allele dropout is important to detect PCR bias due to unexpected variations in the primer sites. In cases where the depth ratio is drastically changed such as 1:5 or more, the primer sets and/or PCR condition may have to be modified. Nevertheless, the newly developed HLA DNA typing method SS-SBT [42] is potentially applicable to the diagnostic laboratory once some of the minor problems described above are solved in future.

Our study is the first direct comparison between the GS Junior and Ion PGM sequencing platforms for HLA genotyping. Although we have as yet to maximize the potential capacity of the Ion PGM to meet our theoretical expectation of sequencing the pooled PCR amplicons for 11 gene loci using 57 barcoded samples, the Ion PGM seems to perform as well as or better than Roche Junior on a number of fronts. However, it is difficult to choose between the two platforms at this stage and further work and comparative analysis will need to be performed before drawing a definite conclusion. Whereas there is little difference in overall performance between the two platforms at this time, the new Ion Torrent 318 chip offers greater capacity for more samples and more accurate reads with read lengths of 400 bp, for which we are presently testing 300 samples. In addition, automation of library preparations and emPCR amplification steps prior to sequencing has improved the overall turn around time from library preparation to allele readouts from four days to two/three days with the sequencing step performed overnight (Figure 2).

Development of better technologies to reduce the complication of the process and running costs is also necessary before the SS-SBT method is introduced into the diagnostic laboratory.

In a previous simulated test of the Ion Torrent PGM system in a clinical laboratory setting, we needed four days for the manual sample preparation and library construction from the time of PCR amplification to HLA allele definition [42]. However, with the use of automated procedures such as the AB Library Builder™ system and Ion OneTouch™ system from Life Technologies we have shortened the workflow significantly to just two days with a running cost of US $17 per locus per sample. In comparison, the workflow for the Roche Junior remains at four days from the time of PCR amplification to HLA allele definition at a running cost of US $40 per locus per sample. Also, a new protocol using the new Ion 318 chip with 32 barcodes for 400 bp-read high sequencing quality has increased sequencing capacity and enabled sequencing reads up to and beyond 400 bp [87]. Although we are at this moment testing the new Ion Torrent protocols with the Ion 318 chip it looks likely to lead to further improvements and further cost reductions. Therefore, a decrease in the running costs of NGS is expected to soon be substantially better than those of the conventional HLA DNA typing methods.

Whereas we have tested the Roche Junior and Ion PGM NGS compact systems, the Illumina MiSeq is another commercially available compact NGS [45]. The Illumina MiSeq sequencer appears to compare well with Roche Junior and Ion PGM for HLA typing [43,72] and sequencing other regions and targets of interest [45]. Other laboratories have favored the Illumina MiSeq system and have published the workflows and results for HLA typing and sequencing haplotypes to high resolution levels [43,72]. The Illumina MiSeq offers some advantages over the Roche and Ion PGM such as low DNA input amount, the pair-end reads (ie., fragments sequenced in both directions) to determine in phase alleles and possibly, a better and more reliable resolution of substitutions and indels [46]. However, the Illumina MiSeq may not perform as well for the middle reads of a 150 bp/200 bp sequence and the generated reads may exhibit rapidly increasing error rates as the read length increases, resulting in lower quality contig assemblies [46]. Also, the HLA DNA data analysis step appears to be a more difficult process [43,72] than that for the Roche Junior and Ion PGM (unpublished data). In cases where the phase of an allele is unresolved by the NGS system and HLA software other approaches may help to resolve the allele ambiguity. For example, one promising approach is to use DNA haplotype-specific extraction of the gene from the sample using a commercially available extraction kit, such as the solid-phase, capture-based EZ1 HaploPrep kit from Qiagen [88], and then resequencing the unresolved haplotype. The DNA haplotype-specific extraction procedure can extract genomic regions of up to 50 kb of contiguous sequence without amplication or concentration of the extracted DNA, and it has been used successfully to genotype and haplotype HLA class I and class II genes [84, 89-93] including adjoining genes such as HLA-B, MICA and HLA-C [89].

HLA in-phase genotyping is important for a variety of applications including for infectious disease studies, transplantation, pharmacogenomics, autoimmune diseases, population diversity and human evolution, and treatment of cancer pathology by vaccination. While we used the genome from whole blood or from peripheral blood mononuclear cells for HLA in phase-genotyping the analysis of HLA cDNA from cells and tissue (fresh or formalin fixed) would also be of value [38,39]. In humans, the HLA-A, -B, and -C locus-specific gene expression patterns were reported in the peripheral blood leukocytes, colon mucosa and larynx mucosa by real-time PCR [94]. Recently, we investigated the relationship between haplotypes and gene expression levels of the class I genes by sequencing the genomic DNA of pigs using the Roche Genome Sequencer 454 FLX and found that the sequence read numbers closely reflected the gene expression levels in white blood cells [95]. The use of the NGS sequencing method in human studies, similar to our MHC locus-specific expression analysis in pigs, could also provide informative data in various biomedical studies on HLA gene expression, such as the detection of expression levels among inter- and intra-populations, and among different tissues, both before and after vaccination against pathogens.

High-resolution donor-recipient HLA matching contributes to the success of unrelated donor organ and marrow transplantation [2,96]. HLA typing also plays critical roles in donor and recipient matching for embryonic (ES) or induced pluripotent stem (iPS) cell transplantation therapy. Currently, an iPS cell bank project is under way, led by Kyoto University, with the participation of one of the co-authors (HI) of this chapter. It was reported that when thirty iPS cell lines that have different combinations of homozygous HLA-A, -B, and -DR are generated, these iPS cells will have matched the three loci in 82.2% of the Japanese population. For fifty iPS cell lines, the chance of a match increases to 90.7% in the Japanese population [97].

In addition to finding new polymorphisms within exons, the SS-SBT method can analyze polymorphisms in introns, promoter, enhancer, and 3'-UTR regions that have largely remained unexplored until now. By analyzing polymorphisms in the entire region of HLA genes, the functional influence of those polymorphisms can be revealed in transplantation, diseases, and adverse effects of medications. For example, it is expected that about one in a thousand people have a null allele (deficient mutant that influences function or expression) in the HLA region. Since null alleles have a profound influence on GVHD or transplant establishment, especially in hematopoietic stem cell transplantation, the detection of null alleles is considered to be of great clinical importance.

The SS-SBT method has been developed to obtain massive and accurate sequencing data easily and cost effectively. Recently, the authors of a critical review of HLA typing by NGS [98] pointed out that the Roche company will discontinue product support for the 454 sequencing systems in 2016, implying that the Roche Junior sequencing platform will be phased out commercially in the near future. However, almost all the materials and reagents required for the Ion PGM™ system are available as kit products, and one Gb of sequencing data can be obtained within 5 hours of running the protocols and data analysis. Up to fifty-seven samples can be multiplexed and eight HLA gene loci analysed at an eight-digit level in a single run. Compared to the Luminex beads method or the SBT method, the SS-SBT is more cost effective. For these reasons, the Ion PGM™ sequencer is potentially the perfect sequencer for HLA genotyping using the SS-SBT method. With an expected increase in throughput and the development of an automated system in the future, we hope that Ion PGM™ will be even easier to use for routine HLA genotyping.

In conclusion, we have developed procedures for massively parallel sequencing of multiplex products that can be used for several benchtop sequencing platforms. We have obtained sequences of sufficient high quality to permit accurate HLA in phase genotypes across the full-length gene from the 5′ promoter/enhancer region to the 3′ UTR for most of the classical class

http://dx.doi.org/10.5772/57556

I and class II genes. The use of sample tags or barcodes allows for optimization of second generation sequencing technologies by pooling samples and sequencing multiple samples in parallel for time- and cost-efficient workflows. We are currently working towards optimizing the Ion PGM/SS-SBT method for HLA in phase genotyping for both the clinical diagnostic and research laboratories.

Erratum

The software Assign MPS 1.0 used in this study was a beta version and still under development at the time of publishing the chapter and not available commercially from Conexio.

Author details

Jerzy K. Kulski[2*], Shingo Suzuki[1], Yuki Ozaki[1], Shigeki Mitsunaga[1], Hidetoshi Inoko[1] and Takashi Shiina[1]

*Address all correspondence to: kulski@me.com

1 Department of Molecular Life Science, Division of Basic Medical Science and Molecular Medicine, Tokai University School of Medicine, Isehara, Kanagawa, Japan

2 Centre for Forensic Science, The University of Western Australia, Nedlands, WA, Australia

References

[1] Zinkernagel RM, Doherty PC. The discovery of MHC restriction. Immunology Today 1997;18(1): 14-7. DOI: 10.1016/S0167-5699(97)80008-4

[2] Sheldon S, Poulton K. HLA typing and its influence on organ transplantation. Methods in Molecular Biology 2006;333: 157-74. DOI: 10.1385/1-59745-049-9:157

[3] Park M, Seo JJ. Role of HLA in hematopoietic stem cell transplantation. Bone Marrow Research 2012;2012: 680841. DOI:10.1155/2012/680841

[4] Shiina T, Inoko H, Kulski JK. An update of the HLA genomic region, locus information and disease associations: 2004.Tissue Antigens 2004;64(6): 631-49. DOI: 10.1111/j.1399-0039.2004.00327.x

[5] Bolton EM, Bradley JA. Transplantation Immunology. In: Eremin O, Sewell H. (ed.) Essential Immunology for Surgeons. Oxford University Press; 2011. Chpt 3, p199-235.

[6] Duquesnoy RJ. Antibody-reactive epitope determination with HLAMatchmaker and its clinical applications. Tissue Antigens 2011;77(6): 525-34. DOI: 10.1111/j.1399-0039.2011.01646.x

[7] Ponticelli C. The mechanisms of acute transplant rejection revisited. Journal of Nephrology 2012;25(2): 150-8. DOI: 10.5301/jn.5000048

[8] Garcia MAA, Yebra BG, Flores ALL, Guerra EG. The Major Histocompatibility Complex in transplantation. Journal of Transplantation. 2012;2012: 842141. DOI: 10.1155/2012/842141

[9] Holoshitz J. The quest for better understanding of HLA-disease association: Scenes from a road less travelled by. Discovery Medicine 2013;16(87): 93-101. www.discoverymedicine.com/Joseph-Holoshitz/2013/08/26/the-quest-for-better-understanding-of-hla-disease-association-scenes-from-a-road-less-travelled-by/ (accessed 18 December 2013).

[10] Shiina T, Hosomichi K, Inoko H, Kulski JK. The HLA genomic loci map: expression, interaction, diversity and disease. Journal of Human Genetics 2009;54(1): 15-39. DOI: 10.1038/jhg.2008.5

[11] Kropshofer H, Hammerling GJ, Vogt AB. The impact of the non-classical MHC proteins HLA-DM and HLA-DO on loading of MHC class II molecules. Immunological Reviews 1999;172: 267-78. DOI: 10.1111/j.1600-065X.1999.tb01371.x

[12] Dawkins R, Leelayuwat C, Gaudieri S, Tay G, Hui J, Cattley S, Martinez P, Kulski J. Genomics of the major histocompatibility complex: haplotypes, duplication, retroviruses and disease. Immunological Reviews 1999;167: 275-304. DOI: 10.1111/j.1600-065X.1999.tb01399.x

[13] Naves EM, Cuadrado JFP, Perez Rosada A, Gomez del Moral M. Structure and function of 'non-classical" HLA class I molecules. Immunologia 2001;20(4): 207-15. http://revista.inmunologia.org/Upload/Articles/5/4/545.pdf (accessed 18 December 2013).

[14] Erlich HA, Opelz G, Hansen J. HLA DNA typing and transplantation. Immunity 2001;14(4): 347-56. DOI: 10.1016/S1074-7613(01)00115-7

[15] Mahdi B M. A glow of HLA typing in organ transplantation. Clinical and Transplantation Medicine 2013;2(1): 6. DOI: 10.1186/2001-1326-2-6

[16] Mack SJ, Sanchez-Mazas A, Single RM, Meyer D, Hill J, Dron HA, Jani AJ, Thomson G, Erlich HA. Population samples and genotyping technology. Tissue Antigens 2007;69(Suppl s1): 188-91. DOI: 10.1111/j.1399-0039.2006.00768.x

[17] Vina MA, Hollenbach JA, Lyke KE et al. Tracking human migrations by the analysis of the distribution of HLA alleles, lineages and haplotypes in closed and open populations. Philosophical Transactions of the Royal Society of London B: Biological Sciences 2012;367(1590): 820-9. DOI: 10.1098/rstb.2011.0320

[18] Nakaoka H, Mitsunaga S, Hosomichi K et al. Detection of ancestry informative HLA alleles confirms the admixed origins of Japanese population. PLoS One 2013;8(4): e60793. DOI: 10.1371/journal.pone.0060793

[19] Grubic Z, Stingl K, Martinez N, Palfi B, Brkljacic-Kerhin, V, Kastelan A. STR and HLA analysis in paternity testing. International Congress Series 2004;1261: 535-7. DOI: 10.1016/S0531-5131(03)01654-6

[20] Alfirevic A, Pirmohamed M. Drug induced hypersensitivity and the HLA complex. Pharmaceuticals 2011;4(1): 69-90. DOI: 10.3390/ph4010069

[21] Mallal S, Nolan D, Witt C et al. Association between presence of HLA-B*5701, HLA-DR7, and HLA-DQ3 and hypersensitivity to HIV-1 reverse-transcriptase inhibitor abacavir. Lancet 2002;359(9308): 727-32. DOI: 10.1016/S0140-6736(02)07873-X

[22] Ota M, Fukushima H, Kulski JK, Inoko H. Single nucleotide polymorphism detection by polymerase chain reaction-restriction fragment length polymorphism. Nature Protocols 2007;2(11): 2857-64. DOI: 10.1038/nprot.2007.407

[23] Argu"ello JR, Madrigal JA. HLA typing by reference strand mediated conformation analysis (RSCA). Reviews in Immunogenetics 1999;1(2): 209-19.

[24] Saiki R, Walsh PS, Levenson CH, Erlich HA. Genetic analysis of amplified DNA with immobilized sequence-specific oligonucleotide probes. Proceedings of the National Academy of Sciences of the United States of America 1989;86(16): 6230-4. www.pnas.org/content/86/16/6230 (accessed 18 December 2013)

[25] Olerup O, Zetterquist H. HLA-DR typing by PCR amplification with sequence-specific primers (PCR-SSP) in 2 hours: an alternative to serological DR typing in clinical practice including donor–recipient matching in cadaveric transplantation. Tissue Antigens 1992;39(5): 225-35. DOI: 10.1111/j.1399-0039.1992.tb01940.x

[26] Santamaria P, Lindstrom AL, Boyce-Jacino MT, Mystera SH, Barbosab JJ, Farasa AJ, Richa SS. HLA class I sequence-based typing. Human Immunology 1993;37(1): 39-50. DOI: 10.1016/0198-8859(93)90141-M

[27] Itoh Y, Mizuki N, Shimada T, Azuma F, Itakura M, Kashiwase K, Kikkawa E, Kulski JK, Satake M, Inoko H. High-throughput DNA typing of HLA-A, -B, -C, and -DRB1 loci by a PCR-SSOP-Luminex method in the Japanese population. Immunogenetics 2005;57(10): 717-29. DOI: 10.1007/s00251-005-0048-3

[28] Itoh Y, Inoko H, Kulski JK, Sasaki S, Meguro A, Takiyama N, Nishida T, Yuasa T, Ohno S, Mizuki N. Four-digit allele genotyping of the HLA-A and HLA-B genes in Japanese patients with Behcet's disease by a PCR-SSOP-Luminex method. Tissue Antigens 2006;67(5): 390-4. DOI: 10.1111/j.1399-0039.2006.00586.x

[29] Hutchison CA III. DNA sequencing: bench to bedside and beyond. Nucleic Acids Research 2007;35(18): 6227-37. DOI: 10.1093/nar/gkm688

[30] Leslie S, Donnelly P, McVean G. A statistical method for predicting classical HLA alleles from SNP data. The American Journal of Human Genetics 2008;82(1): 48-56. DOI: 10.1016/j.ajhg.2007.09.001

[31] Metzger ML. Sequencing technologies – the next generation. Nature Reviews in Genetics 2010;11(1): 31-46. DOI: 10.1038/nrg2626

[32] Rothberg JM, Leamon JH. The development and impact of 454 sequencing. Nature Biotechnology 2008;26(10): 1117-24. DOI: 10.1038/nbt1485

[33] Rothberg JM, Hinz W, Rearick TM et al. An integrated semiconductor device enabling non-optical genome sequencing. Nature 2011;475(7356): 348-52. DOI: 10.1038/nature10242

[34] Sanger F, Nicklen S, Coulson AR. DNA sequencing with chain-terminating inhibitors. Proceedings of the National Academy of Sciences of the United States of America 1977;74(12): 5463-7. www.pnas.org/content/74/12/5463 (accessed 18 December 2013).

[35] Maxam A, Gilbert W. A new method of sequencing DNA. Proceedings of the National Academy of Sciences, USA 1977;74(2): 560-4. www.pnas.org/content/74/2/560 (accessed 18 December 2013).

[36] Gabriel C, Danzer M, Hackl C, Kopal G, Hufnagl P, Hofer K, Polin H, Stabentheiner S, Proll J. Rapid high-throughput human leukocyte antigen typing by massively parallel pyrosequencing for high-resolution allele identification. Human Immunology 2009;70(11): 960-4. DOI: 10.1016/j.humimm.2009.08.009

[37] Holcomb CL, Hoglund B, Anderson MW et al. A multi-site study using high-resolution HLA genotyping by next generation sequencing. Tissue Antigens 2011;77(3): 206-17. DOI: 10.1111/j.1399-0039.2010.01606.x

[38] Lank SM, Golbach BA, Creager HM, Wiseman RW, Keskin DB, Reinherz EL, Brusic V, O'Connor DH. Ultra-high resolution HLA genotyping and allele discovery by highly multiplexed cDNA amplicon pyrosequencing. BMC Genomics 2012;13: 378. DOI: 10.1186/1471-2164-13-378

[39] Lank SM, Wiseman RW, Dudley DM, O'Connor DH. A novel single cDNA amplicon pyrosequencing method for high-throughput, cost-effective sequence-based HLA class I genotyping. Human Immunology 2010;71(10): 1011-7. DOI: 10.1016/j.humimm.2010.07.012

[40] Lind C, Ferriola D, Mackiewicz K et al. Next-generation sequencing: the solution for high-resolution, unambiguous human leukocyte antigen typing. Human Immunology 2010;71(10): 1033-42. DOI: 10.1016/j.humimm.2010.06.016

[41] Erlich H. HLA DNA typing: past, present, and future. Tissue Antigens 2012;80(1): 1-11. DOI: 10.1111/j.1399-0039.2012.01881.x

[42] Shiina T, Suzuki S, Ozaki Y et al. Super high resolution for single molecule-sequence-based typing of classical HLA loci at the 8-digit level using next generation sequencers. Tissue Antigens 2012;80(4): 305-16. DOI: 10.1111/j.1399-0039.2012.01941.x

[43] Hosomichi K, Jinam TA, Mitsunaga S, Nakaoka H, Inoue I. Phase-defined complete sequencing of the HLA genes by next-generation sequencing. BMC Genomics 2013;14: 355. DOI: 10.1186/1471-2164-14-355

[44] Glenn TC. Field guide to next-generation DNA sequencers. Molecular Ecology Resources 2011;11(5): 759-69. DOI: 10.1111/j.1755-0998.2011.03024.x

[45] Liu L, Li Y, Li S, Hu N, He Y, Pong R, Lin D, Lu L, Law M. Comparison of next-generation sequencing systems. Journal of Biomedicine and Biotechnology 2012,2012: 251364. DOI: 10.1155/2012/251364

[46] Loman NJ, Misra RV, Dallman TJ, Constantinidou C, Gharbia SE, Wain J, Pallen MJ. Performance comparison of benchtop high-throughput sequencing platforms. Nature Biotechnology 2012;30(5): 434-9. DOI: 10.1038/nbt.2198

[47] Quail M, Smith M, Coupland P, Otto TD, Harris SR, Connor TR, Bertoni A, Swerdlow HP, Gu Y. A tale of three next generation sequencing platforms: comparison of Ion torrent, pacific biosciences and illumina MiSeq sequencers. BMC Genomics 2012;13: 341. DOI: 10.1186/1471-2164-13-341

[48] Bentley DR, Balasubramanian S, Swerdlow HP et al. Accurate whole human genome sequencing using reversible terminator chemistry. Nature 2008;456(7218): 53-9. DOI: 10.1038/nature07517

[49] Parameswaran P, Jalili R, Tao L, Shokralla S, Gharizadeh B, Ronaghi M, Fire AZ. A pyrosequencing-tailored nucleotide barcode design unveils opportunities for large-scale sample multiplexing. Nucleic Acids Research 2007;35(19): e130. DOI: 10.1093/nar/gkm760

[50] Lennon NJ, Lintner RE, Anderson S et al. A scalable, fully automated process for construction of sequence-ready barcoded libraries for 454. Genome Biology 2010;11(2): R15. DOI: 10.1186/gb-2010-11-2-r15

[51] Margulies M, Egholm M, Altman WE et al. Genome sequencing in microfabricated high-density picolitre reactors. Nature 2005;437(7057): 376-80. DOI: 10.1038/nature03959

[52] Shendure JA, Porreca GJ, Church GM. Overview of DNA Sequencing Strategies. In: Current Protocols in Molecular Biology. Hoboken: John Wiley and Sons; 2008. Vol 8, Ch 7. DOI: 10.1002/0471142727.mb0701s81

[53] Fedurco M, Romieu A, Williams S, Lawrence I, Turcatti G. BTA, a novel reagent for DNA attachment on glass and efficient generation of solid-phase amplified DNA colonies. Nucleic Acids Research 2006;34(3): e22. DOI: 10.1093/nar/gnj023

[54] GS Junior Bench Top System. Roche 454 Sequencing. http://www.gsjunior.com (accessed 17 October 2013).

[55] Ion Personal Genome Machine (PGM) Sequencer. Specification sheet. http://www3.appliedbiosystems.com/cms/groups/applied_markets_marketing/documents/generaldocuments/cms_094139.pdf (accessed 17 October 2013).

[56] Ozaki Y, Suzuki S, Shigenari A, Okudaira Y, Kikkawa E, Oka A, Ota M, Mitsunaga, S, Kulski JK, Inoko H, Shiina T. HLA-DRB1, -DRB3, -DRB4 and -DRB5 genotyping at a super-high resolution level by long range PCR and high-throughput sequencing. Tissue Antigens. 2014 Jan;83(1):10-6. doi: 10.1111/tan.12258. Epub 2013 Nov 30. PubMed PMID: 24355003.

[57] HLA nomenclature. http://hla.alleles.org/nomenclature/naming.html (accessed 17 October 2013).

[58] Ando A, Shigenari A, Ota M et al. SLA-DRB1 and -DQB1 genotyping by the PCR-SSOP-Luminex method. Tissue Antigens 2011;78(1): 49-55. DOI: 10.1111/j.1399-0039.2011.01669.x

[59] Conexio. http://www.conexio-genomics.com (accessed 17 October 2013).

[60] 454 Sequencing system. Guidelines for amplicon experimental design. June 2013. Roche. http://dna.uga.edu/docs/454SeqSys_AmpliconDesignGuide_Jun2013.pdf (accessed 17 October 2013).

[61] Application note. Ion Torrent amplicon sequencing. http://www3.appliedbiosystems.com/cms/groups/applied_markets_marketing/documents/generaldocuments/cms_094273.pdf (accessed 17 October 2013).

[62] Ewing B, Green P. Base-calling of automated sequencer traces using phred. II. Error probabilities. Genome Research 1998;8(3): 186-94. genome.cshlp.org/content/8/3/186.long (accessed 18 December 2013)

[63] Ewing B, Hillier L, Wendl MC, Green P. Base-calling of automated sequencer traces using phred. I. Accuracy assessment. Genome Research 1998;8(3): 175-85. DOI: 10.1101/gr.8.3.175

[64] Technical note: sequencing. Quality scores for next-generation sequencing. Illumina. http://res.illumina.com/documents/products/technotes/technote_q-scores.pdf (accessed 17 October 2013).

[65] Bragg LM, Stone G, Butler MK, Hugenholtz P, Tyson GW. Shining a light on dark sequencing: Characterising errors in Ion Torrent PGM data. PLoS Computational Biology 2013;9(4): e1003031. DOI: 10.1371/journal.pcbi.1003031

[66] Gilles A, Meglecz E, Pech N, Ferreira S, Malausa T, Martin JF. Accuracy and quality assessment of 454 GS-FLX Titanium pyrosequencing. BMC Genomics 2011;12: 245. DOI: 10.1186/1471-2164-12-245

[67] Huse SM, Huber JA, Morrison HG, Sogin ML, Mark Welch D. Accuracy and quality of massively parallel DNA pyrosequencing. Genome Biology 2007;8(7): R143. DOI: 10.1186/gb-2007-8-7-r143

[68] Technical note: sequencing. Estimating sequence coverage. Illumina. http://res.illumina.com/documents/products/technotes/technote_coverage_calculation.pdf (accessed 17 October 2013).

[69] UCSC genome bioinformatics. http://genome.ucsc.edu/ (accessed 17 October 2013).

[70] Omixon. Targeted NGS data analysis. http://www.omixon.com (accessed 17 October 2013).

[71] Erlich RL, Jia X, Anderson S et al. Next-generation sequencing for HLA typing of class I loci. BMC Genomics 2011;12: 42. DOI: 10.1186/1471-2164-12-42

[72] Wang C, Krishnakumar S, Wilhelmy J, Babrzadeh F, Stepanyan L et al. High-throughput, high-fidelity HLA genotyping with deep sequencing. Proceedings of the National Academy of Sciences of the United States of America 2012;109(22): 8676-81. DOI: 10.1073/pnas.1206614109

[73] Cline J, Braman JC, Hogrefe HH. PCR fidelity of pfu DNA polymerase and other thermostable DNA polymerases. Nucleic Acids Research 1996;24(18): 3546-51. DOI: 10.1093/nar/24.18.3546

[74] Robinson J, Halliwell JA, McWilliam H, Lopez R, Parham P, Marsh SGE. The IMGT/HLA database. Nucleic Acids Research 2013;41(D1): D1222-7. DOI: 10.1093/nar/gks949

[75] Robinson J, Mistry K, McWilliam H, Lopez R, Parham P, Marsh SGE. The IMGT/HLA database. Nucleic Acids Research 2011;39 (suppl 1): D1171-6. DOI: 10.1093/nar/gkq998

[76] Cocco E, Meloni A, Murru MR et al. Vitamin D responsive elements within the HLA-DRB1 promoter region in Sardinian multiple sclerosis associated allele. PLoS One 2012;7(7): e41678. DOI: 10.1371/journal.pone.0041678

[77] Thomas R, Apps R, Qi Y et al. HLA-C cell surface expression and control of HIV/AIDS correlate with a variant upstream of HLA-C. Nature Genetics 2009;41(12): 1290-4. DOI: 10.1038/ng.486

[78] Vandiedonck C, Taylor MS, Lockstone HE, Plant K, Taylor JM, Durrant C, Broxholme J, Fairfax BP, Knight JC. Pervasive haplotypic variation in the spliceo-transcriptome of the human major histocompatibility complex. Genome Research 2011;21(7): 1042-54. DOI: 10.1101/gr.116681.110

[79] Elsner HA, Bernard G, Eiz-Vesper B, de Matteis M, Bernard A, Blasczyk R. Non-expression of HLA-A*2901102 N is caused by a nucleotide exchange in the mRNA

splicing site at the beginning of intron 4. Tissue Antigens 2002;59(2): 139-41. DOI: 10.1034/j.1399-0039.2002.590212.x

[80] Curran MD, Williams F, Little AM, Rima BK, Madrigal JA, Middleton D. Aberrant splicing of intron 1 creates a novel null HLA-B*1501 allele. Tissue Antigens 1999;53(3): 244-52. DOI: 10.1034/j.1399-0039.1999.530304.x

[81] Tamouza R, El Kassar N, Schaeffer V et al. A novel HLA-B*39 allele (HLA-B*3916) due to a rare mutation causing cryptic splice site activation. Human Immunology 2000;61(5): 467-73. DOI: 10.1016/S0198-8859(00)00108-7

[82] Dubois V, Tiercy JM, Labonne MP, Dormoy A, Gebuhrer L. A new HLA-B44 allele (B*44020102S) with a splicing mutation leading to a complete deletion of exon 5. Tissue Antigens 2004;63(2): 173-80. DOI: 10.1111/j.1399-0039.2004.00134.x

[83] Bettinotti MP, Mitsuishi Y, Bibee K, Lau M, Terasaki PI. Comprehensive method for the typing of HLA-A, B, and C alleles by direct sequencing of PCR products obtained from genomic DNA. Journal of Immunotherapy 1997;20(6): 425-30. journals.lww.com/immunotherapy-journal/Abstract/1997/11000/Comprehensive_Method_for_the_Typing_of_HLA_A,_B,.1.aspx (accessed 18 December 2013)

[84] Dapprich J, Cleary MA, Gabel HW, Akkapeddi A, Iglehart B, Turino C, Beaudet L, Lian J, Murphy NB. A Rapid, Automatable Method For Molecular Haplotyping. In: J.A. Hansen, (ed.) Immunobiology of the Human MHC: Proceedings of the 13th International Histocompatibility Workshop and Conference. Seattle, WA: IHWG Press; 2006. Volume 2, p93-96.

[85] Eid J, Fehr A, Gray J et al. Real-time DNA sequencing from single polymerase molecules. Science 2009;323(5910): 133-8. DOI: 10.1126/science.1162986

[86] Pacific Biosciences. http://www.pacificbiosciences.com/products/ (accessed 18 October 2013).

[87] Ion 318™ Chip Kit v2 (Ion Torrent™). http://www.lifetechnologies.com/order/catalog/product/4484355 (accessed 18 October 2013).

[88] EZ1 HaploPrep Handbook - Qiagen. http://www.qiagen.com/search.aspx?q=ez1%2520haploprep&c={7B5D5E07-20AE-4E4D-B233-FEFA27C84B5B}#&&p=1 (accessed 22 October 2013).

[89] Dapprich J, Ferriola D, Magira EE, Kunkel M, Monos D. SNP-specific extraction of haplotype-resolved targeted genomic regions. Nucleic Acids Research 2008;36(15): e94. DOI: 10.1093/nar/gkn345

[90] Dapprich J, Magira E, Samonte MA, Rosenman K, Monos D. Identification of a novel HLA-DPB1 allele (DPB1*1902) by haplotype-specific extraction and nucleotide sequencing. Tissue Antigens 2007;69(3): 282-3. DOI: 10.1111/j.1399-0039.2006.00752.x

[91] Dapprich J, Witter K, Gabel H, Murphy NB, Albert ED. Identification of a new HLA-B (B*1576) by haplotype Specific Extraction. Human Immunology 2007;68(5): 418-21. DOI: 10.1016/j.humimm.2007.01.015

[92] Guo Z, Hood L, Malkki M, Petersdorf EW. Long-range multilocus haplotype phasing of the MHC. Proceedings of the National Academy of Sciences of the United States of America 2006;103(18): 6964-9. DOI: 10.1073/pnas.0602286103

[93] Nagy M, Entz P, Otremba P, Schoenemann C, Murphy N, Dapprich J. Haplotype-specific extraction: a universal method to resolve ambiguous genotypes and detect new alleles – demonstrated on HLA-B. Tissue Antigens 2007; 69(2): 176-80. DOI: 10.1111/j.1399-0039.2006.00741.x

[94] García-Ruano AB, Méndez R, Romero JM, Cabrera T, Ruiz-Cabello F, Garrido F. Analysis of HLA-ABC locus-specific transcription in normal tissues. Immunogenetics 2010;62(11-12): 711-9. DOI: 10.1007/s00251-010-0470-z

[95] Kita YF, Ando A, Tanaka K, Suzuki S, Ozaki Y, Uenishi H, Inoko H, Kulski JK, Shiina T. Application of high-resolution, massively parallel pyrosequencing for estimation of haplotypes and gene expression levels of swine leukocyte antigen (SLA) class I genes. Immunogenetics 2012;64(3): 187-99. DOI: 10.1007/s00251-011-0572-2

[96] Lee SJ, Klein J, Haagenson M et al. High-resolution donor-recipient HLA matching contributes to the success of unrelated donor marrow transplantation. Blood 2007;110(13): 4576-83. DOI: 10.1182/blood-2007-06-097386

[97] Nakagawa M, Koyanagi M, Tanabe K, Takahashi K, Ichisaka T, Aoi T, Okita K, Mochiduki Y, Takizawa N, Yamanaka S. Generation of induced pluripotent stem cells without Myc from mouse and human fibroblasts. Nature Biotechnology 2008;26(1): 101-6. DOI:10.1038/nbt1374

[98] Gabriel C, Fürst D, Faé I, Wenda S, Zollikofer C, Mytilineos J, Fischer GF. HLA typing by next-generation sequencing - getting closer to reality. Tissue Antigens. 2014;83(2):65-75. DOI:10.1111/tan.12298

Section 2

HLA-Associated Important Autoimmune Diseases

Chapter 6

The Relationship Between Human Leukocyte Antigen Class II Genes and Type 1 Diabetes, Autoimmune Thyroid Diseases, and Autoimmune Polyendocrine Syndrome Type 3

Masahito Katahira

Additional information is available at the end of the chapter

http://dx.doi.org/10.5772/57498

1. Introduction

Common genetic risk factors have been associated with type 1 diabetes (T1D) and autoimmune thyroid diseases (AITD). Graves' disease (GD) and Hashimoto's thyroiditis (HT) are typical AITD. T1D and AITD are major components of autoimmune polyendocrine syndrome (APS)-2 and/or APS-3. The human leukocyte antigen (HLA) has been extensively studied in these diseases [1]. However, population studies have shown that HLA associations may vary depending on the ethnic origin [2]. In Caucasian populations, the highest-risk HLA haplotype for T1D is DRB1*03:01-DQA1*05-DQB1*02 (DR3) and/or DRB1*04-DQA1*03:01-DQB1*03:02 (DR4) [2, 3], and the corresponding haplotype for AITD is DR3 [4, 5]. DRB1*15-DQB1*06:02 and DRB1*07:01-DQA1*02:01 (DR7) haplotypes confer strong protection against both T1D [2, 3] and AITD [6, 7]. However, in the Japanese population, the DR3 haplotype is absent, and the DR4 and DR7 haplotypes are rare [8–10], which may be more helpful for examining the susceptibility and resistance to T1D and AITD of HLA DR-DQ haplotypes, with the exception of DR3, DR4, and DR7.

DR3 and DR4 haplotypes occur very frequently among Caucasian patients with T1D, and only a small percentage (approximately 10%) of Caucasian patients with T1D carry neither of these haplotypes [11, 12]. At the DQB1 locus, "non-Asp" alleles, which code for an amino acid other than aspartate at codon 57, confer an increased risk for T1D in Caucasian populations [13]. The risk due to DR4 haplotypes is primarily attributable to an association with the DQB1*03:02 allele, which codes for an Ala at codon 57 [14]. The risk conferred by the DR3 haplotype may be associated with DQA1 alleles that encode the amino acid Arg at codon 52, such as

DQA1*05:01 [15]. Recently, a similar mechanism was shown to be important in the etiology of AITD. Tomer et al. identified an Arg at position 74 of the HLA-DRβ1 chain (DRβ-Arg-74), encoded by the DRB1*03:01 allele, as the critical DR amino acid conferring susceptibility to GD [16, 17]. Further analysis has shown that the presence of Gln at position 74 was protective not only for GD [16] but also for APS-3 [18].

In the Japanese population, in contrast to Caucasians and other Asians, the DRB1*04:05-DQA1*03:03-DQB1*04:01 haplotype, which differs from the DR4 haplotype in Caucasians, and the DRB1*08:02-DQA1*03:01-DQB1*03:02, DRB1*09:01-DQA1*03:02-DQB1*03:03 (DR9), and DRB1*13:02-DQA1*01:02-DQB1*06:04 (DR13) haplotypes confer susceptibility to T1D [9, 19]. The DRB1*15:01-DQB1:06:02, DRB1*15:02-DQB1*06:01, and DRB1*08:03-DQB1*06:01 haplotypes confer protection against T1D [9, 10, 19]. On the other hand, the DRB1*08:03-DQB1*06:01 and DR9 haplotypes confers susceptibility to AITD [19–23], whereas the DR13 and DRB1*15:01-DQB1:06:02 haplotypes confer protection against AITD [7, 23–29]. Taken together, regarding susceptibility and resistance to T1D and AITD, the DR3, DR4, DR7, DR9, and DRB1*15:01-DQB1:06:02 haplotypes have the same effect. On the contrary, DRB1*08:03-DQB1*06:01 and DR13 haplotypes have an adverse effect on these diseases.

In this chapter, we will review HLA class II genes that confer susceptibility and resistance to T1D and AITD, and discuss the relationship between HLA class II genes and T1D, AITD, and APS-3. Furthermore, we focus on amino acids at position 74 of the HLA-DRβ1 chain, position 52 of the HLA-DQα1 chain, and position 57 of the HLA-DQβ1 chain as key factors involved in susceptibility and resistance to T1D and AITD, and we discuss key amino acids and their involvement in susceptibility and resistance to T1D and AITD.

2. Nomenclature

In 1980, Neufeld and Blizzard suggested a classification of APS based on clinical criteria alone, and described four main types [30]. Of the four types, APS-2 and APS-3 are mainly associated with AITD and/or T1D. APS-2 is characterized by Addison's disease (AD) associated with AITD and/or T1D. APS-2 is quite rare with an incidence of 1.4-4.5 cases for every 100,000 individuals [31, 32]. While all patients with APS-2 have AD [30, 32–35], AITD and T1D are reported to occur in 69–82% and 30–52% of patients with APS-2, respectively [30, 34, 35]. APS-3 has been defined as an association between a clinical entity of AITD and an additional autoimmune disease such as T1D (Type 3A), chronic atrophic gastritis, pernicious anemia (Type 3B), vitiligo, alopecia, myasthenia gravis (Type 3C). AD and/or chronic hypoparathyroidism were categorically excluded from APS-3 [30]. Although AITD consists of HT, idiopathic myxedema, asymptomatic thyroiditis, GD, endocrine ophthalmopathy, and pretibial myxedema, GD or HT comprise the majority of AITD. Thus, in discussing the relationship between HLA and T1D and/or AITD, it is necessary to focus on APS type 3A (APS-3A) rather than APS-2 or APS type 3B/3C, and GD or HT may be considered as AITD.

In Caucasian populations, including those in Northern Europe, the incidence rates of T1D are high, in excess of 30 cases/100,000 individuals per year. In contrast, the Japanese population has one of the lowest incidence rate of T1D in the world, at 1.6 cases/100,000 individuals per year, suggesting that the Japanese population may either lack an important susceptibility gene or have a unique T1D protective gene [36, 37]. However, AITD is the most frequent autoimmune disease in the population, present in approximately 7–8% of the general population [38, 39]. When thyroid disease is caused by environmental factors such as levels of iodine, incidence rates have been found to vary between locations and over time [40–43]. Studies regarding the incidence rates of AITD have come from a limited range of geographical areas. Therefore, it is difficult to comment on the absence or presence of variances in incidence rates of AITD between different geographical locations. Coexistence of T1D and AITD is common, with 15 to 30% of T1D subjects having AITD [44–46], whereas the prevalence of glutamic acid decarboxylase antibodies (GADAb) in AITD patients is around 5% [47, 48]. There is a need to distinguish T1D with AITD (T1D+AITD, APS-3A) from T1D without AITD (T1D-AITD). Conversely, we may not need to distinguish AITD with T1D from AITD without T1D (AITD-T1D). Abbreviations are listed in Table 1.

Abbreviations		**AITD**		**T1D**
		GD	**HT**	
AITD-T1D	GD-T1D	+	-	-
	HT-T1D	-	+	-
T1D-AITD		-	-	+
T1D+AITD (APS-3A)	T1D+GD	+	-	+
	T1D+HT	-	+	+

+, present; -, absent

Table 1. Relationship among T1D, AITD, and APS-3A

3. T1D

HLA class II genes are closely related to the onset of T1D in all ethnic groups. Recently, Thomson et al. investigated whether HLA DR-DQ haplotypes and genotypes show the same relative predispositional effects across populations and ethnic groups using data from 38 studies worldwide [49]. They introduced a new static, the patient/control (P/C) ratio of haplotype or genotype frequencies within a study that allows comparison of absolute penetrance values within and across studies. Mean P/C ratios are listed in Table 2. When the mean P/C ratio is >1.10, we consider that the haplotype confers susceptibility to T1D, whereas when the mean P/C ratio is <0.90, we consider that the haplotype confers protection against T1D. When the mean P/C ratio is 0.90–1.10, we consider the haplotype as neutral to T1D.

DRB1	DQB1	Mean P/C ratio	Effect on T1D [a]
*01	*05:01	0.85	P
*03:01	*02	3.72	S
*04	*03:01	0.73	P
*04:01	*03:02	6.23	S
*04:02	*03:02	5.10	S
*04:03	*03:02	0.64	P
*04:05	*03:02	7.15	S
*04:05	*04:01	2.35	S
*04:06	*03:02	0.31	P
*07:01	*02	0.66	P
*08	*03:02	3.25	S
*08	*04:02	1.92	S
*08:03	*06:01	0.38	P
*09:01	*03:03	1.12	S
*12	*03:01	0.47	P
*13	*06:04	0.93	N
*14	*03:01	0.25	P
*15	*06:01	0.46	P
*15	*06:02	0.22	P
*16	*05:02	0.95	N

[a] Effect on T1D is classified as: S, susceptible; N, neutral; P, protective.

Table 2. DRB1-DQB1 haplotype P/C ratios with regard to susceptibility to T1D

4. AITD

The results of HLA association studies in AITD have been less consistent than in T1D. Moreover, data on HLA haplotypes in HT have been less definitive than on those in GD. A general methodological problem has been disease definition [50]; though the diagnosis of GD may be relatively straightforward, the definition of HT has been more controversial. Three varieties of thyroid autoantibodies are commonly used and widely available in clinical diagnostic laboratories: anti-thyroglobulin antibodies (TgAb), anti-thyroid peroxidase autoantibodies (TPOAb), and antibodies to thyrotropin receptor (TRAb). TgAb and TPOAb are found in almost 100% of patients with HT, whereas these antibodies are also detectable in 50% to 90% of patients with GD and are common in the general population. The low levels of TPOAb and TgAb found in many individuals are of uncertain significance in the presence of normal thyroid function [51].

Table 3 shows previous reports on the relationship between HLA class II and AITD. The most probable HLA-DR and -DQ haplotypes were deduced from linkage disequilibria [8–10]. Alleles in parentheses following the reference number indicate that the reference reported susceptibility or resistance of the allele, but not the haplotype, to the disease. There is no parenthesis following the reference number if the references reported susceptibility or resistance with 4-digit DRB1-DQB1, DQA1-DQB1, or DRB1-DQA1-DQB1 haplotypes. In cases with more than 2 haplotypes sharing the same allele, the allele is listed redundantly in each haplotype. However, considering the ethnicities that the references examined, the allele is removed from the corresponding haplotypes; for example, the DRB1*08:02-DQA1*03:01-DQB1*03:02 haplotype is rare in Caucasian populations [49] and thus in the reference examining Caucasian populations, the DQA1*03:01 allele is listed only in the DRB1*04:01-DQA1*03:01-DQB1*03:02 haplotype, and not in the DRB1*08:02-DQA1*03:01-DQB1*03:02 haplotype.

DRB1 DQA1 DQB1	**Effect on GD**[a]		**Effect on HT**[a]		**Effect on AITD-T1D**[a]	
		Ref. no.		**Ref. no.**		
*01:01 *01:01 *05:01	P	24 (DR1), 52 (DR1), 21 (DRB1), 26 (DQB1), 27 (DQB1)	–		–	
*03:01 *05:01 *02:01	S	21 (DRB1), 29 (DRB1), 27 (DQA1)	S	53 (DR3), 7 (DQB1)	S	57 (DQB1)
*04:01 *03:01 *03:02	P	54 (DQB1)	S	6 (DQA1), 7	–	
*04:01 *03:03 *03:01	–		S	6 (DQB1), 55 (DRB1*04-DQB1)	–	
*04:05 *03:01 *03:02	–		S	7 (DRB1), 6 (DQA1)	–	
*04:05 *03:03 *04:01	S	56	–		N	58 (DRB1)
*07:01 *02:01 *02:02	P	21 (DRB1), 29 (DRB1)	P	7 (DRB1*07), 6 (DRB1*07-DQA1-DQB1*02)	–	
*08:02 *03:01 *03:02	S	29 (DRB1)	–		–	
*08:02 *04:01 *04:02	S	29 (DRB1)	S	6 (DRB1*08-DQA1-DQB1*04)	–	
*08:03 *01:03 *06:01	S	20-22	S	23[b]	–	
*09:01 *03:02 *03:03	–		S	22, 23[b]	N	58 (DRB1)
*12:02 *06:01 *03:01	P	21 (DRB1), 54 (DRB1)	–		–	
*13:02 *01:02 *06:04	P	21 (DRB1), 29 (DRB1)	P	7 (DQB1), (DRB1*13-DQA1-DQB1*06), 23[b]	–	
*14:03 *05:01 *03:01	S	29 (DRB1), 20	–		–	
*15:01 *01:02 *06:02	S/P	54 (DRB1) / 27 (DQB1)	P	24 (DR2), 25 (DR2), 6 (DRB1*15-DQA1-DQB1*06), 23[b], 26	–	
*15:02 *01:03 *06:01	–		P	24 (DR2), 25 (DR2), 6 (DRB1*15-DQA1-DQB1*06)	–	
*16:02 *01:02 *05:02	S	54 (DRB1), 21	–		–	

[a] Effect on GD, HT, or AITD-T1D is classified as: S, susceptible; N, neutral; P, protective.

[b] HT-T1D

Table 3. Effects of HLA DR-DQ genes on GD, HT, or AITD

With the exception of the DRB1*15:01-DQA1*01:02-DQB1*06:02 haplotype, there are no controversial results concerning susceptibility and resistance to AITD. Additionally, except for the DRB1*04:01-DQA1*03:01-DQB1*03:02 haplotype, no haplotype has been found to have an adverse effect on GD and HT. Chen et al. demonstrated, for the first time, that the DRB1*15:01 allele confers susceptibility to GD and that the DQB1*03:02 allele confers protection against GD in the Taiwan Chinese population [54]. Further investigations in other ethnic groups may be necessary to confirm whether their conclusions are widely applicable.

5. T1D-AITD and T1D+AITD

Few previous reports have been published on the relationship between HLA class II and T1D-AITD. In contrast, there are a number of reports concerning the relationship between HLA class II and T1D+AITD, which includes T1D+GD and T1D+HT. The results are shown in Table 4. As in Table 3, alleles in parentheses following the reference number indicate that the reference reported susceptibility or resistance of the allele, but not the haplotype, to the disease. There is no parenthesis following the reference number if the references reported the susceptibility or resistance of 4-digit DRB1-DQB1, DQA1-DQB1, or DRB1-DQA1-DQB1 haplotypes to the disease. In cases with more than 2 haplotypes sharing the same allele, the allele is listed redundantly in each haplotype. However, with consideration of the ethnicities that the references examined, the allele may be removed from the corresponding haplotypes.

DRB1	DQA1	DQB1	Effect on T1D-AITD [a]		Effect on T1D+AITD [a]	
				Ref no.		Ref no.
*01:01	*01:01	*05:01	S	59	P	18 (DR1), 63[b] (DQB1*05)
*03:01	*05:01	*02:01	S	57 (DQB1), 60	S	18 (DR3), 57 (DQB1), 60
*04:01	*03:01	*03:02	S	57 (DQB1)	S	18 (DR4), 63[b] (DQB1), 57 (DQB1)
*04:05	*03:01	*03:02	S	60	N	60
*04:05	*03:03	*04:01	S/N	61 (DR4) / 60	S	58 (DRB1), 22, 59, 60
*07:01	*02:01	*02:02	–		N	18 (DR7)
*08:02	*03:01	*03:02	S	61 (DQA1)	S	61[c] (DQA1), 22[c], 59
*08:02	*04:01	*04:02	–		S	22
*08:03	*01:03	*06:01	P	61 (DQA1)	P	61 (DQA1)
*09:01	*03:02	*03:03	S	59	S	62 (DR9), 58 (DRB1), 22, 59
*13:02	*01:02	*06:04	S	59	P	18 (DR6), 60 (DR13)
*15:01	*01:02	*06:02	P	62 (DR2), 57 (DQB1), 59	P	18 (DR2), 62 (DR2), 57 (DQB1), 59
*15:02	*01:03	*06:01	P	62 (DR2), 61 (DQA1)	P	62 (DR2), 61[c] (DQA1)

[a] Effect on T1D-AITD or T1D+AITD is classified as: S, susceptible; N, neutral; P, protective.

[b] T1D+HT; [c] T1D+GD

Table 4. Effects of HLA DR-DQ genes on T1D-AITD and T1D+AITD

6. Relationship between GD and amino acid

Badenhoop et al. demonstrated that Arg at position 52 of the DQα1 chain plays an important role in susceptibility to GD [27]. It was recently shown that Arg at position 74 of the DRβ1 chain is important for the development of GD in a significant number of patients [16, 17]. Further analysis has shown that the presence of Gln at position 74 of the DRβ1 chain was protective for GD [16]. Table 5 shows the susceptibility and resistance of HLA DR-DQ genes to GD, and amino acids at position 74 of the DRβ1 chain and position 52 of the DQα1 chain. When more than 2 references reported susceptibility, we considered that the haplotype confers susceptibility to GD (abbreviated as "S"). When more than 2 references reported protection against the disease, we considered that the haplotype confers protection against GD (abbreviated as "P"). When only one reference reported susceptibility, we considered that the haplotype either confers susceptibility or is neutral to GD (abbreviated as "S/N"). When only one reference reported a protective effect, we considered that the haplotype either confers protection against or is neutral to GD (abbreviated as "P/N"). Badenhoop et al. showed that susceptibility to GD is conferred by the DQA1*05:01 allele as well as Arg at position 52 of the DQα1 chain [27]. DRβ-Arg-74 and DRβ-Gln-74 are always present on DR3 and DR7, respectively [16]. These amino acids are indicated in bold. The amino acids at position 52 of the DQα1 chain that are encoded by the haplotypes listed in Table 5 are Arg, Gln, and Ser. The effect on GD of the haplotypes which encode Arg or Ser at position 52 of the DQα1 chain varies from susceptible to protective. Amino acids at position 74 of the DRβ1 chain that are encoded by the haplotypes listed in Table 5 are Ala, Arg, Gln, and Leu. The effect on GD of these haplotypes also varies from susceptible to protective. However, haplotypes that encode Leu at position 74 of the DRβ1 chain, indicated by italics, are virtually all susceptible to GD. Interestingly, DR3 encodes Arg at both position 52 of the DQα1 chain and position 74 of the DRβ1 chain. Moreover, 3 of 4 haplotypes that encode Leu at position 74 of the DRβ1 chain encode Arg at position 52 of the DQα1 chain. These findings may indicate that amino acids at position 74 of the DRβ1 chain, rather than those at position 52 of the DQα1 chain, play an important role in susceptibility or protection for GD.

7. Relationship between T1D±AITD and amino acid

It is well known that DQα-Arg-52 confer susceptibility to T1D [15]. Todd et al. demonstrated that DQβ-Asp-57 is neutral or negatively associated with T1D, and that Ala, Val, or Ser at position 57 of the DQβ1 chain is positively associated with T1D [13]. Table 6 lists the amino acids at position 52 of the DQα1 chain and position 57 of the DQβ1 chain in each haplotype. Although the effect on T1D of haplotypes with both DQα-Arg-52 and DQβ-Asp-57 is usually protective or neutral, DRB1*04:05-DQA1*03:03-DQB1*04:01 and DRB1*09:01-DQA1*03:02-DQB1*03:03 haplotypes confer susceptibility to T1D. In addition, the effect of some haplotypes with Ala, Val, or Ser at position 57 of the DQβ1 chain on T1D is protective or neutral (DRB1*01:01-DQA1*01:01-DQB1*05:01, DRB1*07:01-DQA1*02:01-DQB1*02:02, DRB1*13:02-DQA1*01:02-DQB1*06:04, and DRB1*16:02-DQA1*01:02-DQB1*05:02). In Table 6, areas of the

DRB1	DQA1	DQB1	Effect on GD [a]	Amino acid at position 52 of DQα1 chain	Amino acid at position 74 of DRβ1 chain
*01:01	*01:01	*05:01	P	Ser	Ala
*03:01	*05:01	*02:01	S	**Arg**	**Arg**
*04:01	*03:01	*03:02	P/N	Arg	Ala
*04:05	*03:03	*04:01	S/N	Arg	Ala
*07:01	*02:01	*02:02	P	Gln	**Gln**
*08:02	*03:01	*03:02	S/N	Arg	*Leu*
*08:02	*04:01	*04:02	S/N	Arg	*Leu*
*08:03	*01:03	*06:01	S	Ser	*Leu*
*12:02	*06:01	*03:01	P	Arg	Ala
*13:02	*01:02	*06:04	P	Ser	Ala
*14:03	*05:01	*03:01	S	**Arg**	*Leu*
*15:01	*01:02	*06:02	S/N, P/N	Ser	Ala
*16:02	*01:02	*05:02	S	Ser	Ala

[a] Effect on GD is classified as: S, susceptible; P, protective; S/N, susceptible or neutral; P/N, protective or neutral.

Table 5. Relationship between effect on GD and amino acids

effect on T1D are shaded in the haplotypes that conflict with the theory that DQα-Arg-52 or "non-Asp" at position 57 of the DQβ1 chain confers susceptibility to T1D, and that DQβ-Asp-57 confers protection against T1D.

Table 6 also shows the effects of HLA DR-DQ genes on AITD, T1D-AITD, and T1D+AITD. When more than 2 references reported susceptibility to the disease, we considered that the haplotype confers susceptibility (abbreviated as "S"), regardless of a single report demonstrating that the haplotype confers protection against the disease. When more than 2 references reported protection against the disease, we considered that the haplotype confers protection (abbreviated as "P"), regardless of one report demonstrating to the disease. When only one reference reported susceptibility, we considered that the haplotype confers susceptibility or is neutral (abbreviated as "S/N"). When only one reference reported protection against the disease, we considered that the haplotype confers protection or is neutral (abbreviated as "P/N"). Recently, Menconi et al. demonstrated that amino acids at position 74 of the DRβ1 chain play an important role in susceptibility and resistance to APS-3A, i.e., T1D+AITD as well as GD [18]. DRβ-Tyr-26, DRβ-Leu-67, DRβ-Lys-71, and DRβ-Arg-74 are positively associated with APS-3A, while DRβ-Ala-71 and DRβ-Gln-74 are negatively associated with APS-3A. These amino acids are indicated in bold in Table 6.

http://dx.doi.org/10.5772/57498

DRB1	DQA1	DQB1	Effect of HLA DR-DQ gene				DQα1	DQβ1	DRβ1			
			AITD[a]	T1D-AITD[a]	T1D[b]	T1D+AITD[a]	52	57	26	67	71	74
*01:01	*01:01	*05:01	P	S/N	P	P	Ser	Val	Leu	**Leu**	Arg	Ala
*03:01	*05:01	*02:01	S	S	S	S	**Arg**	Ala	**Tyr**	**Leu**	**Lys**	**Arg**
*04:01	*03:01	*03:02	S	S/N	S	S	Arg	Ala	Phe	**Leu**	**Lys**	Ala
*04:01	*03:03	*03:01	S	–	P	–	Arg	Asp	Phe	**Leu**	**Lys**	Ala
*04:05	*03:01	*03:02	S	S/N	S	N	Arg	Ala	Phe	**Leu**	Arg	Ala
*04:05	*03:03	*04:01	S/N	S/N	S	S	Arg	Asp	Phe	**Leu**	Arg	Ala
*07:01	*02:01	*02:02	P	–	P	N	Gln	Ala	Phe	Ile	Arg	**Gln**
*08:02	*03:01	*03:02	S/N	S/N	S	S	Arg	Ala	Phe	Phe	Arg	Leu
*08:02	*04:01	*04:02	S	–	N	S/N	Arg	Asp	Phe	Phe	Arg	Leu
*08:03	*01:03	*06:01	S	P/N	P	P/N	Ser	Asp	Phe	Ile	Arg	Leu
*09:01	*03:02	*03:03	S	S/N	S	S	Arg	Asp	**Tyr**	Phe	Arg	Glu
*12:02	*06:01	*03:01	P	–	P	–	Arg	Asp	Leu	Phe	Arg	Ala
*13:02	*01:02	*06:04	P	S/N	N	P	Ser	Val	Phe	Ile	Glu	Ala
*14:03	*05:01	*03:01	S	–	P	–	Arg	Asp	Phe	**Leu**	Arg	Leu
*15:01	*01:02	*06:02	P	P	P	P	Ser	**Asp**	Phe	Ile	**Ala**	Ala
*15:02	*01:03	*06:01	P	P	P	P	Ser	Asp	Phe	Ile	**Ala**	Ala
*16:02	*01:02	*05:02	S	–	N	–	Ser	Ser	Phe	**Leu**	Arg	Ala

[a] Effect on AITD, T1D-AITD, or T1D+AITD is classified as: S, susceptible; P, protective; S/N, susceptible or neutral; P/N, protective or neutral.

[b] Effect on T1D is classified as: S, susceptible; N, neutral; P, protective.

Table 6. Effects of HLA DR-DQ genes on AITD, T1D-AITD, T1D, or T1D+AITD

In this section, we discuss the relationship between the above-mentioned HLA DR-DQ genes, amino acids at positions 26, 67, 71, and 74 of the DRβ1 chain, and T1D with or without AITD.

*DRB1*01:01-DQA1*01:01-DQB1*05:01 and DRB1*13:02-DQA1*01:02-DQB1*06:04 haplotypes*

While these haplotypes encode Val at position 57 of the DQβ1 chain, they confer protection or are neutral to T1D. Although they confer protection against AITD and T1D+AITD, they tend to confer susceptibility to T1D-AITD (S/N in Table 6). Since 15 to 30% of subjects with T1D have AITD [44–46], the effect of AITD on T1D may result in resistance of subjects with these haplotypes to T1D.

*DRB1*04:05-DQA1*03:03-DQB1*04:01 and DRB1*09:01-DQA1*03:02-DQB1*03:03 haplotypes*

These haplotypes are the major haplotypes which confer susceptibility to T1D in East Asians, especially in the Japanese population where the DR3 haplotype is absent and the DR4 haplotype is rare [8–10]. While these haplotypes encode Asp at position 57 of the DQβ1 chain, they confer susceptibility to T1D+AITD. DRβ-Leu-67 in the DRB1*04:05-DQA1*03:03-DQB1*04:01 haplotype and DRβ-Tyr-26 in the DRB1*09:01-DQA1*03:02-DQB1*03:03 haplotype might play an important role in susceptibility to T1D+AITD. Since 15 to 30% of subjects with T1D have AITD [44–46], the effect of these amino acids on T1D may be susceptibility, and that on T1D-AITD might be susceptibility or neutrality, which is weaker than that on T1D or T1D+AITD.

*DRB1*07:01-DQA1*02:01-DQB1*02:02 and DRB1*16:02-DQA1*01:02-DQB1*05:02 haplotypes*

There are few reports concerning the effect of HLA DR-DQ genes on T1D-AITD in the Caucasian [57], Japanese [59, 61, 62], and Taiwan Chinese [60] populations (Table 4). The DRB1*07:01-DQA1*02:01-DQB1*02:02 and DRB1*16:02-DQA1*01:02-DQB1*05:02 haplotypes are rare in the Japanese population [8–10, 49]. Therefore, it is difficult to explain the protective or neutral effect of these haplotypes with "non-Asp" at position 57 of the DQβ1 chain on T1D by examining the effect of these haplotypes on T1D-AITD. However, Menconi et al. demonstrated that DRβ-Gln-74 is negatively associated with T1D+AITD, although they failed to demonstrate that the DR7 allele, which encodes Gln at position 74 of the DRβ1 chain, confers protection against T1D+AITD [18] (Table 6). The DR3 and DR4 haplotypes encode Ala at position 57 of the DQβ1 chain, which confers strong susceptibility to T1D [2]. Since the DR7 haplotype also encodes Ala at position 57 of the DQβ1 chain, the effect of this haplotype might potentially result in susceptibility to T1D-AITD. Since 15 to 30% of subjects with T1D have AITD [44–46], DRβ-Gln-74 might play a role in protection against T1D.

There are several reports concerning the effect of HLA DR-DQ genes on T1D+AITD, which also studied Caucasian [18, 57, 63], Japanese [22, 58, 59, 61, 62], and Taiwan Chinese [60] populations (Table 4). The DRB1*16:02-DQA1*01:02-DQB1*05:02 haplotype is rare in the Caucasian population as well as in the Japanese population [49], and Menconi et al. did not examine patients and controls with the DR16 allele [18]. Moreover, the positive effect of DQβ-Ser-57 on T1D is weaker than that of DQβ-Ala-57 or DQβ-Val-57 [2]. To our knowledge, the evidence of the effect of the DRB1*16:02-DQA1*01:02-DQB1*05:02 haplotype on T1D is insufficient.

8. Conclusion

T1D and AITD share common genetic risk factors. The prevalence of given HLA haplotypes varies among populations, but given the same DR and DQ haplotypes, the influence of HLA on T1D and/or AITD is similar on populations throughout the world. By clarifying the region of the diseases on which certain reports were focused, we can explain to some extent and speculate on the relationship between HLA haplotypes, specific amino acids, and T1D and/or AITD.

http://dx.doi.org/10.5772/57498

Author details

Masahito Katahira*

Address all correspondence to: katahira-0034@umin.net

Department of Endocrinology and Diabetes, Ichinomiya Municipal Hospital, Aichi, Japan

References

[1] Betterle C, Zanchetta R. Update on autoimmune polyendocrine syndromes (APS). Acta Biomed 2003;74(1) 9-33.

[2] She JX. Susceptibility to type I diabetes: HLA-DQ and DR revisited. Immunol Today 1996;17(7) 323-329.

[3] Baisch JM, Weeks T, Giles R, Hoover M, Stastny P, Capra JD. Analysis of HLA-DQ genotypes and susceptibility in insulin-dependent diabetes mellitus. N Engl J Med 1990;322(26) 1836-1841.

[4] Mangklabruks A, Cox N, DeGroot LJ. Genetic factors in autoimmune thyroid disease analyzed by restriction fragment length polymorphisms of candidate genes. J Clin Endocrinol Metab 1991;73(2) 236-244.

[5] Heward JM, Allahabadia A, Daykin J, Carr-Smith J, Daly A, Armitage M, Dodson PM, Sheppard MC, Barnett AH, Franklyn JA, Gough SC. Linkage disequilibrium between the human leukocyte antigen class II region of the major histocompatibility complex and Graves' disease: replication using a population case control and family-based study. J Clin Endocrinol Metab 1998;83(10) 3394-3397.

[6] Zeitlin AA, Heward JM, Newby PR, Carr-Smith JD, Franklyn JA, Gough SC, Simmonds MJ. Analysis of HLA class II genes in Hashimoto's thyroiditis reveals differences compared to Graves' disease. Genes Immun 2008;9(4) 358-363.

[7] Kokaraki G, Daniilidis M, Yiangou M, Arsenakis M, Karyotis N, Tsilipakou M, Fleva A, Gerofotis A, Karadani N, Yovos JG. Major histocompatibility complex class II (DRB1*, DQA1*, and DQB1*) and DRB1*04 subtypes' associations of Hashimoto's thyroiditis in a Greek population. Tissue Antigens 2009;73(3) 199-205.

[8] Nakajima F, Nakamura J, Yokota T. Analysis of HLA haplotypes in Japanese, using high resolution allele typing. MHC 2001;8(1) 1-32 [in Japanese].

[9] Katahira M, Segawa S, Maeda H, Yasuda Y. Effect of human leukocyte antigen class II genes on acute-onset and slow-onset type 1 diabetes in the Japanese population. Hum Immunol 2010;71(8) 789-794.

[10] Yasunaga S, Kimura A, Hamaguchi K, Rønningen KS, Sasazuki T. Different contribution of HLA-DR and -DQ genes in susceptibility and resistance to insulin-dependent diabetes mellitus (IDDM). Tissue Antigens. 1996;47(1) 37-48.

[11] Sanjeevi CB, Lybrand TP, DeWeese C, Landin-Olsson M, Kockum I, Dahlquist G, Sundkvist G, Stenger D, Lernmark Å. Polymorphic amino acid variations in HLA-DQ are associated with systematic physical property changes and occurrence of IDDM. Members of the Swedish Childhood Diabetes Study. Diabetes 1995;44(1) 125-131.

[12] Rønningen KS, Spurkland A, Iwe T, Vartdal F, Thorsby E. Distribution of HLA-DRB1, -DQA1 and -DQB1 alleles and DQA1-DQB1 genotypes among Norwegian patients with insulin-dependent diabetes mellitus. Tissue Antigens 1991;37(3) 105-111.

[13] Todd JA, Bell JI, McDevitt HO. HLA-DQβ gene contributes to susceptibility and resistance to insulin-dependent diabetes mellitus. Nature 1987;329(6140) 599-604.

[14] Nepom BS, Palmer J, Kim SJ, Hansen JA, Holbeck SL, Nepom GT. Specific genomic markers for the HLA-DQ subregion discriminate between DR4+ insulin-dependent diabetes mellitus and DR4+ seropositive juvenile rheumatoid arthritis. J Exp Med 1986;164(1) 345-350.

[15] Khalil I, Deschamps I, Lepage V, al-Daccak R, Degos L, Hors J. Dose effect of cis- and trans-encoded HLA-DQαβ heterodimers in IDDM susceptibility. Diabetes. 1992;41(3) 378-84.

[16] Ban Y, Davies TF, Greenberg DA, Concepcion ES, Osman R, Oashi T, Tomer Y. Arginine at position 74 of the HLA-DRβ1 chain is associated with Graves' disease. Genes Immun 2004;5(3) 203-208.

[17] Simmonds MJ, Howson JM, Heward JM, Cordell HJ, Foxall H, Carr-Smith J, Gibson SM, Walker N, Tomer Y, Franklyn JA, Todd JA, Gough SC. Regression mapping of association between the human leukocyte antigen region and Graves disease. Am J Hum Genet 2005;76(1) 157-163.

[18] Menconi F, Osman R, Monti MC, Greenberg DA, Concepcion ES, Tomer Y. Shared molecular amino acid signature in the HLA-DR peptide binding pocket predisposes to both autoimmune diabetes and thyroiditis. Proc Natl Acad Sci USA 2010;107(39) 16899-16903.

[19] Katahira M, Ishiguro T, Segawa S, Kuzuya-Nagao K, Hara I, Nishisaki T. Reevaluation of human leukocyte antigen DR-DQ haplotype and genotype in type 1 diabetes in the Japanese population. Horm Res 2008;69(5) 284-289.

[20] Katsuren E, Awata T, Matsumoto C, Yamamoto K. HLA class II alleles in Japanese patients with Graves' disease: weak associations of HLA-DR and -DQ. Endocr J 1994;41(6) 599-603.

[21] Park MH, Park YJ, Song EY, Park H, Kim TY, Park DJ, Park KS, Cho BY. Association of HLA-DR and -DQ genes with Graves disease in Koreans. Hum Immunol 2005;66(6) 741-747.

[22] Hashimoto K, Maruyama H, Nishiyama M, Asaba K, Ikeda Y, Takao T, Iwasaki Y, Kumon Y, Suehiro T, Tanimoto N, Mizobuchi M, Nakamura T. Susceptibility alleles and haplotypes of human leukocyte antigen DRB1, DQA1, and DQB1 in autoimmune polyglandular syndrome type III in Japanese population. Horm Res 2005;64(5) 253-260.

[23] Katahira M, Hanakita M, Ito T, Suzuki M. Effect of human leukocyte antigen class II genes on Hashimoto's thyroiditis requiring replacement therapy with levothyroxine in the Japanese population. Hum Immunol 2013;74(5) 607-609.

[24] Azuma Y, Sakurami T, Ueno Y, Ohishi M, Saji H, Terasaki PI, Park MS. HLA-DR antigens in Japanese with Hashimoto's thyroiditis and Graves' disease. Endocrinol Jpn 1982;29(4) 423-427.

[25] Sakurami T, Ueno Y, Iwaki Y, Park MS, Terasaki PI, Saji H. HLA-DR specificities among Japanese with several autoimmune diseases. Tissue Antigens 1982;19(2) 129-133.

[26] Tamai H, Kimura A, Dong RP, Matsubayashi S, Kuma K, Nagataki S, Sasazuki T. Resistance to autoimmune thyroid disease is associated with HLA-DQ. J Clin Endocrinol Metab 1994;78(1) 94-97.

[27] Badenhoop K, Walfish PG, Rau H, Fischer S, Nicolay A, Bogner U, Schleusener H, Usadel KH. Susceptibility and resistance alleles of human leukocyte antigen (HLA) DQA1 and HLA DQB1 are shared in endocrine autoimmune disease. J Clin Endocrinol Metab 1995;80(7) 2112-2117.

[28] Zeitlin AA, Heward JM, Newby PR, Carr-Smith JD, Franklyn JA, Gough SC, Simmonds MJ. Analysis of HLA class II genes in Hashimoto's thyroiditis reveals differences compared to Graves' disease. Genes Immun 2008;9(4) 358-363.

[29] Jang HW, Shin HW, Cho HJ, Kim HK, Lee JI, Kim SW, Kim JW, Chung JH. Identification of HLA-DRB1 alleles associated with Graves' disease in Koreans by sequence-based typing. Immunol Invest 2011;40(2) 172-182.

[30] Neufeld M, Blizzard RM. Polyglandular autoimmune diseases. In: Pinchera A, Doniach D, Fenzi GF, Baschieri L. (ed) Symposium on Autoimmune Aspects of Endocrine Disorders. New York: Academic Press; 1980. p357-365.

[31] Chen QY, Kukreja A, Maclaren NK. The autoimmune polyglandular syndromes. In: De Groot LJ, Jameson JL. (ed) Endocrinology 4th Edition. Philadelphia: Saunders; 2001. p587-599.

[32] Betterle C, Volpato M, Greggio AN, Presotto F. Type 2 polyglandular autoimmune disease (Schmidt's syndrome). J Pediatr Endocrinol Metab 1996;9(Suppl 1) 113-123.

[33] Neufeld M, Maclaren NK, Blizzard RM. Two types of autoimmune Addison's disease associated with different polyglandular autoimmune (PGA) syndromes. Medicine (Baltimore) 1981;60(5) 355-362.

[34] Betterle C, Dal Pra C, Mantero F, Zanchetta R. Autoimmune adrenal insufficiency and autoimmune polyendocrine syndromes: autoantibodies, autoantigens, and their applicability in diagnosis and disease prediction. Endocr Rev 2002;23(3) 327-64.

[35] Papadopoulos KI, Hallengren B. Polyglandular autoimmune syndrome type II in patients with idiopathic Addison's disease. Acta Endocrinol (Copenh) 1990;122(4) 472-478.

[36] Tuomilehto J, Virtala E, Karvonen M, Lounamaa R, Pitkäniemi J, Reunanen A, Tuomilehto-Wolf E, Toivanen L. Increase in incidence of insulin-dependent diabetes mellitus among children in Finland. Int J Epidemiol 1995;24(5) 984-992.

[37] Matsuura N, Fukuda K, Okuno A, Harada S, Fukushima N, Koike A, Ito Y, Hotsubo T. Descriptive epidemiology of IDDM in Hokkaido, Japan: the Childhood IDDM Hokkaido Registry. Diabetes Care 1998;21(10) 1632-1636.

[38] Dayan CM, Daniels GH. Chronic autoimmune thyroiditis. N Engl J Med 1996;335(2) 99-107.

[39] Weetman AP. Graves' disease. N Engl J Med. 2000;343(17) 1236-1248.

[40] Perros P, McCrimmon RJ, Shaw G, Frier BM. Frequency of thyroid dysfunction in diabetic patients: value of annual screening. Diabet Med 1995;12(7) 622-627.

[41] Bürgi H, Kohler M, Morselli B. Thyrotoxicosis incidence in Switzerland and benefit of improved iodine supply. Lancet 1998;352(9133) 1034.

[42] Lewiński A, Szybiński Z, Bandurska-Stankiewicz E, Grzywa M, Karwowska A, Kinalska I, Kowalska A, Makarewicz J, Nauman J, Słowińska-Klencka D, Sowiński J, Syrenicz A, Zonenberg A, Huszno B, Klencki M. Iodine-induced hyperthyroidism--an epidemiological survey several years after institution of iodine prophylaxis in Poland. J Endocrinol Invest 2003;26(2 Suppl) 57-62.

[43] Laurberg P, Pedersen KM, Vestergaard H, Sigurdsson G. High incidence of multinodular toxic goitre in the elderly population in a low iodine intake area vs. high incidence of Graves' disease in the young in a high iodine intake area: comparative surveys of thyrotoxicosis epidemiology in East-Jutland Denmark and Iceland. J Intern Med 1991;229(5) 415-420.

[44] Stanbury JB, Ermans AE, Bourdoux P, Todd C, Oken E, Tonglet R, Vidor G, Braverman LE, Medeiros-Neto G. Iodine-induced hyperthyroidism: occurrence and epidemiology. Thyroid 1998;8(1) 83-100.

[45] Umpierrez GE, Latif KA, Murphy MB, Lambeth HC, Stentz F, Bush A, Kitabchi AE. Thyroid dysfunction in patients with type 1 diabetes: a longitudinal study. Diabetes Care 2003;26(4) 1181-1185.

[46] Barker JM, Yu J, Yu L, Wang J, Miao D, Bao F, Hoffenberg E, Nelson JC, Gottlieb PA, Rewers M, Eisenbarth GS. Autoantibody "subspecificity" in type 1 diabetes: risk for organ-specific autoimmunity clusters in distinct groups. Diabetes Care 2005;28(4) 850-855.

[47] Aksoy DY, Yürekli BP, Yildiz BO, Gedik O. Prevalence of glutamic acid decarboxylase antibody positivity and its association with insulin secretion and sensitivity in autoimmune thyroid disease: A pilot study. Exp Clin Endocrinol Diabetes 2006;114(8) 412-416.

[48] Moriguchi M, Noso S, Kawabata Y, Yamauchi T, Harada T, Komaki K, Babaya N, Hiromine Y, Ito H, Yamagata S, Murata K, Higashimoto T, Park C, Yamamoto A, Ohno Y, Ikegami H. Clinical and genetic characteristics of patients with autoimmune thyroid disease with anti-islet autoimmunity. Metabolism 2011;60(6) 761-766.

[49] Thomson G, Valdes AM, Noble JA, Kockum I, Grote MN, Najman J, Erlich HA, Cucca F, Pugliese A, Steenkiste A, Dorman JS, Caillat-Zucman S, Hermann R, Ilonen J, Lambert AP, Bingley PJ, Gillespie KM, Lernmark A, Sanjeevi CB, Rønningen KS, Undlien DE, Thorsby E, Petrone A, Buzzetti R, Koeleman BP, Roep BO, Saruhan-Direskeneli G, Uyar FA, Günoz H, Gorodezky C, Alaez C, Boehm BO, Mlynarski W, Ikegami H, Berrino M, Fasano ME, Dametto E, Israel S, Brautbar C, Santiago-Cortes A, Frazer de Llado T, She JX, Bugawan TL, Rotter JI, Raffel L, Zeidler A, Leyva-Cobian F, Hawkins BR, Chan SH, Castano L, Pociot F, Nerup J. Relative predispositional effects of HLA class II DRB1-DQB1 haplotypes and genotypes on type 1 diabetes: a meta-analysis. Tissue Antigens 2007;70(2) 110-127.

[50] Jacobson EM, Huber A, Tomer Y. The HLA gene complex in thyroid autoimmunity: from epidemiology to etiology. J Autoimmun 2008;30(1-2) 58-62.

[51] Salvatore D, Davies TF, Schlumberger MJ, Hay ID, Larsen PR. Thyroid physiology and diagnostic evaluation of patients with thyroid disorders. In: Melmed S, Polonsky KS, Larsen PR, Kronenberg HM. (ed.) Williams textbook of endocrinology. 12th ed. Philadelphia: Elsevier Saunders; 2011. p327-361.

[52] Dong RP, Kimura A, Okubo R, Shinagawa H, Tamai H, Nishimura Y, Sasazuki T. HLA-A and DPB1 loci confer susceptibility to Graves' disease. Hum Immunol 1992;35(3) 165-172.

[53] Tandon N, Zhang L, Weetman AP. HLA associations with Hashimoto's thyroiditis. Clin Endocrinol (Oxf) 1991;34(5) 383-386.

[54] Chen PL, Fann CS, Chu CC, Chang CC, Chang SW, Hsieh HY, Lin M, Yang WS, Chang TC. Comprehensive genotyping in two homogeneous Graves' disease samples reveals major and novel HLA association alleles. PLoS One 2011;6(1) e16635.

[55] Petrone A, Giorgi G, Mesturino CA, Capizzi M, Cascino I, Nistico L, Osborn J, Di Mario U, Buzzetti R. Association of DRB1*04-DQB1*0301 haplotype and lack of association of two polymorphic sites at CTLA-4 gene with Hashimoto's thyroiditis in an Italian population. Thyroid 2001;11(2) 171-175.

[56] Iwama S, Ikezaki A, Kikuoka N, Kim HS, Matsuoka H, Yanagawa T, Sato H, Hoshi M, Sakamaki T, Sugihara S. Association of HLA-DR, -DQ genotype and CTLA-4 gene polymorphism with Graves' disease in Japanese children. Horm Res 2005;63(2) 55-60.

[57] Santamaria P, Barbosa JJ, Lindstrom AL, Lemke TA, Goetz FC, Rich SS. HLA-DQB1-associated susceptibility that distinguishes Hashimoto's thyroiditis from Graves' disease in type I diabetic patients. J Clin Endocrinol Metab 1994;78(4) 878-883.

[58] Ikegami H, Awata T, Kawasaki E, Kobayashi T, Maruyama T, Nakanishi K, Shimada A, Amemiya S, Kawabata Y, Kurihara S, Tanaka S, Kanazawa Y, Mochizuki M, Ogihara T. The association of CTLA4 polymorphism with type 1 diabetes is concentrated in patients complicated with autoimmune thyroid disease: a multicenter collaborative study in Japan. J Clin Endocrinol Metab 2006;91(3) 1087-1092.

[59] Katahira M, Maeda H, Tosaki T, Segawa S. The human leukocyte antigen class II gene has different contributions to autoimmune type 1 diabetes with or without autoimmune thyroid disease in the Japanese population. Diabetes Res Clin Pract 2009;85(3) 293-297.

[60] Chuang LM, Wu HP, Chang CC, Tsai WY, Chang HM, Tai TY, Lin BJ. HLA DRB1/DQA1/DQB1 haplotype determines thyroid autoimmunity in patients with insulin-dependent diabetes mellitus. Clin Endocrinol (Oxf) 1996;45(5) 631-636.

[61] Chikuba N, Akazawa S, Yamaguchi Y, Kawasaki E, Takino H, Yoshimoto M, Ohe N, Yamashita K, Yano A, Nagataki S. Immunogenetic heterogeneity in type 1 (insulin-dependent) diabetes among Japanese--class II antigen and autoimmune thyroid disease. Diabetes Res Clin Pract 1995;27(1) 31-37.

[62] Chikuba N, Akazawa S, Yamaguchi Y, Kawasaki E, Takino H, Takao Y, Maeda Y, Okuno S, Yamamoto H, Yokota A, Yoshimoto M, Nagataki S. Type 1 (insulin-dependent) diabetes mellitus with coexisting autoimmune thyroid disease in Japan. Intern Med 1992;31(9) 1076-1080.

[63] Sumník Z, Drevínek P, Snajderová M, Kolousková S, Sedláková P, Pechová M, Vavrinec J, Cinek O. HLA-DQ polymorphisms modify the risk of thyroid autoimmunity in children with type 1 diabetes mellitus. J Pediatr Endocrinol Metab 2003;16(6) 851-858.

Chapter 7

Functional Implications of MHC Associations in Autoimmune Diseases with Special Reference to Type1 Diabetes, Vitiligo and Hypoparathyroidism

Rajni Rani and Archana Singh

Additional information is available at the end of the chapter

http://dx.doi.org/10.5772/57494

1. Introduction

Immune cells get educated in the thymus during development to recognize self antigens so that there are no immune responses against self antigens. However, whenever they encounter non-self antigens like bacteria or viruses, they are recognized as non-self and immune response takes place against them to save us from infections. While the basic purpose of the immune response is to save us from infections, something goes awry in some cases such that the self antigens are recognized as foreign by one's own immune cells which attack the cells /organs containing those antigens presuming them to be foreign. This results in auto-immune disorders like Type 1 diabetes, vitiligo or hypoparathyroidism, the focus for the present chapter. All these disorders are complex, multi-factorial, organ specific disorders where auto-immune responses have been implicated due to presence of auto-antibodies and auto-antigen specific T cells in the peripheral circulation of the patients. Although what triggers the autoimmune responses in these disorders is not clearly understood, association with certain major histocompatibility complex (MHC) alleles has been considered a hallmark of autoimmune disorders [1] since they have a role in antigen presentation that orchestrates the antigen specific adaptive immune responses.

Major Histocompatibility Complex (MHC) is a set of glycoprotein molecules present on the cell surface of nucleated cells encoded by several polymorphic genes localized on chromosome 6 of man. In human, MHC is known as Human leukocyte Antigens (HLA). MHC region is spread over 3.84 megabases of chromosome 6p21.3 and is the most gene dense region of the human genome with 224 genes. 128 of these 224 genes are known to be expressed. And 40 % of these genes have immune related functions [2]. HLA constitutes a small part of the MHC region. Major function of HLA molecules is to present antigenic peptides to T cells. HLA can be broadly classified into two major classes: class-I and class-II. HLA class-I genes are HLA-A, -B and –C. These are classical class-I genes which are very polymorphic with 2365, 3005 and 1848 alleles respectively.

The MHC class-I molecules are present on the surface of all nucleated cells and present antigenic peptides to the $CD8^+$ cytotoxic T cells. MHC class-I molecule is a hetero-dimer of a heavy and a light chain. The molecular weight of the heavy alpha chain is about 40-45 KDa and that of the light chain, beta 2 microglobulin (β_2m) is 12 KDa [3]. The genes for the alpha chains are encoded on chromosome 6. However, the gene for β_2m is encoded on human chromosome 15. The heavy chain of the MHC class-I molecule has three domains alpha 1 (α1), alpha 2 (α2) and alpha 3 (α3). Alpha 1 (α1) and alpha 2 (α2) domains are the most polymorphic domains since they constitute the peptide binding groove of the MHC molecule. These polymorphic domains are encoded by exons 2 and 3 of the genes encoding MHC class-I alpha chain which has in total 8 exons. The peptides that are presented by the MHC molecules have allele specific motifs i.e., certain peptides can be presented by certain MHC molecules. The affinity of the peptide to bind to the peptide binding groove is determined by the anchors present on the peptide binding groove where the peptides go and bind through hydrogen bonds. Specific motifs or the amino acid residues present in the pockets of the peptide binding grove which are involved in binding the side chains of complimentary residues of the peptide determine which peptides would bind to which MHC molecule [4, 5]. Pockets B (key residues at positions 9, 45, 63, 67, 70 and 99) and F (key residues at positions 77, 80, 81 and 116) of alpha chain are the main anchors which engage the peptides at their amino acid positions 2 and the C-terminus [6]. However, several alleles of the MHC share peptide binding specificities i.e. similar peptides may be presented by different MHC molecules. These alleles are clustered in supertypes [6].

HLA class-II molecules are expressed on antigen presenting cells like macrophages, dendritic cells, B cells, thymic epithelium and activated T cells [7]. MHC class-II molecules present antigenic peptides to the $CD4^+$ T helper cells (Th cells) which in turn initiate a cascade of immunological events that result in activation of $CD8^+$ cytotoxic T cells and B lymphocytes [2]. $CD4^+$ T helper cells get activated when a non-self antigen is presented to them. T helper cells are of two types T helper 1 (Th1) and Th2. Th1 cells secrete cytokines like Interferon gamma and TNF-alpha which are involved in cell-mediated immune responses as they activate the cytotoxic T cells which have already seen the antigen in the context of MHC class-I. Th2 cells, on the other hand, secrete IL-4, IL-5 and/or IL-6 which are involved in humoral immunity as they activate the B cells to become plasma cells which make the antibodies against antigen they have seen. Thus an immune response takes place which varies in strength depending on the host factors and the peptides being presented.

The classical MHC class-II glycoproteins in humans are HLA-DR, -DP and –DQ. The MHC class-II molecule is a heterodimer of two polypeptide chains: an alpha (25-33 KDa) and a beta chain (24-29KDa) [8, 9]. Unlike MHC class-I, both alpha and beta chains of the class-II molecule are encoded on chromosome 6. DRB1 gene encodes DR beta chain while DRA1 encodes DR alpha chain with 1355 DRB1 alleles and 7 DRA1 alleles. Similarly DQB1 and DPB1 encode beta chains of DQ and DP molecules with 416 and 190 alleles respectively and DQA1 and DPA1 encode the alpha chains of DQ and DP molecules with 51 and 37 alleles respectively [10, 11].

Besides the classical class-I and class-II genes there are several non-classical HLA genes with specialized functions and also pseudo HLA genes present in the MHC region. However, they will not be discussed here since their roles are not very clearly understood in autoimmunity.

A recurring theme of several autoimmune disorders is the aberrant presentation of self antigens to the immune system that triggers downstream perturbations. Under normal circumstances most of the MHC molecules are occupied by self peptides and the T cells are tolerized against them during thymic education so that auto-immune responses do not take place, however, sometimes there is a break in the tolerance resulting in recognition of self as non-self by the immune system which results in an auto-immune response. This break in tolerance could be due to low expression of some antigens in the thymus which may result in self-reactive T cells to reach the peripheral circulation. Or it could be due to escape of self-reactive T cells from clonal deletion during T cell development. Since associations with MHC alleles have been considered a hallmark of autoimmune disorders due to their role in antigen presentation, we have studied HLA alleles in two common and one rare autoimmune disorders: Type1 diabetes, vitiligo and hypoparathyroidism.

2. Patients and controls

DNAs were extracted using standard protocol from 10 ml of blood from type 1 diabetes (N=211), vitiligo (N=1404), hypoparathyroidism patients (N=134) and 902 normal healthy controls from the same ethnic background after obtaining informed consent. All the patients attending diabetes of young clinic were carefully assessed and categorized as type 1, type 2 and fibrocalculous pancreatopathy as per the recent classification by American Diabetes Association expert committee [12, 13]. All of the T1D subjects included in the study required insulin for glycemic control and 51 of them had history of ketosis at presentation. Insulin requiring patients with fibrocalculous pancreatopathy and subjects with diabetes in whom glycemic control was achieved with diet and oral hypoglycemic agent were excluded from the study [12, 14].

Vitiligo group consisted of 1404 North Indian patients enrolled at Dr. Ram Manohar Lohia Hospital (RMLH), and All India Institute of Medical Sciences (AIIMS), New Delhi Diagnosis of vitiligo was based on clinical examination done by dermatologists. Clinically, the cases were classified as having Generalized (Vulgaris, Acrofacial, Universalis) or Localized (Focal, Acral, mucosal and segmental) forms of vitiligo. The replication study was done on 355 vitiligo cases from Gujarat, a state in west of India [15].

Idiopathic hypoparathyroidism group consisted of 134 unrelated patients who attended the endocrine clinics of All India Institute of Medical Sciences during 1998-2011. The diagnosis of IH was based on presence of hypocalcemia, hyperphosphatemia, low serum intact PTH, normal renal function and serum magnesium levels. Patients with post surgical hypoparathyroidism were not included. Patients with clinical features of APECED syndrome indicated by mucocutaneous candidiasis or presence of adrenocortical autoantibody were excluded from the study[16].

Nine hundred and two ethnically matched unaffected controls from North India were used for all three studies and 441 ethnically matched unaffected controls from Gujarat were studied in the replication study for vitiligo only. None of the unaffected controls had personal or family history of T1D, vitiligo, hypoparathyroidism or any other autoimmune or infectious disease.

All Cases and control samples were collected after obtaining informed consent and Institutional Human Ethics Committee's clearance from all the institutes/Hospitals involved, following declaration of Helsinki protocols.

3. Study of *HLA-A, HLA-B* and *HLA–DRB1* alleles

DNA extraction was carried out by standard procedures from fresh whole blood samples collected in anticoagulant EDTA. Alleles of *HLA-A, HLA-B* and *HLA-DRB1* were studied using Polymerase chain reaction followed by hybridization with sequence specific oligonucleotide probes (SSOPs) as described earlier [17] using a bead-based technology (Luminex, Austin, Tx) following Manufacturer's instructions (Labtype SSO kit from One Lambda, Canoga Park, USA). The latest nomenclature for the *HLA* system was used to designate the alleles of the three loci studied [18].

4. Statistical analysis

Frequencies of alleles in the patient samples were compared with their respective unaffected controls using Chi-square analysis and the strength of associations was estimated by odds ratio (OR) and 95% confidence interval using Stata 9.2 statistical program. Fisher's exact test was used when the numbers were five or less in any group i.e. in cases or controls for any allele. In such cases, Odds ratios were calculated using Woolf's method [19] with Haldane's [20] modification as described earlier [21].

5. Type 1 diabetes

Type 1 diabetes (T1D) is an incurable, multi-factorial and complex autoimmune disorder characterized by the loss of insulin producing beta cells of the pancreas. This results in abnormal metabolism of glucose that may be detrimental for several other complications like ketoacidosis, retinopathy, nephropathy and even cardio-vascular diseases and pre-mature deaths [22]. World-wide disease affects 1 in 300-400 children [23]. The incidence in South India has been reported to be 10.5/100,000/year [24]. In North India, a higher prevalence in urban

(26.6/100,000) as compared to rural areas (4.27/100,000) has been reported with a total prevalence of 10.20/100,000. T1D develops as a result of complex interaction of many genetic and environmental factors leading to autoimmune destruction of the insulin producing Pancreatic Beta cells. While 20 genomic intervals have been implicated for the manifestation of the disease [22], role of an intricate network of the products of these genes cannot be ruled out. However, unraveling different factors involved and how they interact in integrated networks is like solving a zig-saw puzzle which is the aim of our studies [12, 14, 17]. However, in this chapter we will be concentrating on MHC associations and their implications only.

When the patients report to the clinician, he is left with no option but to give daily insulin injections since most of their pancreatic beta cells are already destroyed. So, if we want to stop autoimmune responses in the people who are predisposed to get T1D, we need to identify the prediabetics before the onset of the disease and device ways to inhibit autoimmunity in them. This is possible by using genetic predisposition criteria to get the disease.

We have studied the frequencies of MHC class-I alleles for HLA-B locus and MHC class-II alleles for HLA-DRB1 and DQB1 loci in patients with Type 1 diabetes and normal healthy controls using polymerase chain reaction followed by hybridization with sequence specific oligonucleotide probes (PCR-SSOP). DNAs were isolated from peripheral blood mononuclear cells (PBMCs) from patients and healthy controls using standard protocol. The second and third exons of the HLA-B gene and second exons of HLA-DRB1 and DQB1 genes were amplified using PCR and hybridized with oligonucleotide probes and the hybridization pattern with different probes was used to identify the alleles present in a sample. The results showed that *HLA-B*08* ($p<7.8X10^{-13}$, Odds Ratio (OR) = 3.3), *HLA-B*50* ($p< 4.2 X 10^{-21}$, OR= 7.5), *HLA-B*58* ($p< 3.3 X 10^{-6}$, OR= 2.6), *HLA- DRB1*03:01* ($p<1.7x10^{-35}$, OR= 13.2), *DRB1*04:01* ($p<0.00001$, OR= 5.4), *and DRB1*04:05* ($p<0.00001$, OR=16.01), were significantly increased in the patients (Figure 1a, b) as compared to controls. We had earlier compared the results of the T1D patients with 91 healthy controls [14], however, now we have compared the results of T1D samples with 902 healthy controls, with the same results reinforcing our earlier data. These results were in concordance with earlier studies in North Indians [25-29]. However, we also observed *DRB1*07:01*($p<8x10^{-6}$, OR= 0.19) to be significantly decreased in the patients as compared to controls. In our earlier study when we had less number of controls, we observed *DRB1*04:03* ($p< 0.02$, OR=0.25) and *DRB1*04:04* ($p< 0.05$, OR= 0.2) also to be significantly reduced in the patients [14], however, when we increased the number of controls to 902, this finding did not remain significant, although *DRB1*04:03* and *DRB1*04:04* were reduced in the patients but not significantly. We did not find any significant reduction of HLA-DR2 which has been shown to confer strong protection from T1D in most ethnic groups [30, 31] probably because the DR2 haplotype which has been shown to be protective i.e., *DRB1*15:01-DQB1*06:02,* was observed with a low frequency of only 1.06% in North Indians [21]. On the other hand, we observed a marginally increased frequency of *DRB1*15:01* and reduced frequency of *DRB1*15:06* in patients as compared to controls, which did not remain significant when p was corrected for the number of alleles tested for DRB1 locus. *DRB1*04:03* has been shown to be associated with protection in a Belgian study on T1D [32]. Our results are in concordance with studies on T1D patients from Sardinia, black population from Zimbabwe,

Lithuania, Czecks, Lebanese, Brazilians and African Americans where *DRB1*03:01*, *DRB1*04:01* and *DRB1*04:05* have been shown to be associated with the disease [33-40].

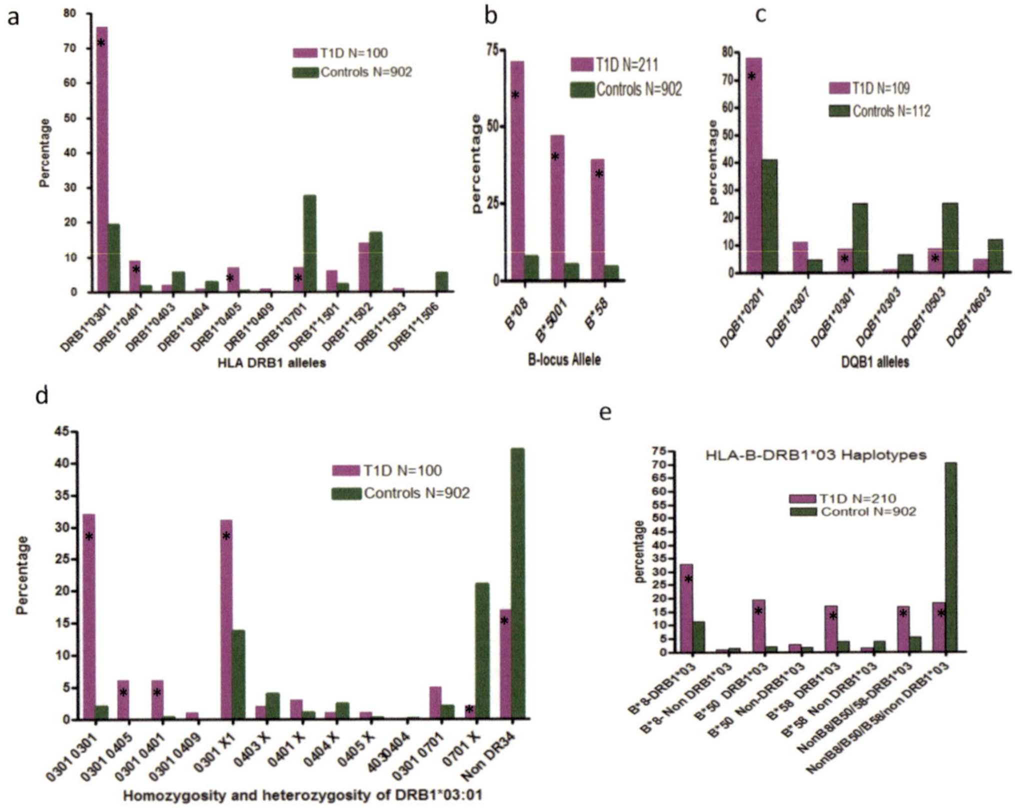

Rani et al., Tissue Antigens, 2004, Kumar et al., Tissue Antigens , 2007

Figure 1. Distribution of *HLA-DRB1*, *HLA-B* and *DQB1* alleles in Type 1 diabetes and healthy controls. a. *HLA-DRB1* alleles significantly increased or decreased in T1D are shown. *DRB1*03:01*, **04:01* and **04:05* are significantly increased and *DRB1*07:01*is significantly reduced in T1D as compared to controls. b. *HLA-B*08*, *B*50:01* and *B*58* are significantly increased in T1D as compared to controls c. *DQB1*02:01* is significantly increased and *DQB1*03:01* and *DQB1*05:03* are significantly reduced in T1D as compared to controls. d. Homozygous *DRB1*03:01* and heterozygous *DRB1*03:01* with **04:01*, **04:05* or any other allele (*0301,X) are significantly increased in T1D as compared to controls. e. *HLA-B-DRB1*03* haplotypes in T1D patients and controls. * denotes alleles that show statistically significant increase or decrease in the frequencies of the depicted alleles.

HLA-DRB1 and DQB1 are in strong linkage disequilibrium. We also studied the alleles of *DQB1* locus. *DQB1*02:01* which is linked to *DRB1*03:01* was significantly increased ($p<1x10^{-8}$, OR=5.08) in patients (Figure 1c). However *DQB1*03:02* and *DQB1*03:07*, alleles linked with *DRB1*04:01, DRB1*04:03, DRB1*04:04* and *DRB1*04:05* were not significantly increased in the patients because two of these alleles *DRB1*04:01* and *DRB1*04:05* were increased in the patients and the other two DR4 alleles *DRB1*04:03* and *DRB1*04:04* were reduced in the patients. *DQB1*03:01* ($p<6x10^{-4}$, OR=0.27) and *DQB1*05:03* ($6x10^{-4}$, OR=0.28) were reduced in the patients [14].

Figure 1d shows the homozygosity and heterozygosity of *DRB1*03:01* and *DRB1*04* alleles significantly increased in T1D. Homozygous *DRB1*03:01* ($p<4.6X10^{-39}$, OR=23.1), heterozygous *DRB1*03:01/*04:05* ($p<5.5X10^{-6}$, OR =124.2) and *DRB1*03:01/*04:01* (p<0.0001, OR =17.6) were significantly increased in the patients as compared to controls. Heterozygous *03:01*/X (i.e. any other allele) ($p<5.9X10^{-6}$, OR = 2.8) was also significantly increased in the patients as compared to controls. Heterozygous *DRB1*07:01/X* ($p < 1.3X10^{-7}$, OR = 0.09) were significantly reduced in the T1D patients as compared to controls suggesting their protective role. Thirty two percent of the patients studied were homozygous for *DRB1*0301* as compared to 2% of the controls and this difference was highly significant. Homozygosity of *DQB1*02:01* was significantly ($p<1x10^{-5}$, OR=5.4) increased in the patients. *DQB1*03:02* which was not significantly increased in the patients, showed a significant increase in heterozygous combination with *DQB1*0201* ($p<3x10^{-5}$, OR=34.16) [14]. In fact none of the controls had *DQB1*0201/*0302* heterozygous combination [14]. In a Swedish study, *DQA1*0301/DQB1*0302* and heterozygous combinations of *DQA1*0301/DQB1*0302* and *DQA1*0201/DQB1*0501* have been shown to confer the highest susceptibility [41]

Figure 1 e shows the *HLA-B-DRB1* haplotypes that were significantly increased in T1D patients. HLA alleles are very closely linked to each other in such a way that the haplotypes are inherited en-bloc. Three *HLA-DRB1*03* haplotypes, *B*08-DRB1*03:01*($p<1x10^{-14}$, OR=3.7), *B*50-DRB1*03:01*($p<8x10^{-24}$, OR=11.2) and *B*58-DRB1*03:01* ($p<1.4x10^{-12}$, OR=5.1) and *DRB1*03:01* haplotypes with non *B*8/ B*50/ B*58* alleles ($p<2.8x10^{-8}$, OR=3.4) were significantly increased in the patients as compared to controls. On the other hand non- *B*8/ B*50/ B*58-non DRB1*03:01* haplotypes were significantly reduced ($p<1.5x10^{-44}$, OR=0.09) in T1D patients as compared to controls [12].

Thus our studies show a significant increase of HLA class-I and II alleles which may have a role in auto-antigen presentation to $CD8^+$ and $CD4^+$ T cells respectively.

6. Vitiligo

Vitiligo is a depigmenting disorder of the skin caused by autoimmune destruction of pigment producing cells called melanocytes. It effects 0.5-1 % of the world population [42], while in India the incidence varies from 0.25 to 2.5% [43, 44] in most ethnic groups, however, it has been reported to be 8.8% in populations from western states of Gujarat and Rajasthan [45]. Vitiligo manifests in several forms which can be broadly classified in two clinical subtypes: generalized and localized [42]. While precise etiology of vitiligo is not very well understood, several hypotheses have been proposed which include autoimmune [46], neural [47], auto-cytotoxic [48] and genetic hypotheses [49]. However, autoimmune hypothesis gets credence due to co-occurrence of other autoimmune diseases in vitiligo patients in some cases, presence of auto reactive T cells and circulating auto-antibodies in the patients [46, 50-55]. The role of genetic factors has been suggested due to the fact that 7% of first-degree relatives of vitiligo develop the disease. [56, 57].

Recent genome wide studies [58, 59] have shown that several *single nucleotide polymorphisms* (*SNPs*) in the *MHC* region were significantly associated with the disease. Using imputation based on the previous studies done on associations of HLA, the authors showed that certain *HLA-class-I* alleles were associated with vitiligo but they could not impute *HLA class-II* alleles. [58]. As mentioned before MHC is the most polymorphic system of the human genome. With such a great diversity at each locus, linkage disequilibrium (LD) of *HLA* alleles with di-allelic *SNPs* may not be appropriate since several *HLA* alleles may be in LD with one or the alternate *SNP*. Thus the derivation based on these LDs may not be accurate especially in the populations from where no previous *HLA* data is available i.e. if there is no HLA data available it would be impossible to determine the linkage disequilibrium of HLA alleles with di-allelic SNPs. So, we conducted a very robust study on a sample size of 1404 vitiligo cases consisting of 1097 generalized and 307 localized vitiligo cases and 902 unaffected controls from North India for the alleles at *HLA-A, -B,*(class-I) and *-DRB1* (Class-II) loci using molecular methods and also replicated the study on 355 cases (250 generalized and 105 localized) and 441 controls from Gujarat, a state in west of India [15]. We also reported differences in the amino acid signatures of peptide binding pockets of the HLA molecules in vitiligo patients as compared to controls [15].

Our study showed a lot of diversity in number and frequencies of HLA alleles in patients and controls, with 78, 160 and 106 alleles in cases and 68, 111 and 94 alleles in controls for *HLA-A, -B* and *-DRB1* loci respectively from North India. Similar diversity was observed in the replication study as well. However, *HLA-A*33:01*($p<1.21x10^{-15}$, OR=2.57 in North Indians and $p<0.008$, OR=1.69 in Gujaratis), *B*44:03* ($p<7.05x10^{-27}$, OR=3.53 in North Indians and $p<1.54x10^{-8}$, OR=3.13 in Gujaratis) and *DRB1*07:01* ($p<3.16x10^{-30}$, OR=2.8 in North Indians and $p<9.81x10^{-15}$, OR=3.19 in Gujaratis) were significantly increased in both initial and replication study (Figure 2), suggesting these alleles are the markers for Vitiligo in both North India and Gujarat. These associations were significant irrespective of the age at onset or the gender of the cases. So, to determine which *HLA* alleles have primary association, we sequentially deleted samples having *DRB1*07:01, A*33:01*and *B*44:03* from both the case and control groups and then analysed the data for remainder alleles. The analysis showed that association of *DRB1*07:01* with vitiligo seemed to be primary because in the absence of *DRB1*07:01,* the class-I alleles *A*33:01* and *B*44:03* did not remain significantly increased. However, in the absence of *A*33:01*and *B*44:03, DRB1*07:01* still remained significantly increased in both the populations studied. The basic predisposing alleles in both localized and generalized vitiligo are same; however, similarities with the controls in terms of allele frequencies of some alleles and amino acid signature of the DR beta chain (figure 3) seem to be protective from generalized distribution of the lesions in localized vitiligo[15].

Removal of *DRB1*07:01* from both patients and control groups resulted in removal of all the samples that had *A*33:01* and *B*44:03,* suggesting that these alleles being on the same chromosome may be making a haplotype, such that when samples with *DRB1*07:01* are removed they also get removed simultaneously. To prove that we estimated the *HLA* haplotype frequencies using the expectation-maximization (EM) algorithm [60, 61] using Arlequin Ver 3.5 (http://cmpg.unibe.ch/software/arlequin35/). Haplotype analysis for three loci showed

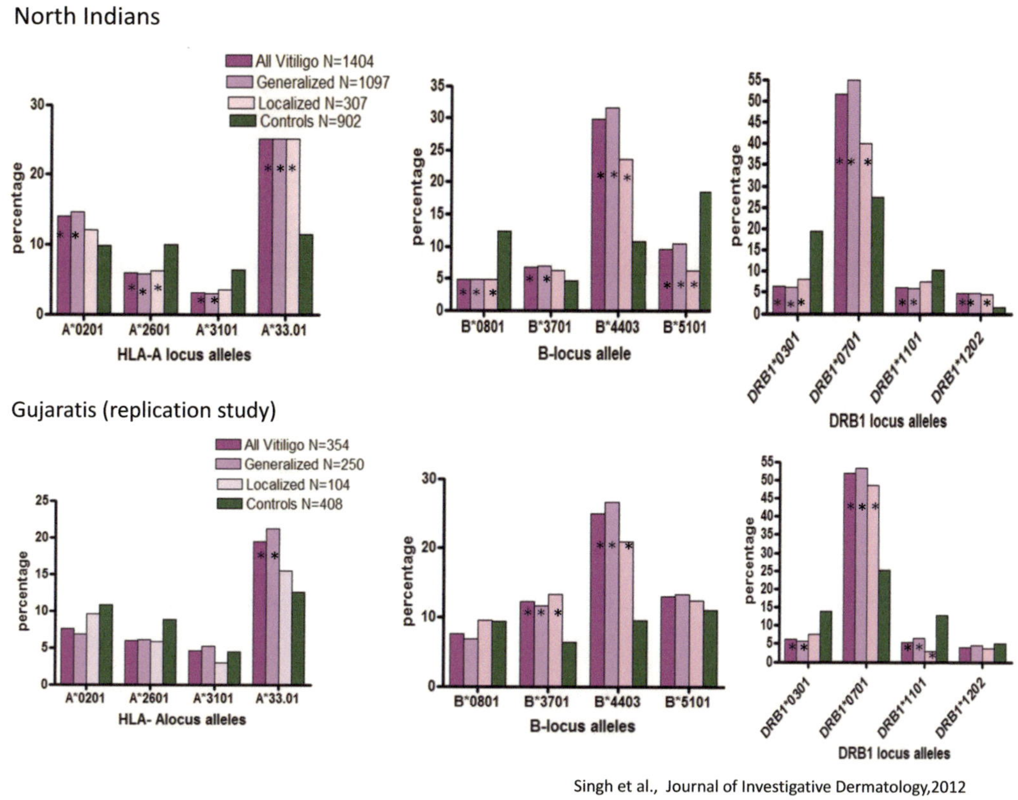

Figure 2. HLA-A, B and DRB1 loci alleles significantly increased in all vitiligo, generalized vitiligo and localized vitiligo patients when compared with healthy controls in North Indian and Gujarat patients. * denotes alleles that show statistically significant increase or decrease in the frequencies of the depicted alleles.

haplotypes *A*33:01-B*44:03-DRB1*07:01* ($p<8.75 \times 10^{-23}$, OR=6.21 in North Indians and p<0.000016, OR=3.65 in Gujaratis) and *A*24:02-B*44:03-DRB1*07:01* (p<0.0019, OR=3.83 in North Indians and p<0.0034, OR=7.73 in Gujaratis) were significantly increased and *A*26:01-B*08:01-DRB1*03:01* was significantly reduced (p<0.00005, OR=0.33 in North Indians and p<0.0007, OR=0.15 in Gujaratis) in vitiligo patients in both the initial study as well as in the replication study. Analysis of two-locus haplotypes revealed haplotypes *A*33:01-DRB1*07:01* ($p<6.97 \times 10^{-26}$, OR=6.55 in North Indians and p<0.00001, OR=3.59 in Gujaratis) and *B*44:03-DRB1*07:01* ($p < 2.4 \times 10^{-29}$, OR=4.01 in North Indians and $p<1.84 \times 10^{-14}$, OR=6.34 in Gujaratis) was significantly increased and *A*26:01-DRB1*03:01* was significantly reduced (p<0.00005, OR=0.33 in North Indians and p<0.0007, OR=0.15 in Gujaratis) in vitiligo cases in both initial and replication study[15].

We further studied the amino acid signatures of the peptide binding pockets of DRB1 in vitiligo cases and unaffected controls Eleven residues representing integral parts of peptide binding pockets of DR beta chain were analysed at positions 26, 28, 30, 37, 47, 67, 70, 71, 74, 77 and 86 [62]. The protein sequences were downloaded for all the alleles observed from the HLA database (http://www.ebi.ac.uk/cgi-bin/imgt/HLA/align.cgi) and the amino acids present at

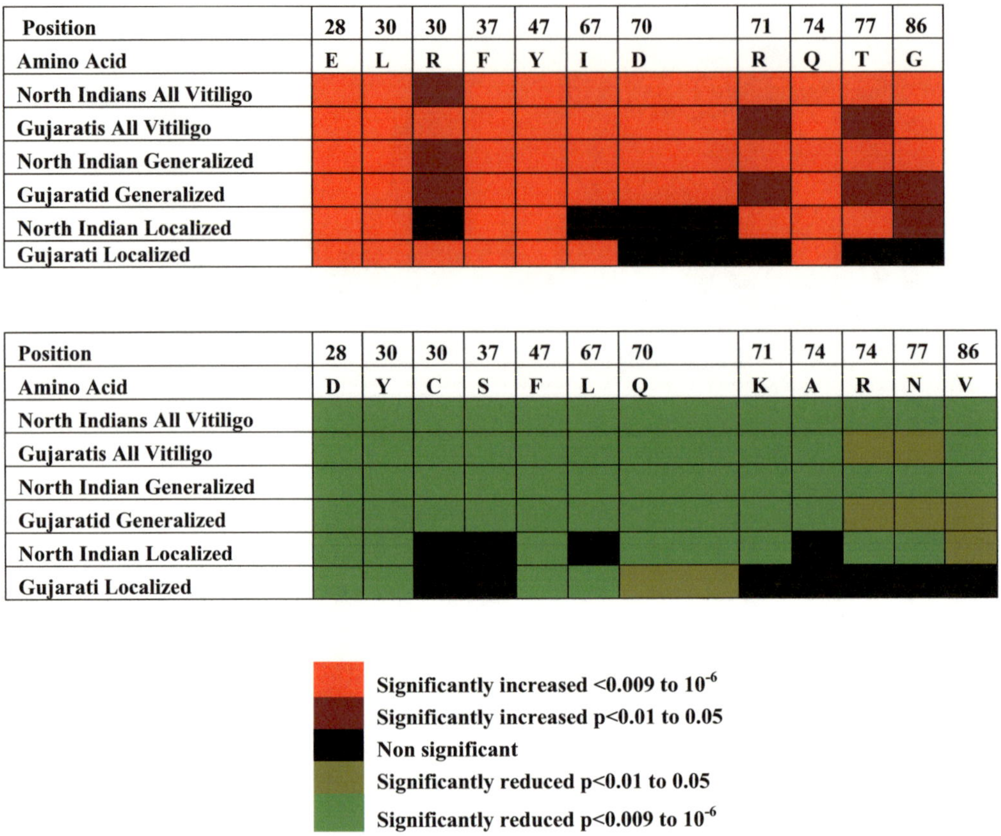

Figure 3. Amino acid signatures for the peptide binding pockets of HLA molecules for DR beta1 chain in all vitiligo, generalized vitiligo and localized vitiligo patients from North India and Gujarat. Amino acids shown in red are significantly increased in vitiligo patients while amino acids shown in green are significantly reduced in vitiligo patients as compared to controls and those in black are not significantly different from controls (Singh et al., JID, 2012).

the aforesaid positions were compared in patients with controls. Figure 3 shows the amino acid residues at the aforesaid positions that were either significantly increased or decreased in all vitiligo patients, generalized and localzed vitiligo patients when compared with controls. The results show that Glu$^{28\beta}$, Leu$^{30\beta}$/Arg$^{30\beta}$ Phe$^{37\beta}$, Tyr$^{47\beta}$, Ile$^{67\beta}$, Asp$^{70\beta}$, Arg$^{71\beta}$, Gln$^{74\beta}$, Thr$^{77\beta}$ and Gly$^{86\beta}$ make the molecular signature of the peptide binding pockets of DRB1 for predisposition to develop vitiligo in both the initial as well as in the replication study (Figure 3). Asp$^{28\beta}$, Tyr$^{30\beta}$/Cys$^{30\beta}$, Ser$^{37\beta}$, Phe$^{47\beta}$, Leu$^{67\beta}$, Gln$^{70\beta}$, Lys$^{71\beta}$, Ala/Arg$^{74\beta}$, Asn$^{77\beta}$ and Val$^{86\beta}$ make the molecular signature for the protection from Vitiligo in both North India and Gujarat. [15].

We observed subtle differences in the molecular signatures of the peptide binding pockets of DR beta chain in localized and generalized vitiligo. Localized vitiligo patients show similarities in the amino acid signatures with not only generalized vitiligo but also with healthy controls probably responsible for localized distribution of the lesions in them. Amino acid signature at positions Glu$^{28\beta}$, Leu$^{30\beta}$, Phe$^{37\beta}$, Tyr$^{47\beta}$ and Gln$^{74\beta}$ in the localized vitiligo patients is similar to generalized vitiligo in both the initial and replication study. However, the amino acid signature similar to healthy controls were observed at positions $Arg^{30\beta}/Cys^{30\beta}$, $Ser^{37\beta}$, $Ile^{67\beta}/Leu^{67\beta}$ $Asp^{70\beta}$, $Ala^{74\beta}$ in North Indians and $Cys^{30\beta}$, $Ser^{37\beta}$, $Asp^{70\beta}$, $Arg^{71\beta}$/Lys $Ser^{71\beta}$, $Ala^{74\beta}$/ $Arg^{74\beta}$ and $Thr^{77\beta}$ / $Asn^{77\beta}$ in Gujaratis [15].

Most of the studies previously have been done on Generalized vitiligo which has been considered to be an autoimmune disease. We showed for the first time that both generalized and localized vitiligo have the same predisposing MHC alleles i.e., *B*44:03 and DRB1*07:01* in both the populations studied. Association of *MHC* alleles with localized vitiligo clearly suggests an autoimmune etiology of the disease due to antigen presenting function of the MHC molecules. Thus there seems to be a need to re-look at the aetiopathogenesis of localized vitiligo in light of our results. While it may be an autoimmune disorder, similarities with unaffected controls in terms of *HLA* alleles and amino acid signature of the peptide binding pockets of DR beta chain may be contributing to the localized distribution of the lesions [15].

7. Idiopathic hypoparathyroidism

Idiopathic hypoparathyroidism (IH) is a rare endocrine disease where parathyroid gland is functionally impaired resulting in subnormal PTH secretion, hypocalcemia, hyperphosphatemia and associated complications [63]. While it may be an autoimmune disorder [63], there is hardly any evidence to confirm the autoimmune etiology of the disease. Since there was no comprehensive study on the immunogenetic basis of IH, we studied the association of *HLA class-I* and *II* alleles in a large group of North Indian patients (N=134) with IH [16, 64-70] and compared them to 902 healthy controls from the same ethnic background. We also reported significant differences in the amino acid signatures of peptide binding pockets of the HLA molecules in patients with IH as compared with controls [16].

Just like vitiligo, we observed diversity in number and frequencies of HLA alleles with 23, 40 and 44 alleles in patients for *HLA-A, -B, and -DRB1* loci, respectively. However, specific alleles at these loci were found to be predisposing. *HLA-A*26:01* ($p<1.71\times10^{-34}$, OR = 9.29), *HLA-B*08:01* ($p<8.19\times10^{-6}$, OR = 2.59), and *HLA-DRB1*03:01* ($p<0.013$, OR = 1.67) and *HLA-DRB1*12:02* ($p<0.0046$, OR = 3.52) were significantly increased in IH when compared with healthy controls. However, alleles *HLA-A*01:01* ($p<0.039$, OR = 0.60), *HLA-A*03:01* ($p<0.004$, OR=0.33), *HLA-B*15:01* ($p<0.0038$, OR=0.17) and *HLA-B*57:01* ($p<0.0074$, OR=0.3) were significantly reduced in IH as compared with controls (Figure 4a). Since *HLA-A*26:01* showed the highest significance, we studied whether any other allele was significantly increased in the absence of *HLA-A*26:01*. So, all the samples with *A*26:01* were removed from both cases and controls and then analysis was done for significant differences in frequencies of the remainder alleles. In the absence of *HLA-A*26:01*, no other allele showed any significant differences [16].

Associations of *A*26:01* and *B*08:01* with IH were significant irrespective of the gender and age at onset of the disease. To investigate whether there was any association of HLA alleles with associated clinical autoimmunity in IH, patients were categorized into two groups, those with associated clinical autoimmunity and those without. While *HLA-A*26:01* was significantly increased in both the groups as compared with controls, *HLA-B*08:01* and *DRB1*12:02* were significantly increased in patients without any associated clinical autoimmunity when compared with controls [16].

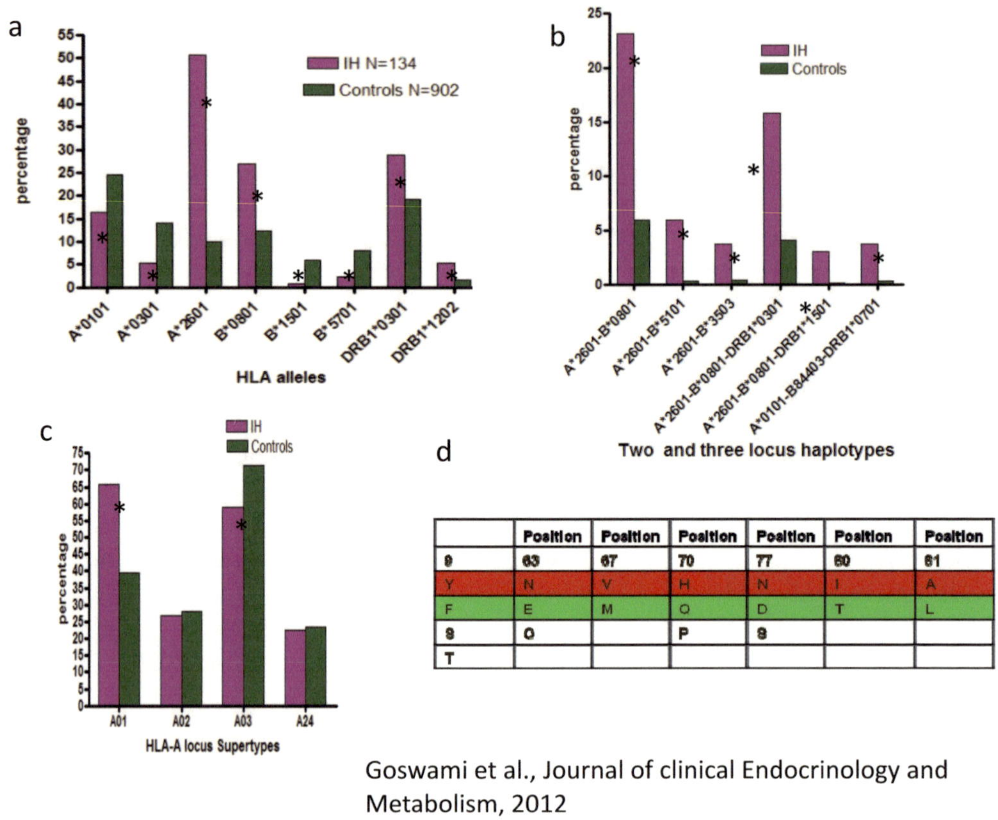

Figure 4. *HLA-A, B* and *DRB1* loci alleles significantly increased in idiopathic hypoparathyroidism patients when compared with healthy controls in North Indian patients. * denotes alleles that show statistically significant increase or decrease in the frequencies of the depicted alleles.

We constructed HLA haplotypes for HLA-A-B-DRB1 and HLA-A-B and HLA-A-DRB1 for 133 cases and 902 controls using Arlequin 3.5 program (http://cmpg.unibe.ch/software/arlequin35/). Haplotype *HLA-A*26:01-B*08:01-DRB1*03:01* (p<4.47x10^{-8}, OR = 4.38), was significantly increased in cases as compared with controls. Two locus haplotype analysis (figure 4b) showed haplotypes *A*26:01-B*08:01*(p<1.48x10^{-11}, OR = 4.72), *A*26:01-B*51:01* (p<7.59x10^{-6}, OR = 17.26), *A*26:01-B*35:03* (p<0.0028, OR = 8.48), and *A*11:01-B*40:06* (p<0.0009, OR = 4.46), were significantly increased in IH as compared to controls. However, the association of *A*26:01* with IH seems to be primary since in the absence of *A*26:01*, none of the other alleles like *B*08:01, B*51:01* or *DRB1*03:01* remained significantly different suggesting that the significant increase in these alleles is due to their being in linkage disequilibrium with the *A*26:01*[16].

MHC molecules are extremely polymorphic, however, alleles with similar peptide binding pockets may be clustered in one group [6], called supertypes, such that HLA molecules in one supertype may present similar peptides[16]. Assignment of alleles in the supertypes have been done based on published motifs, binding data, shared repertoires of binding peptides and the amino acid sequences of different alleles at the peptide binding pockets [6]. Supertype A01 (which includes *A*26:01*) was significantly increased in IH with 65.67% of the patients as compared to 39.36% of the controls having this supertype (figure 4 c). However, *A*26:01* was observed only in 50.75% of the patients as compared to 9.98% of the controls. About 15% of the IH cases had different alleles of A01 supertype (other than *A*26:01*), which did not show statistically significant differences due to small numbers. Significant increase of A01 supertype suggests that similar auto-antigenic peptides may be getting presented by different MHC molecules which belong to the supertype [6, 16].

While the amino acid residue at a particular position in different alleles in a supertype may not be the same, they would be similar in nature such that they would bind similar peptides. For instance, all the alleles falling in supertype A01 will bind small and aliphatic residues in the B pocket and aromatic and large hydrophobic residues in F pocket [6]. Thus, the nature of the shared amino acids and not amino acid per se constitutes the molecular signatures of the peptide binding groove of different alleles in a supertype.

The peptide binding groove of the MHC class-I molecules contain small pockets where the side chains of complimentary residues of the peptide bind [4]. Pockets B (key residues at positions 9, 45, 63, 67, 70 and 99) and F (key residues at positions 77, 80, 81 and 116) of alpha chain are the main anchors which engage the peptides at its amino acid position 2 and the C-terminus [6]. Since we observed a significant increase in an HLA-A locus allele (*HLA-A*26:01*), we analysed the amino acid signatures of the peptide binding groove of the alleles of A-locus to check for shared peptide binding specificity. For this purpose, the protein sequences of the *HLA-A* locus alleles were downloaded from the HLA database as mentioned for the vitiligo study and the amino acids present at the aforesaid positions were compared in patients with controls. We observed that $Tyr^{9\alpha}$, $Asn^{63\alpha}$, $Val^{67\alpha}$, $His^{70\alpha}$, $Asn^{77\alpha}$, $Ile^{80\alpha}$ and $Ala^{81\alpha}$ make the molecular signature for HLA-A peptide binding pockets for predisposition to IH, however, $Phe^{9\alpha}$, $Glu^{63\alpha}$, $Met^{67\alpha}$, $Gln^{70\alpha}$, $Asp^{77\alpha}$, $Thr^{80\alpha}$ and $Leu^{81\alpha}$ make the molecular signature for negative association with the disease (Figure 4d). While the most significant association was derived from *HLA-A*26:01*, peptide binding grooves of other alleles shared some of the residues with the peptide binding grove of *HLA-A*26:01* (Figure 5)[16].

MHC is the most polymorphic system of the man with more than 6000 alleles for different loci. With such a great diversity, association of particular *MHC* alleles with a disease has functional implications due to the antigen presenting function of the MHC. The peptides presented by the MHC molecules have allele specific motifs [4]. The affinity of the peptide to a particular MHC molecule is determined by the amino acid residues present in peptide binding pockets of the peptide binding groove. Shared amino acids in the peptide binding pockets have been demonstrated in autoimmune diseases like Type 1 diabetes [71], rheumatoid arthritis [72] and thyroiditis [62]. Investigation of amino acid signatures for the peptide binding pockets of HLA-A and HLA-B alpha chain and HLA-DR beta chain revealed specific molecular signatures for

HLA-A	N=259	Position	Position	Position	Position	Position	Position	Position	supertypes
*Alleles	No.	9	63	67	70	77	80	81	
A*26:01	68	Y	N	V	H	N	I	A	A01
A*0101	22	F	E	M	H	N	T	L	A01
A*29:01	5	T	Q	V	Q	N	T	L	A01
A*30:01	4	S	E	V	Q	D	T	L	A01
A*32:01	3	F	E	V	H	S	I	A	A01
A*26:25N	1	Y	N	V	P	N	T	L	A01
A*11:01	42	Y	E	V	Q	D	T	L	A03
A*68:01	18	Y	N	V	Q	D	T	L	A03
A*24:02	28	S	E	V	H	N	I	A	A24
A*23:01	1	S	E	V	H	N	I	A	A24
A*23:15	1	S	E	V	H	N	I	A	A24
A*24:07	1	S	E	V	Q	N	I	A	A24
A*02:06	4	Y	E	V	H	D	T	L	A02
A*02:05	3	Y	E	V	H	D	T	L	A02
A*33:01	10	T	N	V	H	D	T	L	A03
A*33:03	2	T	N	V	H	D	T	L	A03
A*30:36	1	S	E	V	Q	D	T	L	A03
A*02:01	13	F	E	V	H	D	T	L	A02
A*02:11	12	F	E	V	H	D	T	L	A02
A*02:03	6	F	E	V	H	D	T	L	A02
A*03:01	7	F	E	V	Q	D	T	L	A03
A*31:01	6	T	E	V	H	D	T	L	A03
A*03:02	1	F	E	V	Q	D	T	L	A03

$p < 0.017$ to $1.06\text{x}10^{-10}$, Significantly increased in IH as compared to controls

$p < 0.017$ to $4.79\text{x}10^{-10}$, Significantly reduced in IH as compared to controls

Figure 5. Amino acid signatures (single letter codes) of the peptide binding pockets and HLA supertypes of 23 HLA-A locus alleles observed in IH cases showing significant increase or decrease in the number of amino acids. N=259 indicates 259 alleles were observed in 134 patients which were compared with amino acid signatures of 1698 alleles from 902 controls.

predisposition and protection from these diseases. Our data shows that haplotypes *B*8-DRB1*03:01*, *B*50-DRB1*03:01* and *B*58-DRB1*03:01* were significantly increased in T1D patients [12]. *A*26:01-B*08:01-DRB1*03:01* and *A*26:01* with other B-locus alleles were significantly increased in hypoparathyroidism [16]. And in yet another autoimmune disorder, vitiligo, *A*33:01-B*44:03-DRB1*07:01* is the predisposing haplotype and *A*26:01-B*08:01-DRB1*03:01* seems to be protective haplotype, with *DRB1*07:01* having primary association with the disease [15]. While in T1D and vitiligo it is the MHC class-II alleles*DRB1*03:01* and*DRB1*07:01* respectively, which had primary association, in hypoparathyroidism it is the MHC class-I allele *HLA-A*26:01* which has primary association. Interestingly, in T1D *DRB1*03:01* is predisposing and *DRB1*07:01* is protective from the disease. However, in vitiligo it is exactly the opposite i.e., *DRB1*07:01* is predisposing and DRB1*03:01 is protective.

http://dx.doi.org/10.5772/57494

These data suggest the autoantigenic peptides presented by different MHC molecules are restricted by these common alleles in a population which are associated with the autoimmune disorders. Of about 350 alleles that were observed in the three patient groups and healthy controls, *A*26:01* (9.98%), *A*33:01* (11.53%), *B*08:01* (12.42%), *B*44:03* (10.75%), DRB1*03:01* (19.29%) and *DRB1*07:01* (27.49%), were quite common alleles in the healthy North Indians that were associated with the three autoimmune disorders discussed above.

Our results suggest affinity of auto-antigenic peptides for predisposing MHC class-II and class-I molecules which may be involved in orchestrating (through $CD4^+$ T cells) and implementing the autoimmune responses (through $CD8^+$ T cells) in Type 1 diabetes, vitiligo and hypoparathyroidism.

Acknowledgements

We are thankful to the study participants: cases and the controls that provided blood samples for the study. Authors are thankful to Dr. Mitali Mukerji, IGIB, Delhi, for providing access to the Indian Genome Variation Consortium samples that have been used as unaffected controls in these studies. The projects were funded in part by grants from Department of Science and Technology (DST), Department of Biotechnology (DBT), Ministry of Science and Technology, Government of India and partly by Core funds of National Institute of Immunology, New Delhi, India. Diabetes work was supported by Department of Science & Technology, New Delhi, India, grant No. SP/SO/B54/98. Vitiligo work was supported by grants for 'Genetic and autoimmune factors associated with vitiligo' (Grant number BT/PR6653/Med/12/258/2005) and the 'Program support for Skin pigmentation and melanocyte-keratinocyte biology' (grant number BT/01/COE/07/07) from the Department of Biotechnology, India. The hypoparathyroidism work was sponsored by Department of Biotechnology, grant number BT/PR15022/Med/30/589/2010. The patient sample for this work came from All India Institute of Medical Sciences (AIIMS), New Delhi and Dr. Ram Manohar Lohia Hospital (RMLH), New Delhi, India. We would like to thank Dr. R. Goswami, Department of Endocrinology and Metabolism, (AIIMS) for T1D and hypoparathyroidism samples. We would like to acknowledge Dr. H. Kar (RMLH), Dr. V. K. Sharma (AIIMS) and Dr. Somesh Gupta (AIIMS), the dermatologists for providing the vitiligo samples. We thankfully acknowledge Dr. Rasheedunnisa Begum and her team for providing vitiligo samples for the replication study from Gujarat. We would like to acknowledge the students and project fellows who have been involved in doing this work. Mr. Kapoor Chand's technical support is acknowledged.

Author details

Rajni Rani and Archana Singh

Molecular Immunogenetics Group, National Institute of Immunology, New Delhi, India

References

[1] Bowcock AM, Fernandez-Vina M Targeting skin: vitiligo and autoimmunity. J Invest Dermatol 2012; 132:13-15

[2] Horton R, Wilming L, Rand V, Lovering RC, Bruford EA, Khodiyar VK, Lush MJ, Povey S, Talbot CC, Jr., Wright MW, Wain HM, Trowsdale J, Ziegler A, Beck S Gene map of the extended human MHC. Nat Rev Genet 2004; 5:889-899

[3] Bjorkman PJ, Saper MA, Samraoui B, Bennett WS, Strominger JL, Wiley DC Structure of the human class I histocompatibility antigen, HLA-A2. Nature 1987; 329:506-512

[4] Falk K, Rotzschke O, Stevanovic S, Jung G, Rammensee HG Allele-specific motifs revealed by sequencing of self-peptides eluted from MHC molecules. Nature 1991; 351:290-296

[5] Garrett TP, Saper MA, Bjorkman PJ, Strominger JL, Wiley DC Specificity pockets for the side chains of peptide antigens in HLA-Aw68. Nature 1989; 342:692-696

[6] Sidney J, Peters B, Frahm N, Brander C, Sette A HLA class I supertypes: a revised and updated classification. BMC Immunol 2008; 9:1

[7] Holling TM, Schooten E, van Den Elsen PJ Function and regulation of MHC class II molecules in T-lymphocytes: of mice and men. Hum Immunol 2004; 65:282-290

[8] de Vries RR, van Rood JJ Immunobiology of HLA class-I and class-II molecules. Introduction. Prog Allergy 1985; 36:1-9

[9] Brown JH, Jardetzky TS, Gorga JC, Stern LJ, Urban RG, Strominger JL, Wiley DC Three-dimensional structure of the human class II histocompatibility antigen HLA-DR1. Nature 1993; 364:33-39

[10] Robinson J, Waller MJ, Fail SC, McWilliam H, Lopez R, Parham P, Marsh SG The IMGT/HLA database. Nucleic Acids Res 2009; 37:D1013-1017

[11] Robinson J, Mistry K, McWilliam H, Lopez R, Parham P, Marsh SG The IMGT/HLA database. Nucleic Acids Res 39:D1171-1176

[12] Kumar R, Goswami R, Agarwal S, Israni N, Singh SK, Rani R Association and interaction of the TNF-alpha gene with other pro- and anti-inflammatory cytokine genes and HLA genes in patients with type 1 diabetes from North India. Tissue Antigens 2007; 69:557-567

[13] Report of the expert committee on the diagnosis and classification of diabetes mellitus. Diabetes Care2003; 26 Suppl 1:S5-20

[14] Rani R, Sood A, Goswami R Molecular basis of predisposition to develop type 1 diabetes mellitus in North Indians. Tissue Antigens 2004; 64:145-155

[15] Singh A, Sharma P, Kar HK, Sharma VK, Tembhre MK, Gupta S, Laddha NC, Dwivedi M, Begum R, Gokhale RS, Rani R HLA Alleles and Amino-Acid Signatures of

the Peptide-Binding Pockets of HLA Molecules in Vitiligo. J Invest Dermatol 2012; 132:124-134

[16] Goswami R, Singh A, Gupta N, Rani R Presence of Strong Association of the Major Histocompatibility Complex (MHC) Class I Allele HLA-A*26:01 with Idiopathic Hypoparathyroidism. J Clin Endocrinol Metab 06/2012; 97(9):E1820-4. DOI:10.1210/jc. 2012-1328

[17] Israni N, Goswami R, Kumar A, Rani R Interaction of vitamin D receptor with HLA DRB1 0301 in type 1 diabetes patients from North India. PLoS One 2009; 4:e8023

[18] Marsh SG, Albert ED, Bodmer WF, Bontrop RE, Dupont B, Erlich HA, Fernandez-Vina M, Geraghty DE, Holdsworth R, Hurley CK, Lau M, Lee KW, Mach B, Maiers M, Mayr WR, Muller CR, Parham P, Petersdorf EW, Sasazuki T, Strominger JL, Svejgaard A, Terasaki PI, Tiercy JM, Trowsdale J Nomenclature for factors of the HLA system, 2010. Tissue Antigens 2010; 75:291-455

[19] Woolf B On estimating the relation between blood group and disease. Ann Hum Genet 1955; 19:251-253

[20] Haldane JB The estimation and significance of the logarithm of a ratio of frequencies. Ann Hum Genet 1956; 20:309-311

[21] Rani R, Fernandez-Vina MA, Stastny P Associations between HLA class II alleles in a North Indian population. Tissue Antigens 1998; 52:37-43

[22] Pociot F, McDermott MF Genetics of type 1 diabetes mellitus. Genes Immun 2002; 3:235-249

[23] Todd JA Genetic analysis of type 1 diabetes using whole genome approaches. Proc Natl Acad Sci U S A 1995; 92:8560-8565

[24] Ramachandran A, Snehalatha C, Krishnaswamy CV Incidence of IDDM in children in urban population in southern India. Madras IDDM Registry Group Madras, South India. Diabetes Res Clin Pract 1996; 34:79-82

[25] Gupta MM, Raghunath D, Kher SK, Radhakrishnan AP Human leucocyte antigen and insulin dependent diabetes mellitus. J Assoc Physicians India 1991; 39:540-543

[26] Sanjeevi CB, Kanungo A, Shtauvere A, Samal KC, Tripathi BB Association of HLA class II alleles with different subgroups of diabetes mellitus in Eastern India identify different associations with IDDM and malnutrition-related diabetes. Tissue Antigens 1999; 54:83-87

[27] Mehra NK, Kaur G, Kanga U, Tandon N Immunogenetics of autoimmune diseases in Asian Indians. Ann N Y Acad Sci 2002; 958:333-336

[28] Witt CS, Price P, Kaur G, Cheong K, Kanga U, Sayer D, Christiansen F, Mehra NK Common HLA-B8-DR3 haplotype in Northern India is different from that found in Europe. Tissue Antigens 2002; 60:474-480

[29] Kanga U, Vaidyanathan B, Jaini R, Menon PS, Mehra NK HLA haplotypes associated with type 1 diabetes mellitus in North Indian children. Hum Immunol 2004; 65:47-53

[30] Pugliese A, Gianani R, Moromisato R, Awdeh ZL, Alper CA, Erlich HA, Jackson RA, Eisenbarth GS HLA-DQB1*0602 is associated with dominant protection from diabetes even among islet cell antibody-positive first-degree relatives of patients with IDDM. Diabetes 1995; 44:608-613

[31] Baisch JM, Weeks T, Giles R, Hoover M, Stastny P, Capra JD Analysis of HLA-DQ genotypes and susceptibility in insulin-dependent diabetes mellitus. N Engl J Med 1990; 322:1836-1841

[32] Van der Auwera B, Van Waeyenberge C, Schuit F, Heimberg H, Vandewalle C, Gorus F, Flament J DRB1*0403 protects against IDDM in Caucasians with the high-risk heterozygous DQA1*0301-DQB1*0302/DQA1*0501-DQB1*0201 genotype. Belgian Diabetes Registry. Diabetes 1995; 44:527-530

[33] Ei Wafai RJ, Chmaisse HN, Makki RF, Fakhoury H Association of HLA class II alleles and CTLA-4 polymorphism with type 1 diabetes. Saudi J Kidney Dis Transpl 2011; 22:273-281

[34] Alves C, Toralles MB, Carvalho GC HLA class II polymorphism in patients with type 1 diabetes mellitus from a Brazilian racially admixtured population. Ethn Dis 2009; 19:420-424

[35] Weber P, Meluzinova H, Kubesova H, Ambrosova P, Polcarova V, Cejkova P, Cerna M Type 1 diabetes and LADA--occurrence of HLA-DRB1 *03 and DRB1 *04 alleles in two age different groups of diabetics. Adv Gerontol 2010; 23:243-248

[36] Skrodeniene E, Marciulionyte D, Padaiga Z, Jasinskiene E, Sadauskaite-Kuehne V, Sanjeevi CB, Ludvigsson J HLA class II alleles and haplotypes in Lithuanian children with type 1 diabetes and healthy children (HLA and type 1 diabetes). Medicina (Kaunas) 2010; 46:505-510

[37] Cucca F, Lampis R, Frau F, Macis D, Angius E, Masile P, Chessa M, Frongia P, Silvetti M, Cao A, De Virgiliis S, Congia M The distribution of DR4 haplotypes in Sardinia suggests a primary association of type I diabetes with DRB1 and DQB1 loci. Hum Immunol 1995; 43:301-308

[38] Garcia-Pacheco JM, Herbut B, Cutbush S, Hitman GA, Zhonglin W, Magzoub M, Bottazzo GF, Kiere C, West G, Mvere D, et al. Distribution of HLA-DQA1, -DQB1 and DRB1 alleles in black IDDM patients and controls from Zimbabwe. Tissue Antigens 1992; 40:145-149

[39] Fernandez-Vina M, Ramirez LC, Raskin P, Stastny P Genes for insulin-dependent diabetes mellitus (IDDM) in the major histocompatibility complex (MHC) of African-Americans. Tissue Antigens 1993; 41:57-64

[40] Tait BD, Drummond BP, Varney MD, Harrison LC HLA-DRB1*0401 is associated with susceptibility to insulin-dependent diabetes mellitus independently of the DQB1 locus. Eur J Immunogenet 1995; 22:289-297

[41] Sanjeevi CB, Landin-Olsson M, Kockum I, Dahlquist G, Lernmark A Effects of the second HLA-DQ haplotype on the association with childhood insulin-dependent diabetes mellitus. Tissue Antigens 1995; 45:148-152

[42] Taieb A, Picardo M The definition and assessment of vitiligo: a consensus report of the Vitiligo European Task Force. Pigment Cell Res 2007; 20:27-35

[43] Handa S, Kaur I Vitiligo: clinical findings in 1436 patients. J Dermatol 1999; 26:653-657

[44] Das SK, Majumder PP, Chakraborty R, Majumdar TK, Haldar B Studies on vitiligo. I. Epidemiological profile in Calcutta, India. Genet Epidemiol 1985; 2:71-78

[45] Shajil EM, Chatterjee S, Agrawal D, Bagchi T, Begum R Vitiligo: pathomechanisms and genetic polymorphism of susceptible genes. Indian J Exp Biol 2006; 44:526-539

[46] Kemp EH, Waterman EA, Weetman AP Immunological pathomechanisms in vitiligo. Expert Rev Mol Med 2001; 3:1-22

[47] Dell'anna ML, Picardo M A review and a new hypothesis for non-immunological pathogenetic mechanisms in vitiligo. Pigment Cell Res 2006; 19:406-411

[48] Lerner AB On the etiology of vitiligo and gray hair. Am J Med 1971; 51:141-147

[49] Bhatia PS, Mohan L, Pandey ON, Singh KK, Arora SK, Mukhija RD Genetic nature of vitiligo. J Dermatol Sci 1992; 4:180-184

[50] Kovacs SO Vitiligo. J Am Acad Dermatol 1998; 38:647-666; quiz 667-648

[51] Lang KS, Caroli CC, Muhm A, Wernet D, Moris A, Schittek B, Knauss-Scherwitz E, Stevanovic S, Rammensee HG, Garbe C HLA-A2 restricted, melanocyte-specific CD8(+) T lymphocytes detected in vitiligo patients are related to disease activity and are predominantly directed against MelanA/MART1. J Invest Dermatol 2001; 116:891-897

[52] Wankowicz-Kalinska A, van den Wijngaard RM, Tigges BJ, Westerhof W, Ogg GS, Cerundolo V, Storkus WJ, Das PK Immunopolarization of CD4+ and CD8+ T cells to Type-1-like is associated with melanocyte loss in human vitiligo. Lab Invest 2003; 83:683-695

[53] Waterman EA, Gawkrodger DJ, Watson PF, Weetman AP, Kemp EH Autoantigens in vitiligo identified by the serological selection of a phage-displayed melanocyte cDNA expression library. J Invest Dermatol 130:230-240

[54] van den Boorn JG, Konijnenberg D, Dellemijn TA, van der Veen JP, Bos JD, Melief CJ, Vyth-Dreese FA, Luiten RM Autoimmune destruction of skin melanocytes by perilesional T cells from vitiligo patients. J Invest Dermatol 2009; 129:2220-2232

[55] Schwartz RA, Janniger CK Vitiligo. Cutis 1997; 60:239-244

[56] Majumder PP, Nordlund JJ, Nath SK Pattern of familial aggregation of vitiligo. Arch Dermatol 1993; 129:994-998

[57] Alkhateeb A, Fain PR, Thody A, Bennett DC, Spritz RA Epidemiology of vitiligo and associated autoimmune diseases in Caucasian probands and their families. Pigment Cell Res 2003; 16:208-214

[58] Quan C, Ren YQ, Xiang LH, Sun LD, Xu AE, Gao XH, Chen HD, Pu XM, Wu RN, Liang CZ, Li JB, Gao TW, Zhang JZ, Wang XL, Wang J, Yang RY, Liang L, Yu JB, Zuo XB, Zhang SQ, Zhang SM, Chen G, Zheng XD, Li P, Zhu J, Li YW, Wei XD, Hong WS, Ye Y, Zhang Y, Wu WS, Cheng H, Dong PL, Hu DY, Li Y, Li M, Zhang X, Tang HY, Tang XF, Xu SX, He SM, Lv YM, Shen M, Jiang HQ, Wang Y, Li K, Kang XJ, Liu YQ, Sun L, Liu ZF, Xie SQ, Zhu CY, Xu Q, Gao JP, Hu WL, Ni C, Pan TM, Yao S, He CF, Liu YS, Yu ZY, Yin XY, Zhang FY, Yang S, Zhou Y, Zhang XJ Genome-wide association study for vitiligo identifies susceptibility loci at 6q27 and the MHC. Nat Genet 2010; 42:614-618

[59] Jin Y, Birlea SA, Fain PR, Gowan K, Riccardi SL, Holland PJ, Mailloux CM, Sufit AJ, Hutton SM, Amadi-Myers A, Bennett DC, Wallace MR, McCormack WT, Kemp EH, Gawkrodger DJ, Weetman AP, Picardo M, Leone G, Taieb A, Jouary T, Ezzedine K, van Geel N, Lambert J, Overbeck A, Spritz RA Variant of TYR and autoimmunity susceptibility loci in generalized vitiligo. N Engl J Med 2010; 362:1686-1697

[60] Excoffier L, Laval G, Schneider S Arlequin (version 3.0): an integrated software package for population genetics data analysis. Evol Bioinform Online 2005; 1:47-50

[61] Excoffier L, Slatkin M Maximum-likelihood estimation of molecular haplotype frequencies in a diploid population. Mol Biol Evol 1995; 12:921-927

[62] Menconi F, Osman R, Monti MC, Greenberg DA, Concepcion ES, Tomer Y Shared molecular amino acid signature in the HLA-DR peptide binding pocket predisposes to both autoimmune diabetes and thyroiditis. Proc Natl Acad Sci U S A 2010; 107:16899-16903

[63] Rose NR Is idiopathic hypoparathyroidism an autoimmune disease? J Clin Invest 1996; 97:899-900

[64] Goswami R, Brown EM, Kochupillai N, Gupta N, Rani R, Kifor O, Chattopadhyay N Prevalence of calcium sensing receptor autoantibodies in patients with sporadic idiopathic hypoparathyroidism. Eur J Endocrinol 2004; 150:9-18

[65] Goswami R, Goel S, Tomar N, Gupta N, Lumb V, Sharma YD Prevalence of clinical remission in patients with sporadic idiopathic hypoparathyroidism. Clin Endocrinol (Oxf) 2010; 72:328-333

[66] Goswami R, Marwaha RK, Goswami D, Gupta N, Ray D, Tomar N, Singh S Prevalence of thyroid autoimmunity in sporadic idiopathic hypoparathyroidism in comparison to type 1 diabetes and premature ovarian failure. J Clin Endocrinol Metab 2006; 91:4256-4259

[67] Goswami R, Bhatia M, Goyal R, Kochupillai N Reversible peripheral neuropathy in idiopathic hypoparathyroidism. Acta Neurol Scand 2002; 105:128-131

[68] Goswami R, Mohapatra T, Gupta N, Rani R, Tomar N, Dikshit A, Sharma RK Parathyroid hormone gene polymorphism and sporadic idiopathic hypoparathyroidism. J Clin Endocrinol Metab 2004; 89:4840-4845

[69] Goswami R, Gupta N, Ray D, Rani R, Tomar N, Sarin R, Vupputuri MR Polymorphisms at +49A/G and CT60 sites in the 3' UTR of the CTLA-4 gene and APECED-related AIRE gene mutations analysis in sporadic idiopathic hypoparathyroidism. Int J Immunogenet 2005; 32:393-400

[70] Sarin R, Tomar N, Ray D, Gupta N, Sharma YD, Goswami R Absence of pathogenic calcium sensing receptor mutations in sporadic idiopathic hypoparathyroidism. Clin Endocrinol (Oxf) 2006; 65:359-363

[71] Todd JA, Bell JI, McDevitt HO HLA-DQ beta gene contributes to susceptibility and resistance to insulin-dependent diabetes mellitus. Nature 1987; 329:599-604

[72] Winchester R The molecular basis of susceptibility to rheumatoid arthritis. Adv Immunol 1994; 56:389-466

Chapter 8

HLA in Gastrointestinal Inflammatory Disorders

M.I. Torres, T. Palomeque and P. Lorite

Additional information is available at the end of the chapter

http://dx.doi.org/10.5772/57497

1. Introduction

1.1. HLA GENE

The human leukocyte antigen (HLA) region is located on chromosome 6p21.3 and encodes genes for the major histocompatibility complex (MHC). MHC genes are among the most polymorphic genes in the vertebrate genome. HLA region contains hundreds of genes with immunological function that is characterized by a high gene density, variability and extensive linkage disequilibrium [1]. HLA encodes proteins with critical role in immunity, including antigen processing and presentation, and self-recognition by immune cells, as ligands receptors, cytokines, signaling factors, heat shock proteins, and transcription regulators. The HLA region is involved in many biological processes such as histocompatibility, inflammation, ligands for immune cell receptors, and the complement cascade [2].

HLA genes have many possible variations, allowing each person's immune system to react to a wide range of foreign invaders. Some HLA genes have hundreds of identified versions (alleles); more than 100 diseases involving abnormal immune function and some forms of cancer have been associated with different alleles of HLA genes [3,4]. Is paradoxical that genes evolved to protect the host against infectious diseases are cause of many genetic disorders themselves. It is often unclear what role HLA genes play in the risk of developing these diseases.

The MHC is the most gene-dense region of the mammalian genome playing a key role in immune defense and autoimmunity [5]. The complex is divided into three subgroups (MHC classes I, II, and III). The class I region is located at the telomeric end of the MHC and encodes heterodimeric peptide-binding proteins as well as antigen processing molecule. The class I family is divided into classical (HLA-A, -B, -C) and non-classical (HLA-E, -F and –G) genes. The classical genes are highly polymorphic and constitutively expressed by most somatic cells, and are co-dominantly expressed on the cell surface and responsible for presenting intracellularly derived peptides to CD8-positive T cells. On the cell surface, these proteins are bound to protein fragments (peptides) that have been exported from within the cell. MHC class I proteins display these peptides to the immune system.

The human MHC class I chain-related genes (MICA and MICB) are located within the HLA class I region of chromosome 6. MICA/MICB organization, expression and products differ considerably from classical HLA class I genes. [6] Mapping studies identified seven MIC loci (MICA–MICG), of which only MICA and MICB encode transcripts, while MICC, MICD, MICE, MICF, and MICG are pseudogenes. MICA gene is located 47 kb centromeric to HLA-B [7] in the MHC class I region and MICB gene is located near to MICA, shares identical structures, functions, and patterns of expression. These genes are highly polymorphic, with several MICA and MICB alleles recognized [8]. A high degree of linkage disequilibrium exists between MICA, MICB, and HLA-B. MICA and MICB gene polymorphisms have been found associated with autoimmune diseases [9] including insulin-dependent diabetes mellitus [10], Addison's disease [11], celiac disease [12, 13], rheumatoid arthritis [14, 15], Behcet's disease [16], and IBD [17–19]

These molecules do not bind β2 microglobulin or peptide typical of HLA class I. The highly polymorphic MICA and MICB encode stress-inducible glycoproteins expressed on a variety of epithelial cells including intestinal epithelial cells. Interaction with the receptor NKG2D is likely to provide an important costimulatory signal for the activation of natural killer (NK) cells, macrophages, CD8+αβ, and gδT cells [20]. MICA/MICB encodes proteins that interact with different T-cell receptors in response to stress as infection, as heat-shock, oxidative stress or neoplastic transformation. Gamma/delta T cells are concentrated in the intestinal mucosa and appear to have a prominent role in recognizing small bacterial phosphoantigens and other antigens presented by MICA/MICB proteins. Gamma/delta T cells have potent cytotoxic activity and have been considered a link between innate and adaptative immunity [20].

MHC class II encodes heterodimeric peptide-binding proteins, and proteins that modulate peptide loading onto MHC class II proteins in the lysosomal compartment. Among the most studied MHC genes are the four classes of human leukocyte antigen (HLA) genes that encode cell-surface antigen-presenting proteins. The class II region lies at the centromeric end of the MHC and encodes HLA class genes HLA-DRA, -DRB1, -DRB3, -DRB4, -DRB5, -DQA1, -DQB1, -DPA1 and -DPB1. HLA class II expression is limited to cells involved in immune responses, where these molecules present extracellularly derived peptides to CD4-positive T cells.

In HLA-DR, the polymorphic variation is provided by the β-chain alone as the α-chain is monomorphic. However, in DQ and DP, both the α-chains and the β-chains are polymorphic. As a result, unique DQ and DP molecules can be formed with α- and β-chains encoded on the same chromosome (*i.e.* encoded in *cis*) or on opposite chromosomes (*i.e.* encoded in *trans*) [21]. The occurrence of *trans*-encoded HLA class II molecules is well documented in the literature [22]. However, evidence suggests that not every α- and β-chain pairing will form a stable heterodimer [23, 24]. It is generally considered that alleles of DQ-α- and DQ-β-chains pair up predominantly in *cis* rather than in *trans* [23, 25].

Located between the class I and class II regions lies the class III region where a number of non-HLA genes with immune function are located. These genes are located on the 1100 kb section between class I and class II genes inside the MHC, and contain about 70 genes. The complement gene block is inherited as a genetic unit known as complotype. Each complotype codifies for the synthesis of complement classic pathway C2, C4A, C4b factors, and alternative pathway B factor, which may suggest that alterations within the region might affect the host's defense system and introduce a complement deficiency [26].

HLA-G is a non-classical MHC class I molecule displaying restricted tissue expression and low polymorphism. Under normal conditions expression of the HLA-G protein is restricted to the feto-maternal interface on the extravillous cytotrophoblast protecting the fetal semi-allograft against the maternal immune system and to the thymus in adults, creating a general state of tolerance. HLA-G exhibit tolerogenic properties via interaction with inhibitory receptors presented in natural killer (NK) cells, T cells and antigen-presenting cells (APC) [27].

HLA-G expression is up-regulated under pathological conditions in inflammatory diseases such as psoriasis [28] and atopic dermatitis [29], IBD [30], celiac disease [31], in viral infection [32], and organ transplants [34]. The main function of HLA-G is suppression of several immune processes carrying out inhibitory effects on cytolysis by NK cells and CTL, T cell proliferative responses and maturation of dendritic cells. These inhibitory effects are mediated by ligation of HLA-G and inhibitory receptors such as ITL2, ITL4 and KIR2DL4 on the surface of immunocompetent cells [34].

HLA-G exhibits low allelic polymorphism in comparison with the classical MHC class I molecules. HLA-G alleles are known at the nucleotide level resulting in seven different proteins [35, 36]. Seven protein isoforms, four membrane bound (HLAG1,-G2, -G3 and -G4) and three soluble (HLA-G5, -G6 and -G7), are generated by alternative splicing [37, 38]. Further nucleotide polymorphisms have been described within the non-coding region of the HLA-G gene, 18 single-nucleotide polymorphisms (SNPs) in the promoter region and a 14-bp deletion polymorphism in exon 8 (rs16375) encoding for the 3'untranslated region [39,40]. The latter polymorphism is potentially functional influencing transcript levels and splicing [41]. In addition to the allelic polymorphism the HLA-G gene shows a deletion/insertion polymorphism of a 14 base pairs sequence (14bp) in the exon 8 at the 3 untranslated region.

2. Inflammatory bowel disease (IBD)

2.1. HLA class I and class II

Inflammatory bowel diseases (IBDs) are complex, multifactorial disorders that comprise Crohn's disease (CD) and ulcerative colitis (UC). Genome-wide association (GWA) studies have identified approximately 100 loci that are significantly associated with IBD [42-44]. These loci implicate a diverse array of genes and pathophysiologic mechanisms, including microbe recognition, lymphocyte activation, cytokine signaling, and intestinal epithelial defense. Although CD and UC are both associated with genomic regions that implicate products of genes involved in leukocyte trafficking, there is evidence for association patterns that are distinct between CD and UC [45].

Evidence from family and twin studies suggests that genetics plays an important role in predisposing an individual to develop ulcerative colitis and Crohn's disease. Further evidence of a genetic predisposition comes from studies of the association between the human leukocyte antigen (HLA) system and IBD [46]. The immunogenetic predisposition may be considered an important requirement for the development of IBD, as several markers of human major histocompatibility complex. HLA complex on chromosome 6 is the most extensively studied genetic region in inflammatory bowel disease [46]. Although it is difficult to estimate the importance of this region in determining overall genetic susceptibility, calculations derived from studies of HLA allele sharing within families suggest that this region contributes between 10%-33% of the total genetic risk of crohn's disease[47] and 64%-100% of the total genetic risk of ulcerative colitis[48].

Antigen presentation by intestinal epithelial cells (IEC) is crucial for intestinal homeostasis [49]. Results from Bisping et al. [50] showed an activation of CD8+effector T cells during active IBD, a process related to MHC I. These data emphasize the importance of the MHC I and II-associated antigen presentation by IEC for the homeostasis of the gut. Disturbances MHC I and II-related presentation pathways in IEC appear to be involved in an altered activation of CD4(+) and CD8(+) T cells in inflammatory bowel disease [51]

The mechanism by which classical HLA class II genes exert their influence in IBD is unclear, although a number of hypotheses have been postulated. Polymorphism in these molecules is concentrated around specific pockets of the binding groove that interact with critical side-chains or 'anchor' residues of a peptide. Thus different HLA molecules may bind preferentially to different peptides, or bind the same peptide with varying affinity. In IBD, cross reactivity (known as "molecular mimicry") may exist between the peptides derived from bacterial luminal flora and from self- antigens present in the gut. This may lead to the generation of auto reactive T cells which contribute to disease pathogenesis through either stimulation or inhibition of the immune system [46].

The recent developments in IBD research point clearly to a defect in the mucosal barrier of the gut as the pivotal and primary pathogenic mechanism [52]. Subsequently, mucosal tolerance is disturbed and effector T cells are stimulated constantly, perpetuating the inflammatory process. In CD, inflammation is driven by CD4+ T helper type 1 (Th1) and Th17 cells that, among others, secrete IFN-γ, TNF-α, IL-17, IL-21, IL-22 and IL-26. The immune response in UC appears to be less polarized, but reveals a strong Th2 component with IL-4, IL-5 and IL-13. The role of CD8+ effector T cells is still uncertain. Activated DC is considered to play the major role in antigen presentation and activation of the afore-mentioned effector T cells [49].

HLA genes are the most extensively studied genetic regions in ulcerative colitis (UC). There is consistent evidence that supports the variable incidence of the disease among ethnic groups, familial aggregation, monozygotic twins and the increased frequency of UC in certain genetic syndromes. There are several HLA alleles associated with different clinical features in UC patients, but they may change according to the ethnic group, such as HLADRB52 and HLA-

http://dx.doi.org/10.5772/57497

DRB1*02 in Japanese [53], HLADRB1*03 in Caucasians [26, 46, 53–56,], the HLA-B35 in Jews [56], HLA-A19, HLA-A33 in Asians [26, 57] and HLADRB1*04 in the Amerindian population in Mexico [58].

The HLA-DRB1 allele is the most studied in inflammatory bowel disease (IBD). There are existing data that some of these alleles may confer risk as well as protective characteristics. There is a consistent association between HLA-DRB1*0103 and severe UC in American and European populations. It is one of the most remarkable allelic associations that provides evidence about the association between HLA-DRB1*0103 and extensive colitis, a severe course of disease, extra-intestinal manifestations (EIMs) and disease activity [59]. A number of HLA associations have been described with the extra-intestinal manifestations of IBD. It is known the association between DRB1*0103 and the extra-intestinal manifestation in patients with colonic Crohn's disease. In this sense, symmetrical arthritis is associated with HLA-B*44 [60]. Uveitis has also been associated with DRB1*0103 and HLA-B*27, and erythema nodosum with the TNF promoter SNP TNF-1031C [61].

Okada Y et al. [62] have demonstrated that a particular HLA haplotype, HLA-Cw*1202-B*5201 DRB1*1502, independently confers a susceptible effect on UC, but has a protective effect on CD in Japanese population. This study showed that one haplotype extending throughout the MHC class I, III, and II regions confers opposite directions of effects on UC and CD. This haplotype accounted for two thirds of the difference of the genetic risks between UC and CD in the MHC region, suggesting its substantial role in the etiology of IBD. The specific pathogens recognized by HLA-Cw*1202-B*5201-DRB1*1502 haplotype will promote the inappropriate proliferation and differentiation of naïve CD4_ T cells and induce the Th1/Th2/Treg imbalance in the intestinal immune response. This imbalance will contribute to the opposite directions of the susceptibility to UC and CD. Contrary to these results, the comparative study for IBD in European populations did not demonstrate the distinct effects in the MHC region. One probable explanation for this discrepancy would be the ethnic differences of haplotype frequencies [62, 63].

Among HLA class I genes, *B52* conferred the greatest risk for UC, whereas *Cw8* and *B21* conferred the greatest risk for CD [64]. GWAS studies have highlighted the importance of the HLA region in IBD, with greater association evidence of HLA variations to risk with UC than CD. A recent meta-analysis of nearly 7000 cases of UC and 20,000 controls reported the strongest association with SNP rs9268853, near HLA DR9.9 In contrast, a meta-analysis of 6300 cases of CD and 15000 controls found a relatively modest level of association for CD within the HLA region, strongest with SNP rs1799964; 21 loci outside the HLA region had more robust significance [65].

Clinical importance of differential diagnosis of UC and CD has been recognized, and incorporation of genetic markers in the diagnosis is proposed as a promising clue [66, 67].The identified HLA haplotype distinguishes UC and CD, which would have more impacts than the previously evaluated variants [67].Thus, utilization of the genotype information of the HLA haplotype, or alternatively the SNP(s) in LD with it, might contribute to improvements of diagnostic approaches on UC and CD.

2.2. Non classical I genes

Intestinal epithelia cells express several non-classical MHC I molecules and are regulated by distinct signals, supporting the hypothesis that these may be involved in local immunoregulation in the intestine [68]. The expression of non-classical MHC I molecules is altered in IBD (all absent in ulcerative colitis [UC] and selective absence of CD1d in Crohn's disease [CD]), providing further evidence for the scenario that non-classical MHC I molecules are involved in T-cell regulation. Distinct regulatory T-cell populations may be regulated by different non-classical class I molecules and that there may be differential regulation of these molecules on intestinal epithelial cells

2.3. MICA/MICB

Some not classical genes related to the class I genes such as MHC class I chain-related gene A (MICA) and MHC class I-related chain B (MICB), are expressed in the basolateral cells in the gastric epithelium, fibroblasts, endothelial and dendritic cells. It is known that its expression rises during viral and bacterial infections [69]. Some genetic studies in patients with IBD have found associations with MICA-A6 and HLA-B52 in Japanese patients with UC [70], MICA*010 and HLA-B*1501 in English patients with fistulous CD [71]. MICA and MICB bind to an activating receptor natural killer group 2D (NKG2D) which is expressed on NK cells, T cells and macrophages and the interactions between these receptors may directly stimulate cell cytotoxicity as well as providing co-stimulation for NK and T cell activation. Several MICA alleles have been shown to alter the binding affinity with NKG2D suggesting they may exert a functional effect on immune activation [26]

Several works showed differences in ethnic and regional living environment that would influence on the MICA/MICB gene distribution. Japanese UC patients showed an increased frequency of allele A6 of the MICA exon 5 trinucleotide microsatellite polymorphism as compared with unaffected controls [72], although a follow up study by this group suggested that the significant increase previously seen was attributable to linkage disequilibrium with HLA-B52 [73]. While Orchard et al. [74] related the MICA × 007 with susceptibility to UC in a British population, Glas et al. [75] failed to show a similar association in their German cohort.

López-Hernández et al. [76] have studied allele polymorphism and the functionally relevant dimorphism (129val/met) of MICA gene in IBD patients in Spanish population. The presence of MICA-129 met/met and MICA-129 val/met genotypes may modify NK, $T\gamma\delta$, and T CD8 lymphocytes activation, and thereby may allow an exacerbated immune response in intestinal environment with a strong inflammatory component. This study showed that MICA-129 val/met genotype was less common in IBD patients than in controls, suggesting that it could be also associated with protection against the disease in these patients. Also, The MICA-129 gene polymorphism was associated with UC in Chinese patients, and the soluble MICA levels in UC patients were higher than those in healthy controls. Based on the role of the *MICA-129* gene in NKG2D-receptor activation, these findings might indicate that the host innate immune response is associated with UC [77].

In recent studies on MIC genes susceptible to UC, MICA*007 [78], MICA*00801, and MICA-A6 [79] were shown to be associated with UC onset in Japan. MICA-A5.1/A5.1 homozygous genotype MICA-A5.1 [80] and MICB-CA18 [81] alleles were associated with UC in the Chinese Han population. Li et al. [82] showed that the frequency of MICB0106 allele was significantly higher in the UC group in a limited population in central China, especially in patients over the age of 40 years with extensive colitis, moderate and severe disease, and in those with extra-intestinal manifestations. The comparison of MICB alleles in the Chinese Han population with those in England and Spain populations showed significant differences in the distribution of the exon2–4 of MICB alleles. Also, significant differences in the distribution of the intron 1 of MICB alleles were also observed between the Chinese and other populations [82].

2.4. HLA-G

A differential pattern of HLA-G expression in CD and UC has been shown. By immunohistochemistry, increased HLA-G surface expression has been only detected in UC, whereas HLA-G expression was absent in CD and also in healthy controls [83]. HLA-G was highly expressed in intestinal tissues of UC, regardless of the intestinal location (ascending, transverse, descending colon, or ileum), and of the medical history and regimen of the patients. The expression of HLA-G was restricted to the apical surface of intestinal epithelial cells (IECs) in the epithelial layer in the intestinal mucosa and Lieberkun crypts. IECs showed intense apical staining and no immunoreactivity was found in the other mucosal cell types such as lymphocytes, macrophages or endothelial cells [83]

Torres et al. [83] suggest a role of HLA-G in the immunopathogenesis of IBD, and proposed that the analysis of HLA-G expression possibly can be used for diagnostic purposes to distinguish between CD and UC in cases of indeterminate colitis In this sense, the study of Rizzo et al. [84] also has documented a clear difference in the production of soluble HLA-G molecules in IBD patients, confirming the presence of a different etiology and immune response mechanisms in UC and CD. HLA-G expression in UC might reflect a down-regulation of the immune response against inflammation. HLA-G expression is likely to be insufficient to protect the intestine from the inflammation after aggression is stopped. HLA-G potentially functions as a shield against inflammatory aggression. It might contribute to tissue protection by inhibiting NK cell activity and tissue infiltration by T cells and monocytes shifting the balance between T_h1 and T_h2 cells toward the T_h2 pathway. A potential role of HLA-G in the pathogenesis of UC is in line with the T_h2 pathway rather characteristic for UC. In UC, the increased expression of HLA-G might reduce clearing of intestinal micro-organisms and therefore promote a secondary chronic inflammation [83].

This differential expression pattern of HLA-G is possibly influenced by genetic variations within the HLA-G gene. The *HLA-G* gene is located in IBD3, a linkage region for inflammatory bowel disease (IBD). A 14-bp deletion polymorphism (Del+/Del−) within exon 8 of the *HLA-G* gene might influence transcription activity and is therefore of potential functional relevance.

Glas et a.l [85] have found that the 14-bp deletion polymorphism in the HLA-G gene displays significant differences between ulcerative colitis and Crohn's disease and is associated with ileocecal resection in Crohn's disease. The allele, genotype and phenotype frequencies of the 14- bp deletion polymorphism in UC or CD displayed no significant differences when compared with a healthy controls [85]. The allele frequencies in the control group found herein were similar to those detected in the control groups of other studies [87-89]. When the UC and CD groups were compared among each other, the Del+ phenotype and the heterozygous Del +/ _ genotype were significantly increased in UC, whereas the frequency of the homozygous genotype Del_/_ was significantly lower in UC than in CD.

The CD patients were stratified for disease behavior, for disease location/extent and for the need of ileocecal resection [85]. In CD patients with ileocecal resection, the frequency of the Del+/Del+ genotype was 47.0% compared with 27.3% in patients without ileocecal resection, whereas the two other genotypes were decreased, showing a significant association of the 14-bp deletion polymorphism. The frequency of the Del+ allele was significantly increased in CD patients with in relation to those patients without ileocecal resection (69.7 versus 52.7%), but not in the comparison of healthy controls. In this sense, HLA-G may play a role in modulating the course of CD rather than determining overall susceptibility. The differences of the 14-bp deletion HLA-G polymorphism between UC and CD found gives evidence for a contribution of the HLA-G gene in the pathogenesis of IBD. The findings of Glas et al. [85] are consistent with the differential expression pattern of HLA-G in UC compared with CD as shown by Torres et al. [83], and in agreement with the work of O'Brien et al. [89], where decreased HLA-G expression was observed in placenta samples of cases with homozygous Del - genotype.

2.5. MHC class III genes

The proteins produced from MHC class III genes exhibiting functions in immunological processes such as the cytokines TNF-α, TNF-β and the heat shock proteins [26]. The functions of some MHC genes are unknown. This raises attention when TNF-α is thought to play an important role in the pathogenesis of IBD, acting as a potent pro-inflammatory cytokine with elevated serum and tissue levels in patients with IBD [59, 90-91], and evidence show that there are specific genetic polymorphisms involving TNF-α that influence the amount of cytokine produced.

Bouma et al. [92] and Louis et al. [93] studied the allelic frequency of TNF-α gene polymorphisms at -308 position finding that polymorphism in allele 2 was decreased in UC patients as compared to normal controls. In a Mexican population with UC, the presence of TNF*2 allele was associated with the presence of this disease as compared with healthy subjects [94]. In Mexican patients with UC, an association was found between complotype SC30 (Bf*S-C2*C-C4A*3-C4B*0) and UC [95], which might suggest that activation of complement system could interfere with the disease pathogenesis.

3. Celiac disease

3.1. HLA class II

HLA is a master piece in the pathogenesis of celiac disease, as first evidenced by the strong genetic association existent between celiac disease susceptibility and certain HLA alleles [96,

97]. Celiac disease is a chronic gluten intolerance that occurs in genetically predisposed individuals. Is a chronic inflammatory disease which is a T cell-mediated inflammatory disorder with autoimmune features and it has environmental and immunologic components. It is characterized by an immune response to ingested wheat gluten and related proteins of rye and barley that leads to inflammation, villous atrophy crypt hyperplasia and lymphocyte infiltration, leading to nutrient malabsorption. A wide spectrum of clinical phenotypes is present, ranging from classical gastrointestinal manifestations to only atypical signs [96].

The prevalence of celiac disease is estimated at about 1:100 in Caucasian population but many cases remain undiagnosed, especially among adult individuals, because of the wide variability of symptoms [98, 99]. As for other autoimmune diseases, celiac disease occurs more often in female than in male subjects with a gender ratio of about 2:1 [98,100,101]. Furthermore, gluten intolerance is more frequent in at-risk groups, such as first-degree relatives of patients as well as individuals with specific genetic syndromes (Down, Turner, Williams) or autoimmune diseases (mainly type 1 diabetes, thyroiditis and multiple sclerosis) [102,103]. Celiac disease has a multifactorial inheritance, so it does not depend on specific mutations of a single gene but it is caused by a combination of environmental factors and variations in multiple genes [104,105]. Familial aggregation (10-12%) and higher concordance rates of celiac disease in monozygotic than in dizygotic twins (83-86% vs. 11%) have been confirmed, indicating that a strong genetic contribution is involved in the disease occurrence [106, 107]. Furthermore, the association with other autoimmune conditions in the same individual or in different members of the same family suggests the existence of common predisposing genes to autoimmunity [108].

The HLA is the most important genetic factor in celiac disease, and carriage of certain HLA alleles is a necessary, but not sufficient, factor for disease development HLA influence on celiac disease susceptibility showing a dose effect that implies the existence of different celiac disease risk categories attending to their HLA constitution [109]. This pathology presents a strong genetic susceptibility: approximately 90 % of celiac patients carry the HLA-DQ2 heterodimer (encoded by DQA1 * 05 and DQB1 * 02 alleles), whereas a smaller percent of subjects carry the HLA-DQ8 heterodimer (encoded by DQA1* 03 and DQB1* 0302 alleles) [110]. The HLA-DQ2 coding alleles can be encoded in *cis* on the DR3-DQ2 haplotype or in *trans* on the DR5-DQ7 / DR7-DQ2 heterozygotes [110,111], whereas the HLA-DQ8 heterodimer is encoded in *cis* on the DR4-DQ8 haplotype. DQ alleles, however, account only for 40 – 50 % of the genetic contribution for CD [112]. It has been reported that not all the HLA DR3 / DQ2 haplotypes confer equal susceptibility to CD, suggesting that DQ2 is not the only HLA-linked genetic risk factor [113].

Individuals can be classified in high or intermediate CD risk according to the number of DQA1*05- and DQB1*02-carrying alleles. Homozigosity for DQ2.5 *cis* and heterozigosity for DQ2.5 *cis* with a chromosome possessing a second DQB1*02allele (DQ2.2) confer the highest risk to develop CD. Heterozigosity or DQ2.5 *cis* in individuals with a single copy of DQB1*02 (non-DQ2.2) or presence of DQ2.5 *trans* confer intermediate risk [109]. The influence of HLADQ8 (genetically DQA1*03, DQB1*03:02) on the disease is already known. This molecule is present in almost all the celiac patients without DQ2.5. However, the genetic influence of the HLA region in CD is not limited to the factors coding DQ2 or DQ8, and several works have attempted to discover new susceptibility factors [109].

In celiac disease, T cell stimulation due to gluten-derived peptides depends on the number and type of HLA-DQ2 molecules expressed. DQ2.5 molecules can bind a high repertoire of gluten peptides, but only a restricted subset is bound to DQ2.2 molecules, which reduce the immunogenicity of DQ2.2. Additionally, the number of these DQ molecules is also a relevant factor in T cell stimulation and this depends on the number of specific alleles in DQA1 and DQB1 loci, which determines the possible αβ-chain combinations constituting the DQ heterodimers [114].

The HLA dose effect is also influenced by differences in the kinetic stability of the interaction between HLA molecules and gluten derived peptides, key factor for development of T cell responses against gluten [115,116]. For most peptide ligands, DQ2.5 shows higher binding stability than DQ2.2.The high kinetic stability of peptide-MHC is a key factor for establishment of antigluten T-cell responses and the development of celiac disease. Kinetic stability of peptide-MHC complexes has been shown to be decisive for antigen-presenting cells to successfully activate naïve T cells in the lymph node [117]. Polymorphism in DQ2.2 results in a lower kinetic binding stability of commonly recognized DQ2.5-restricted T-cell epitopes when tested for binding to DQ2.2. The authors suggest that this phenomenon might explain the large difference in risk of celiac disease for these homologous DQ molecules [118]. Moreover, gluten epitopes recognized by DQ2.2 patients would be peptides that form stable peptide-MHC complexes and T cells reactive with known DQ2.5-restricted gluten epitopes with fast off-rate would be rarely found [116].

Bodd et al. [119] have reported the presence of DQ9-restricted gluten reactive T cells recognizing the DQ8-glut-1 epitope, an epitope previously described to be recognized by DQ8 patients, in the small intestine of a celiac patient expressing DQ9. This epitope appears to be the dominant DQ9-restricted epitope in this patient and binds particularly well to DQ9 compared with other DQ8 gluten epitopes. These authors found that DQ9-restricted gluten-reactive CD4_ T cells could be isolated from the small intestine of a CD patient expressing DQ9 and DQ2.2.

HLA typing does not have an absolute diagnostic value but allows asses the CD relative risk; a positive test is indicative of genetic susceptibility but does not necessarily mean the disease development [97]. A negative test has a more significant value because gluten intolerance rarely occurs in the absence of specific HLA predisposing alleles. HLA genes are stable markers throughout life, so their typing can discriminate genetically CD-susceptible or not susceptible individuals before any clinical or serological signs. HLA test is increasingly considered as a solid support in the diagnostic algorithm of CD. New European Society for Pediatric Gastroenterology, Hepatology and Nutrition (ESPGHAN) guidelines for the diagnosis of CD have established that duodenal biopsy can be omitted in cases with elevated serum anti-TG2 antibodies positive and at-risk HLA [120].

3.2. MICA/MICB

MICA and MICB are interesting candidates as susceptibility genes in celiac disease. It has been demonstrated that peptides from gliadin could induce the expression of MICA in gut epithelium of celiac patients [121]. Moreover, the participation of the MICA/NKG2D pathway in the destruction of intestinal epithelium by intraepithelial T lymphocytes in celiac disease has been revealed [122].

Aberrant MICA responses have been implicated in celiac disease. MICA/B expression was reduced in duodenal samples from patients under a gluten-free diet, reflecting a possible link between the ongoing inflammatory process induced by gluten ingestion and MICA/B expression. Therefore, considering the pattern of MICA/B expression in different cell lineages observed, signals for induction of MICA/B may be part of a more general mechanism associated to the ongoing inflammatory process in the small intestine in untreated celiac patients. Several studies on intestinal tissue, isolated cells from intestinal mucosa or epithelial cell lines support a link between cellular (heat, oxidative and ER) stress and mucosal damage. In their study, the authors also observed expression of MICA/MICB in B and T lymphocytes [123,124]. MICA expression in activated T lymphocytes confers susceptibility to NK cell-mediated cytotoxicity [125].Cell surface MICA/B expression may act to negatively regulate T cell function by decreasing of IFN-c production and cytotoxicity and reduce tissue damage by regulatory mechanisms via NK/T cell interaction.

High production of IL-15 in intestinal mucosa in active celiac disease has been shown to trigger enterocyte apoptosis via the induction of cell surface MICA, which in turn interacts with the activating NKG2D receptor present in intestinal epithelial lymphocytes. Cytotoxic activity of IELs is also potentiated by IL-15 through activation of JNK and ERK pathways [126-128], Though MICA/B confers susceptibility to NKG2D-mediated killing of enterocytes by intraepithelial NK and $CD8^+$ T cells in untreated celiac disease, these results suggest that MICA/B expression may also regulate cell survival of other cells in the intestinal mucosa.

Allegretti et al [129] observed a more ubiquitous distribution of MICA/B expression. In enterocytes, the expression was mainly found in the cytoplasm as peri- and/or supra-nuclear aggregates. The analysis of the intraepithelial compartment, which contains different lymphocytes, most of them $CD7^+$ cells, revealed the expression of MICA/B in lymphocytes in celiacs and control samples. The authors found coarse MICA/B aggregates in the cytoplasma of $CD7^+$ cells; which were more frequently observed in mild enteropathy samples.the intracellular location of MICA in intraepithelial and lamina propria T cells may hinder their recognition by NKG2D-expressing cells avoiding the control of over activated T cells [129]. The results of these authors suggest that expression of MICA/B in the intestinal mucosa of celiac patients is linked to deregulation of mucosa homeostasis in which the stress response plays an active role. MICA/B may play a more general role than previously thought in gut immunobiology.

Rodríguez- Rodero et al. [130] have found that the MICB promoter is polymorphic and some of them were seen to be associated with celiac disease. The variants 45944--, 46219G, and 46286G, as parts of the MICB*008 and MICB*002 promoters (Haplotype 3), were found to be significantly overrepresented in celiac patients. In addition to the MICB*008 allele, the

MICB*002 allele is included in the extended haplotypes EH62.1, EH60.1, EH51.1, and EH18.2 [131], which are frequently found in Caucasian populations. These haplotypes carry one or two susceptibility chains (DQA1*0501, DQB1*0201, DQB1*0202, DQA1*03, and DQB1*0302). MICA-A5.1 transmembrane polymorphism (MICA*00801) is associated with a risk of atypical CD and that this was found to be independent of the known susceptibility extended haplotype EH8.1 [132]. A double dose of the MICA 5.1 allele could also predispose to the onset of gastrointestinal symptoms-celiac disease [133].

3.3. HLA-G

Celiac disease is always associated with the HLADQ heterodimer encoded by DQA1*0501 and DQB1*0201 alleles, although this gene do not explain the entire genetic susceptibility to gluten intolerance [96, 97]. Therefore, it has been suggested that other genes might predispose to celiac disease. HLA-G is a molecule of immune tolerance implicated in several inflammatory diseases. Consequently, it is interesting to study the effect of this molecule in the development of celiac disease.

Torres et al. [134] have demonstrated an association of celiac disease with HLA-G expression. They have described the expression of soluble HLA-G in biopsy samples and in serum from patients with celiac disease. Conversely, membrane HLA-G molecules were not expressed in celiac patients. The lack of membrane HLA-G expression may be linked to a specific regulatory process in the alternative splicing of the primary HLA-G transcript, which could favour selection of the soluble isoforms. The enhancer expression of soluble HLA-G in celiac disease could be due as part of a mechanism to try restore the tolerance process towards oral antigens in a disease caused by loss of tolerance to dietary antigens. A powerful anti-inflammatory response to gliadin might occur during the development of the disease with uncontrolled production of HLA-G that counteract the inflammation or/and may cause recruitment of intra-epithelial lymphocytes, maintaining the intestinal lesions [31].

A number of functional HLA-G gene polymorphisms have been identified, including a 14 bp deletion/ insertion polymorphism (located at the 3 ′ UTR of the gene, in exon 8; rs1704) associated with differences in the pattern of alternatively spliced mRNA isoforms and in concentration of sHLA-G; moreover, the inserted allele affects the mRNA stability [134, 135]. Fabriset et al. [136] have analyzed the 14 bp deletion / insertion polymorphism in a group of celiac patients and healthy individuals, stratified for the presence of HLA-DQ2 genotype, to evaluate the possible association of the HLA-G 14 bp deletion/ insertion polymorphism with the disease. These authors found significant differences in the frequencies of both the 14 bp inserted (I) / deleted (d) alleles and genotypes when comparing celiac patients with healthy controls. The higher frequency of the I allele in celiac patients as compared to healthy controls allowed to hypothesize that HLA-G molecules are involved in the susceptibility to celiac disease, as the presence of the inserted allele associated with an increased susceptibility to this pathology. The presence of the I allele confers an increased risk of celiac disease in addition to the risk conferred by HLADQ2 alone and that subjects that carry both DQ2 and HLA-G I alleles have an increased risk of celiac disease than subjects that carry DQ2 but not the I allele [136].

The 14 bp inserted allele can affect the HLA-G synthesis that is induced in celiac disease, by influencing the pattern of mRNA HLA-G splicing and by affecting the mRNA stability [135, 136]. In healthy individuals the intestinal immunity is set toward tolerance to ingested antigens, and high concentrations of anti-inflammatory cytokines are normally found in the intestine. Celiac disease is instead associated with production of pro-inflammatory cytokines such as IFN- γ and IL-15. In addition, HLA-G is induced by IFN- γ in mononuclear cells, indicating that HLA-G might constitute a pathway to protect tissues from the infiltration of T cells [137].

4. Conclusions

Today, the HLA complex occupies a central position in basic and clinical immunology. This chapter reviews current knowledge of the role of HLA complex genes in IBD and celiac disease susceptibility and phenotype, and shows the factors currently limiting the translation of this knowledge to clinical practice. Interest in the HLA complex in IBD and celiac disease has traditionally focused on association with the classical class II HLA alleles, but recent insights into the biological function of other genes encoded within this region have led investigators to a more diverse exploration of this region. The well characterization of these genes potentially will lead to the identification of therapeutic agents and clinical assessment of phenotype and prognosis in patients with these intestinal disorders.The HLA region represents the genome's highest concentration of potential biomarkers for most studied diseases. Specific HLA genotypes have already been associated with sensitivities to five marketed drugs and arecurrently being investigated as biomarkers in several clinical trials [138].

Author details

M.I. Torres, T. Palomeque and P. Lorite

Department of Experimental Biology, University of Jaén, Spain

References

[1] Medrano LM, Dema B, López-Larios A, *et al.* HLA and Celiac Disease Susceptibility: New Genetic Factors Bring Open Questions about the HLA Influence and Gene-Dosage Effects. Plos One 7 (10) e48403. 2012

[2] Torres AR, Westover JB, Rosenspire AJ. HLA immune function genes in autism. Autism Res Treat. 2012;2012:959073

[3] Horton R, Wilming L, Rand V, *et al*. Gene map of the extended human MHC. Nat Rev Genetics 5: 889–899. 2004

[4] Robinson J, Halliwell JA, McWilliam H, *et al*. The IMGT/HLA database. Nucl Acids Res 41: 1222-27. 2013

[5] Howell WM. HLA and disease: guilt by association. Int J Immunogenet. 2013

[6] Rodriguez-Rodero S, Rodrigo L, Fernandez-Morera JL, *et al*. MHC Class I Chain-Related Gene B Promoter Polymorphisms and Celiac Disease. Hum Immunol 67: 208–214. 2006.

[7] Bahram S, Bresnahan M, Geraghty DE, *et al*. A second lineage of mammalian major histocompatibility complex class I genes. Proc. Natl Acad. Sci.USA 91: 6259-6263. 1994.

[8] Marsh SG, Albert ED, Bodmer WF, *et al*. Nomenclature for factors of the HLA system, 2004. Tissue Antigens 65:301-369. 2005

[9] Stephens HA.MICA and MICB genes: can the enigma of their polymorphism be resolved?. Trends Immunol. 22(7): 378-85. 2001

[10] Gambelunghe G, Ghaderi CA, Cosentino A, *et a*l. Association of MHC Class I chain-related A (MIC-A) gene polymorphism with Type I diabetes. Diabetologia 43: 507–514. 2000

[11] Park YS, Sanjeevi CB, Robles D, *et al*.Additional association of intra-MHC genes, MICA and D6S273, with Addison's disease. Tissue Antigens 60: 155–163. 2002

[12] Rueda B, Pascual M, Lopez-Nevot MA *et al*. Association of MICA-A5. 1 allele with susceptibility to celiac disease in a family study. Am J Gastroenterol 98: 359–362. 2003

[13] González S, Rodrigo L, López-Vázquez A, *et al*. Association of MHC class I related gene B (MICB) to celiac disease. Am J Gastroenterol 99:676–680. 2004

[14] Mok JW, Lee YJ, Kim JY, *et al*. Association of MICA polymorphism with rheumatoid arthritis patients in Koreans. Hum Immunol 64: 1190–1194. 2003

[15] Lopez-Arbesu R, Ballina-Garcia FJ, Alperi-Lopez M, *et al*. MHC class I chain-related gene B (MICB) is associated with rheumatoid arthritis susceptibility. Rheumatology 46: 426–430. 2007

[16] Hughes EH, Collins RW, Kondeatis E, *et al*. Associations of major histocompatibility complex class I chain-related molecule polymorphisms with Behcet's disease in Caucasian patients. Tissue Antigens 66:195–199. 2005

[17] Fernández-Morera JL, Rodrigo L, Lopez-Vazquez A, *et al*. MHC class I chain-related gene A transmembrane polymorphism modulates the extension of ulcerative colitis. Hum Immunol 64: 816–822. 2003

[18] Ahmad T, Marshall SE, Mulcahy-Hawes K, *et al.* High resolution MIC genotyping: design and application to the investigation of inflammatory bowel disease susceptibility. Tissue Antigens 60: 164–179. 2002

[19] Sugimura K, Ota M, Matsuzawa J, *et al.* A close relationship of triplet repeat polymorphism in MHC class I chain-related gene A (MICA) to the disease susceptibility and behavior in ulcerative colitis. Tissue Antigens 57: 9–14.2001

[20] Groh V, Steinle A, Bauer S, *et al.* Recognition of stress induced MHC molecules by intestinal epithelial gamma delta T cells. Science 279: 17–40. 1998

[21] Tollefsen S, Hotta K, Chen X, *et al.* Structural and Functional Studies of *trans*-Encoded HLA-DQ2.3 (DQA1*03:01/DQB1*02:01) Prot Mol J Biol Chem 287(17): 13611–13619. 2012

[22] Charron DJ, Lotteau V, Turmel P. Hybrid HLA-DC antigens provide molecular evidence for gene *trans*-complementation. Nature 312: 157–159. 1984

[23] Kwok WW, Nepom GT. Structural and functional constraints on HLA class II dimers implicated in susceptibility to insulin dependent diabetes mellitus. Baillieres Clin. Endocrinol. Metab. 5: 375–393. 1991

[24] Kwok WW, Kovats S, Thurtle P, *et al.* HLA-DQ allelic polymorphisms constrain patterns of class II heterodimer formation. J Immunol. 150: 2263–2272. 1993

[25] McFarland BJ, Beeson C. Binding interactions between peptides and proteins of the class II major histocompatibility complex. Med Res Rev. 22: 168–203. 2002

[26] Rodríguez-Bores L, Fonseca GC, Villeda MA, *et al.* Novel genetic markers in inflammatory bowel disease. World J Gastroenterol. 13(42): 5560-5570. 2007

[27] Carosella ED, Moreau P, Le Maoult P, *et al.* HLA-G molecules: from maternal-fetal tolerance to tissue acceptance. Adv Immunol 81:199-252. 2003

[28] Aractingi S, Briand N, Le Danff C, *et al.* HLA-G and NK receptor are expressed in psoriatic skin: a possible pathway for regulating infiltrating T cells? Am J Pathol 159: 71–77. 2001

[29] Khosrotehrani K, Le Danff C, Reynaud-Mendel B, *et al.* HLA-G expression in atopic dermatitis. J Invest Dermatol 117(3):750-2. 2001

[30] Torres MI, Le Discorde M, Lorite P, *et al.* Expression of HLA-G in inflammatory bowel disease provides a potential way to distinguish between ulcerative colitis and Crohn's disease. Int Immunol 16(4):579-583. 2004

[31] Torres MI, López-Casado MA, Luque J, *et al.* New advances in coeliac disease: serum and intestinal expression of HLA-G. Int Immunol 18(5):713-718. 2006

[32] Lozano JM, González R, Kindelán JM, *et al.* Monocytes and T lymphocytes in HIV-1-positive patients express HLA-G molecule. AIDS 16(3):347-51. 2002

[33] Carosella ED. The tolerogenic molecule HLA-G. Immunol Lett 138(1):22-24. 2011

[34] Luque J, Torres MI, Aumente MD, et al. Soluble HLA-G in heart transplantation: their relationship to rejection episodes and immunosuppressive therapy. Hum Immunol 67(4-5):257-63. 2006

[35] Kirszenbaum M, Djoulah S, Hors J, *et al.* HLA-G gene polymorphism segregation within CEPH reference families. Hum Immunol 53: 140-147. 1997

[36] Hiby S, E King, Sharkey A, *et al.* Molecular studies of trophoblast HLA-G: polymorphism, isoforms, imprinting and expression in preimplantation embryo. Tissue Antigens 53:1-13. 1999

[37] Kirszenbaum M, Moreau P, Gluckman E, *et al.* An alternatively spliced form of HLA-G mRNA in human trophoblasts and evidence for the presence of HLA-G transcript in adult lymphocytes. Proc. Natl Acad. Sci.USA 91:4209-4213. 1994

[38] Paul P, Cabestre FA, Ibrahim EC, *et al.* Identification of HLA-G7 as a new splice variant of the HLA-G mRNA and expression of soluble HLA-G5, -G6, and -G7 transcripts in human transfected cells. Hum Immunol. 61: 1138-1149. 2000

[39] Harrison GA, Humphrey KE, Jakobsen IB, *et al.* A 14-bp deletion polymorphism in the HLA-G gene. Hum Mol Genet. 2: 2200. 1993

[40] Ober C, Aldrich CL, Chervoneva I, *et al.* Variation in the HLA-G promoter region influences miscarriage rates. Am J Hum Genet. 72:1425-1435. 2003

[41] O'Brien M, McCarthy T, Jenkins D, *et al.* Altered HLA-G transcription in pre-eclampsia is associated with allele specific inheritance: possible role of the HLA-G gene in susceptibility to the disease. Cell Mol Life Sci 58:1943-1949. 2001

[42] Anderson CA, Boucher G, Lees CW, *et al.* Meta-analysis identifies 29 additional ulcerative colitis risk loci, increasing the number of confirmed associations to 47. Nat Genet 43:246–252. 2011

[43] Stokkers PC, Reitsma PH, Tytgat GN, *et al.* HLA-DR and –DQ phenotypes in inflammatory bowel disease: a meta- analysis. Gut 45:395–401 1999.

[44] Franke A, McGovern DP, Barrett JC, *et al.* Genome-wide meta-analysis increases to 71 the number of confirmed Crohn's disease susceptibility loci. Nat Genet 42:1118–1125. 2010

[45] Cho JH, Brant SR. Recent Insights Into the Genetics of Inflammatory Bowel Disease. Gastroenterology 140:1704–1712. 2011

[46] Ahmad T, Marshall SE, Jewell D. Genetics of inflammatory bowel disease: The role of the HLAComplex. World J Gastroenterol 12(23): 3628-3635. 2006

[47] Yang H, Plevy SE, Taylor K, *et al*. Linkage of Crohn's diseaseto the major histocompatibility complex region is detected by multiple non-parametric analyses. Gut 44: 519-526. 1999

[48] Satsangi J, Welsh KI, Bunce M, *et al*. Contribution of genes of the major histocompatibility complex to susceptibility and disease phenotype in inflammatory bowel disease. Lancet 347: 1212-1217. 1996

[49] Bär F, Sina C, Hundorfean G, *et al*. Inflammatory bowel diseases influence major histocompatibilitycomplex class I (MHC I) and II compartments in intestinal epithelial cells. Clinical and Experimental Immunology, 172: 280–289. 2012

[50] Bisping G, Lügering N, Lütke-Brintrup S, *et al*. Patients with inflammatory bowel disease (IBD) reveal increased inductioncapacity of intracellular interferon-gamma (IFN-gamma) in peripheral CD8+ lymphocytes co-cultured with intestinal epithelial cells. Clin Exp Immunol 123:15–22. 2001

[51] Powrie F, Leach MW, Mauze S, *et al*. Phenotypically distinct subsets of CD4+ T cells induce or protect from chronic intestinal inflammation in C. B-17 Scid mice. Int Immunol 5: 1461-1471. 1993

[52] Rosenstiel P, Sina C, Franke A, *et al*. Towards a molecular risk map – recent advances on the etiology of inflammatory bowel disease. Semin Immunol 21:334–45. 2009

[53] Duerr RH, Neigut DA. Molecularly defined HLA-DR2 alleles in ulcerative colitis and an anti-neutrophil cytoplasmic antibody positive subgroup. Gastroenterology 108: 423–427. 1995

[54] Toyoda H, Wang SJ, Yang H. Distinct association of HLA class II genes with inflammatory bowel disease. Gastroenterology 104: 741–748. 1993

[55] Satsangi J, Welsh KI, Bunce M, *et al*. Disease phenotype in inflammatory bowel disease. Lancet 347: 1212–1217. 1996

[56] Delpre G, Kadish U, Gazit E. HLA antigens in ulcerative colitis and Crohn's disease in Israel. Gastroenterology 78: 1452–1457. 1980

[57] Habeeb MA, Rajalingam R, Dhar A, *et al*. HLA association and ocurrence of autoantibodies in Asian Indian patients with ulcerative colitis. Am J Gastroenterol 92: 772–776. 1997

[58] Yamamoto-Furusho JK, Uscanga LF, Vargas-Alarcón G, *et al.* Clinical and genetic heterogeneity in Mexican patients with ulcerative colitis. Hum Immunol 64: 119–123. 2003

[59] Yamamoto-Furusho JK, Rodríguez-Bores L, Granados J. HLA-DRB1 alleles are associated with the clinical course of disease and steroid dependence in Mexican patients with ulcerative colitis. Colorectal Disease. 12: 1231–1235. 2010

[60] Orchard TR, Thiyagaraja S, Welsh KI, *et al*. Clinical phenotype is related to HLA genotype in the peripheral arthropathies of inflammatory bowel disease. Gastroenterology 118: 274-278. 2000

[61] Orchard TR, Chua CN, Ahmad T, *et al*. Uveitis and erythema nodosum in inflammatory bowel disease: clinical features and the role of HLA genes. Gastroenterology 123: 714-718. 2002

[62] Okada Y, Yamazaki K, Umeno J, *et al*. HLA-Cw*1202-B*5201-DRB1*1502 Haplotype Increases Risk for Ulcerative Colitis but Reduces Risk for Crohn's Disease. Gastroenterology 141:864–871. 2011

[63] Asano K, Matsushita T, Umeno J, *et al*. A genome-wide association study identifies three new susceptibility loci for ulcerative colitis in the Japanese population. Nat Genet 41:1325– 1329. 2009

[64] Fernando MM, Stevens CR, Walsh EC, *et al*. Defining the role of the MHC in autoimmunity: a review and pooled analysis. PLoS Genet 4:e1000024. 2008

[65] Yamazaki K, McGovern D, Ragoussis J, *et al*. Single nucleotide polymorphisms in TNFSF15 confers susceptibility to Crohn's disease. Hum Mol Genet 14:3499–3506. 2005

[66] Geboes K, Colombel JF, Greenstein A, *et al*. Indeterminate colitis: a review of the concept—what's in a name? Inflamm Bowel Dis 14:850–857. 2008

[67] Vermeire S, Van Assche G, Rutgeerts P. Role of genetics in prediction of disease course and response to therapy. World J Gastroenterol 16:2609–2615. 2010

[68] Perera L, Shao L, Patel A, *et al*. Expression of Nonclassical Class I Molecules by Intestinal Epithelial Cells. Inflamm Bowel Dis 13:298 –307. 2007

[69] Lee N, Llano M, Carretero M, *et al*. HLA-E is a major ligand for the natural killer inhibitory receptor CD94/NKG2A. Proc Natl Acad Sci US A. 95:5199 –5204. 1998

[70] Braud VM, Allan DS, O'Callaghan CA, *et al*. HLA-E binds to natural killer cell receptors CD94/NKG2A, B and C. Nature. 391:795–799. 1998

[71] Roberts AI, Blumberg RS, Christ AD, *et al*. Staphylococcalentero toxin B induces potent cytotoxic activity by intraepithelial lymphocytes. Immunology 101:185–190. 2000

[72] Sugimura K, Ota M, Matsuzawa J, *et al*. A close relationship of triplet repeat polymorphism in MHC class I chain-related gene A (MICA) to the disease susceptibility and behavior in ulcerative colitis. Tissue Antigens 57: 9–14. 2001

[73] Seki SS, Sugimura K, Ota M, *et al*. Stratification analysis of MICA triplet repeat polymorphisms and HLA antigens associated with ulcerative colitis in Japanese, Tissue Antigens 58: 71– 76. 2001

[74] Orchard TR, Dhar A, Simmons JD, *et al.* Jewell MHC class I chain-like gene A (MICA)and its associations with inflammatory bowel disease and peripheral arthropathy, Clin Exp Immunol 126: 437–440. 2001

[75] Glas J, Martin K, Brunnler G, *et al.* MICA, MICB and C1 4 1 polymorphism in Crohn's disease and ulcerative colitis, Tissue Antigens 58: 243–249. 2001

[76] López-Hernández R, Valdés M, Lucas D, *et al.* Association analysis of MICA gene polymorphism and MICA-129 dimorphism with inflammatory bowel disease susceptibility in a Spanish population. Hum Immunol 71: 512–514. 2010

[77] Zhao J, Jiang Y, Lei Y, *et al.* Functional MICA-129 polymorphism and serum levels of soluble MICA are correlated with ulcerative colitis in Chinese patients. J Gastroenterol Hepatol 26: 593–598. 2011

[78] Sugimura K, Ota M, Matsuzawa J, *et al.* A close relationship of triplet repeat polymorphism in MHC class I chain-related gene A (MICA) to the disease susceptibility and behavior in ulcerative colitis. Tissue Antigens 57:9–14. 2001

[79] Ahmad T, Armuzzi A, Neville M, *et al.* The contribution of human leucocyte antigen complex genes to disease phenotype in ulcerative colitis. Tissue Antigens 62:527–35. 2003

[80] Ding YJ, Xia B, Lü M et al. MHC class I chain-related geneA-A5.1 allele is associated with ulcerative colitis in Chinese population. Clin Exp Immunol 142:193–198. 2005

[81] Lü M, Xia B, Li J, *et al.* MICB microsatellite polymorphism is associated with ulcerative colitis in Chinese population. Clin Immunol 120:199–204. 2006

[82] Li Y, Xia B, Lü M, *et al.* MICB0106 gene polymorphism is associated with ulcerative colitis in central China. Int J Colorectal Dis 25:153–159. 2010

[83] Torres MI, Le Discorde M, Lorite P, *et al.* Expression of HLA-G in inflammatory bowel disease provides a potential way to distinguish between ulcerative colitis and Crohn's disease. Int Immunol 16:579-. 2004

[84] Rizzo R, Melchiorri L, Simone L, *et al.* Different Production of Soluble HLA-G Antigens by Peripheral Blood Mononuclear Cells in Ulcerative Colitis and Crohn's Disease: A Noninvasive Diagnostic Tool?. Inflamm Bowel Dis 14:100 –105. 2008

[85] Glas J, Török H-P, Tonenchi L, *et al.* The 14-bp deletion polymorphism in the HLA-G gene displays significant differences between ulcerative colitis and Crohn's disease and is associated with ileocecal resection in Crohn's disease. Int Immunol. 19 (5): 621–626. 2007

[86] Harrison GA, Humphrey KE, Jakobsen IB, *et al.* A 14-bp deletion polymorphism in the HLA-G gene. Hum Mol Genet 2: 2200. 1993

[87] Hviid TV, Hylenius S, Hoegh AM, *et al.* HLA-G polymorphisms in couples with recurrent spontaneous abortions. Tissue Antigens 60:122-132. 2002

[88] Hviid TV, Hylenius S, Lindhard A, *et al.* Association between human leukocyte antigen-G genotype and success of in vitro fertilization and pregnancy outcome. Tissue Antigens 64:66-69. 2004

[89] O'Brien M, McCarthy T, Jenkins D, *et al.* Altered HLA-G transcription in pre-eclampsia is associated with allele specific inheritance: possible role of the HLA-G gene in susceptibility to the disease. Cell Mol Life Sci 58:1943-1949. 2001

[90] Murch SH, Lamkin VA, Savage MO, *et al.* Serum concentrations of tumour necrosis factor alpha in childhood chronic inflammatory bowel disease. Gut 32: 913-917. 1991

[91] Reimund JM, Wittersheim C, Dumont S, *et al.* Mucosal inflammatory cytokine production by intestinal biopsies in patients with ulcerative colitis and Crohn's disease. J Clin Immunol 16: 144-150. 1996

[92] Bouma G, Xia B, Crusius JB, *et al.* Distribution of four polymorphisms in the tumour necrosis factor (TNF) genes in patients with inflammatory bowel disease (IBD). Clin Exp Immunol 103: 391-396. 1996

[93] Louis E, Satsangi J, Roussomoustakaki M, *et al.* Cytokine gene polymorphisms in inflammatory bowel disease. Gut 39: 705-710. 1996

[94] Yamamoto-Furusho JK, Uscanga LF, Vargas-Alarcon G, *et al.* Polymorphisms in the promoter region of tumor necrosis factor alpha (TNF-alpha) and the HLA-DRB1 locus in Mexican mestizo patients with ulcerative colitis. Immunol Lett 95: 31-35. 2004

[95] Yamamoto-Furusho JK, Cantu C, Vargas-Alarcon G. Complotype SC30 is associated with susceptibility to develop ulcerative colitis in Mexicans. J Clin Gastroenterol 27: 178-179. 1998

[96] Torres MI, López Casado MA, Ríos A. New aspects in celiac disease. World J Gastroenterol. 13(8):1156-61. 2007

[97] Megiorni F, Pizzuti A. HLA-DQA1 and HLA-DQB1 in Celiac disease predisposition: practical implications of the HLA molecular typing. J Biomed Science 19:88. 1-5. 2012

[98] Kagnoff MF. Celiac disease: pathogenesis of a model immunogenetic disease. J Clin Invest 117:41–49. 2007

[99] Tack GJ, Verbeek W, Schreurs M, *et al.* The spectrum of celiac disease: epidemiology, clinical aspects and treatment. Nat Rev Gastroenterol Hepatol 7:204–213. 2010

[100] Llorente-Alonso MJ, Fernandez-Acenero MJ, Sebastian M. Gluten intolerance: sex and age-related features. Can J Gastroenterol 20:719–722. 2006

[101] Megiorni F, Mora B, Bonamico M, *et al.* HLA-DQ and susceptibility to celiac disease: evidence for gender differences and parent-of-origin effects. Am J Gastroenterol 103:997–1003. 2008

[102] Bonamico M, Mariani P, Danesi HM, *et al.* Prevalence and clinical picture of celiac disease in Italian down syndrome patients: a multicenter study. J Pediatr Gastroenterol Nutr 33:139–143. 2001

[103] Ventura A, Magazù G, Gerarduzzi T, *et al.* Coeliac disease and the risk of autoimmune disorders. Gut 51:897-898. 2002

[104] Wolters VM, Wijmenga C. Genetic background of celiac disease and its clinical implications. Am J Gastroenterol 103:190–195. 2008

[105] Fasano A. Zonulin and its regulation of intestinal barrier function: the biological door to inflammation, autoimmunity, and cancer. Physiol Rev 91:151–175. 2011

[106] Greco L, Romino R, Coto I, *et al.* The first large population based twin study of coeliac disease. Gut 50:624–628. 2002

[107] Bonamico M, Ferri M, Mariani P, *et al.* Serologic and genetic markers of celiac disease: a sequential study in the screening of first degree relatives. J Pediatr Gastroenterol Nutr 42:150–154. 2006

[108] Dubois PC, Trynka G, Franke L, *et al.* Multiple common variants for celiac disease influencing immune gene expression. Nat Genet 42:295–302. 2010

[109] Medrano LM, Dema B, López-Larios A, *et al.* HLA and Celiac Disease Susceptibility: New Genetic Factors Bring Open Questions about the HLA Influence and Gene-Dosage Effects. Plos One 7 (10) e48403. 2012

[110] Sollid LM, Thorsby E. HLA susceptibility genes in coeliac disease: genetic mapping and role in pathogenesis. Gastroenterology 105 : 910 – 22. 1993

[111] Mazzilli MC, Ferrante P, Mariani P, *et al.* A study of Italian paediatric coeliac disease patients confirms that the primary HLA association is to the DQ (α 1*0501, β 1*0201) heterodimer. Hum Immunol 33: 133 – 139. 1992

[112] Sollid LM, Lie BA. Celiac disease genetics: current concepts and practical applications. Clin Gastroenterol Hepatol 3: 843 – 51. 2005

[113] Karell K, Holopainen P, Mustalahti K, *et al.* Not all HLA DR3 DQ2 haplotypes confer equal susceptibility to coeliac disease: transmission analysis in families. Scand J Gastroenterol 37: 56 – 61. 2002

[114] Vader W, Stepniak D, Kooy Y, *et al.* The HLADQ2 gene dose effect in celiac disease is directly related to the magnitude and breadth of gluten-specific T cell responses. Proc Natl Acad Sci U S A 100: 12390–12395. 2003

[115] Fallang LE, Bergseng E, Hotta K, *et al.* Differences in the risk of celiac disease associated with HLA-DQ2.5 or HLADQ2.2 are related to sustained gluten antigen presentation. Nat Immunol 10: 1096–1101. 2009

[116] Bodd M, Kim CY, Lundin KE, *et al.* T-Cell Response to Gluten in Patients With HLA-DQ2.2 Reveals Requirement of Peptide-MHC Stability in Celiac Disease. Gastroenterology 142: 552–561. 2012

[117] Henrickson SE, Mempel TR, Mazo IB, *et al.* T cell sensing of antigen dose governs interactive behavior with dendritic cells and sets a threshold for T cell activation. Nat Immunol 9: 282–291. 2008

[118] Fallang LE, Bergseng E, Hotta K, *et al.* Differences in the risk of celiac disease associated with HLA-DQ2.5 or HLA-DQ2.2 are related to sustained gluten antigen presentation. Nat Immunol 10:1096–1101. 2009

[119] Bodd M, Tollefsen S, Bergseng E, *et al.* Evidence that HLA-DQ9 confers risk to celiac disease by presence of DQ9-restricted gluten-specific T cells. Hum Immunol 73: 376-381. 2012.

[120] Hill ID, Horvath K. Non biopsy diagnosis of celiac disease: are we nearly there yet? J Pediatr Gastroenterol Nutr 54:310–311. 2012

[121] Martin-Pagola A, Perez-Nanclares G, Ortiz L, *et al.* MICA response to gliadin in intestinal mucosa from celiac patients. Immunogenetics 56:549-554. 2004.

[122] Mention Hüe J, Monteiro R, Zhang S, *et al.* A Direct Role for NKG2D/MICA Interaction in Villous Atrophy during Celiac Disease. Immunity 21:367-377. 2004.

[123] Kim CY, Quarsten H, Bergseng E, *et al.* Structural basis for HLA-DQ2-mediated presentation of gluten epitopes in celiac disease. Proc Natl Acad Sci U S A. 101:4175–4179. 2004

[124] Schmitt L, Kratz JR, Davis MM, *et al.* Catalysis of peptide dissociation from class II MHC-peptide complexes. Proc Natl Acad Sci U S A. 96:6581–6586.1999

[125] Kropshofer H, Vogt A, Stern LJ, Hämmerling G. Self-release of CLIP in peptide loading of HLA-DR molecules. Science. 270:1357–1359. 1995

[126] Hue S, Mention JJ, Monteiro RC, *et al.* A direct role for NKG2D/MICA interaction in villous atrophy during celiac disease. Immunity 21: 367–377. 2004

[127] Meresse B, Chen Z, Ciszewski C, *et al.* Coordinated induction by IL15 of a TCR-independent NKG2D signaling pathway converts CTL into lymphokine-activated killer cells in celiac disease. Immunity 21(3): 357–66. 2004

[128] Mention JJ, Ben Ahmed M, Begue B, *et al.* Interleukin 15: a key to disrupted intraepithelial lymphocyte homeostasis and lymphomagenesis in celiac disease. Gastroenterology 125: 730–745. 2003

[129] Allegretti YL, Bondar C, Guzman L, *et al.* Broad MICA/B Expression in the Small Bowel Mucosa: A Link between Cellular Stress and Celiac Disease. PLoS One. 8(9): e73658. 2013

[130] Rodríguez-Rodero S, Rodrigo L, Fernández-Morera JL, *et al.* MHC Class I Chain-Related Gene B Promoter Polymorphisms and Celiac Disease Human Immunology 67: 208–214. 2006

[131] Ahmad T, Neville M, Marshall SE, *et al.* Haplotype-specific linkage disequilibrium patterns define the genetic topography of the human MHC. Hum Mol Genet 12: 647-656. 2003.

[132] Lopez-Vazquez A, Rodrigo L, Fuentes D, *et al.* MHC class I chain related gene A (MICA) modulates the development of coeliac disease in patients with the high risk heterodimer DQA1*0501/DQB1*0201 Gut 50: 336-340. 2002

[133] Tinto N, Ciacci C, Calcagno G, *et al.* Increased prevalence of celiac disease without gastrointestinal symptoms in adults MICA 5.1 homozygous subjects from the Campania area. Dig Liver Dis 40:248–52. 2008

[134] Rebmann V, Van der Ven K, Pässler M *et al.* Association of soluble HLA-G plasma levels with HLA-G alleles. Tissue Antigens 7: 15–21. 2001

[135] Rousseau P, Le Discorde M, Mouillot G, *et al.* The 14 bp deletion-insertion polymorphism in the 3 ′ UTR region of the HLA-G gene influences HLA-G mRNA stability. Hum Immunol 64: 1005–10. 2003

[136] Fabris A, Segat L, Catamo E, *et al.* HLA-G 14 bp Deletion / Insertion Polymorphism in Celiac Disease. Am J Gastroenterol 106:139–144. 2011

[137] Lefebvre S, Moreau P, Guiard V, *et al.* Molecular mechanisms controlling constitutive and IFN- γ -inducible HLA-G expression in various cell types. J Reprod Immunol 43 : 213 – 24. 1999

[138] Trowsdale J. The MHC, disease and selection. Immunol Lett 137: 1–8. 2011

Chapter 9

Association Between HLA Gene Polymorphism and Antiepileptic Drugs-Induced Cutaneous Adverse Reactions

Yuying Sun and Yongzhi Xi

Additional information is available at the end of the chapter

http://dx.doi.org/10.5772/57513

1. Introduction

Epilepsy is a chronic, recurrent, and transient brain dysfunction syndrome caused by recurrent seizures due to abnormal firing of brain neurons, and it is one of the most common neurological disorders. The incidence of epilepsy is associated with age; the highest prevalence is generally thought to be under 1 year of age, followed by a gradual reduction after1–10 years. In China, the male to female ratio of epilepsy is between 1.15:1 and1.7:1, and no significant differences associated with race have been found.

The main treatment for epilepsy is medication, with antiepileptic drugs (AEDs) as the principal method. After systemic long-term treatment, most epilepsy patients can be cured by medication. Because new AEDs have come into the market, adverse effects have been significantly reduced, and thus, AEDs treatments have become more acceptable to most epilepsy patients. Among the AEDs, aromatic antiepileptic drugs (AAEDs) are the most commonly used. This class of drugs was named for their similar chemical structures and their possession of benzene rings. Currently, commonly used AAEDs in the clinicinclude carbamazepine (CBZ), oxcarbazepine (OXC), phenobarbital (PB), lamotrigine (LTG), and phenytoin (PHT), mainly used in treatments foridiopathic generalized epilepsy with good efficacy. However, adverse reactions such as rash, fever, and organ damagecan occur. The most common reaction is cutaneous adverse drug reactions (CADRs), which includes mild maculopapular eruptions (MPE);drug hypersensitivity syndrome (HSS),as well as life-threatening reactions such as severe cutaneous reactions (SCRs)(Stevens-Johnson syndrome[SJS] and toxic epidermal necrolysis [TEN]), the mortality rate of which is as high as 40%, resulting in serious socio-economic and family burdens.

In individuals taking AEDs, the overall MPE incidence rate is 2.8%; incidence rates of rash caused by PHT, LG, and CBZ are higher at 5.9%, 4.7%, and 3.7%, respectively. In comparison, the incidence rates of SCRs(including HHS, SJS, and TEN) caused by the above drugs are lower. A population survey in Germany indicated that in patients who had just began AEDs treatment, the incidence rate of CBZ-SJS/TEN was 1.4/10,000, whereas the incidence rates of LTG-SJS/TEN, PB-SJS/TEN, and PHT-SJS/TEN were 2.5/10,000, 8.1/10,000, and 8.3/10,000, respectively. SJS and TEN are considered forms of the same disease at different stages, manifesting as blister-like rashes with skin peeling, and affecting the skin, mucous membranes, organs, visceral trunk, and limbs. SJS is characterized by total area of skin detachment of less than 10%, whereas TEN is defined by an area of detachment greater than 40%, and rates in between are considered SJS/TEN overlap. TEN is more severe, with mortality as high as 40%. Although the incidence rates of SJS and TEN are low, mortality rates nevertheless reach 10–50%. Thus, avoiding SJS/TEN is one of the major challenges during AEDs treatment. Recent studies have indicated that SCRs such as SJS and TEN induced by AAEDs are associated with the *HLA-B*1502* allele.

2. Current cADRs prevalence in various countries and regions

In-depth genetics studies on AEDs-induced adverse reactions suggest that incidence rates of AEDs-induced SJS and TEN vary among ethnic groups and that the associations with relevant loci are different. In Europe, CBZ is the most common drug causing cADRs, with an incidence rate of 8.2%, followed by PB at 5.3%, and PHT at 5.0%. The prevalence rates of cADRs induced by CBZ are different depending on the country and/or region, at 5.88% in Australia, 6.60% in Japan, 27.70% in Singapore, 35.70% in Malaysia, 19.00% in India, and 26.00% in Taiwan. The prevalence rates of cADRs induced by PHT are also largely variable among different countries and regions, at 5.00% in Europe, 5.88% in Australia, 14.20% in Malaysia, 19.00% in India, and 4.30% in Taiwan. A similar phenomenon has also been observed in the prevalence of cADRs induced by other drugs in different countries and regions. CBZ is the main SJS/TEN-inducing drug in Southeast Asian countries and regions. The incidence rate of CBZ-SJS/TEN in Taiwan is approximately 59/10,000 each year, 41/10, 000 in Malaysia, and 55/10,000 in the Philippines, while it is relatively low in the United States and Europe, at 2/10,000 in the U.S.A., 9/10,000 in the United Kingdom, and 5/10,000 in France.

3. Association between AEDs-induced cutaneous adverse reactions and HLA alleles

Detailed studies in human genomics and pharmacogenomics have demonstrated a relationship between drug-induced cADRs and human leucocyte antigen (HLA) genes. HLA genes are located on human chromosome 6p21.3, and are a group of closely linked multiple alleles that include more than 100 loci and a total of 554 alleles, spanning 3,600 k band representing 1/3,000 of the entire human genome. It is a major gene system that regulates human-specific immune responses and individual differences in disease susceptibility, with apparent specificity in different ethnicities or populations of the same ethnicity.HLA genes can be divided into three classes: HLA class I, class II, and class III, on the basis of the structural expression, tissue distribution, and functions of the encoded proteins. HLA-I genes include A, B, and C loci; HLA-II genes consist of DR, DQ, and DP subregions; and HLA-III genes reside between HLA-I and HLA-II genes, and are mainly related to the complement system. Disease-related studies have generally been focused on HLA-I and HLA-II genes.

3.1. Correlation between cADRs incidence and the *HLA-B*1502* allele in different countries and regions

Recent studies have shown that the incidence of CBZ-SJS/TEN is strongly associated with *HLA-B*1502* in Han Chinese, while its frequency is low in Japanese and Caucasians and not associated with the *HLA-B*1502* allele. Chung *et al.*in Taiwan first reported the association between the *HLA-B*1502* allele and CBZ-SJS/TEN. In 2004, they published a study in *Nature* on HLA gene polymorphisms in 44 cases of CBZ-SJS/TEN in Han Chinese living in Taiwan, which also included 101 CBZ-tolerant patients and 93 cases with a positive CBZ history as study controls. The results indicated that all CBZ-SJS/TEN cases were positive for *HLA-B*1502* (100%), whereas only 3% and 9% were positive, respectively, in the other two groups. This finding revolutionized the research field on cADRs and AEDs, and prompted further studies on the *HLA-B*1502* allele. A study in Thailand revealed that among 42 cases of SJS/TEN caused by CBZ, 37 were positive for *HLA-B*1502*, which implies that the *HLA-B*1502* allele is a high-risk factor for CBZ-SJS/TEN occurrence. In the Han Chinese population, *HLA-B*1502* genotyping in CBZ-SJS/TEN patients showed 100% sensitivity and 97% specificity. Avoiding oral CBZ in *HLA-B*1502*-positive patients decreased SJS/TEN incidence, while *HLA-B*1502*-negative patients rarely show adverse reactions and the risk of CBZ-SJS/TEN is low. Thus, *HLA-B*1502* genetic screening in the clinic is important for the use of AEDs. Some experts have suggested that in Asian populations, *HLA-B*1502* genetic screening should be performed before taking CBZ and related AAEDs, and CBZ should be avoided in those positive for *HLA-B*1502*; valproic acid, levetiracetam, or topiramate should be used instead as alternative treatments.

A study by Hung *et al.* on the Han Chinese population found that the *HLA-B*1502*-positive rate is as high as 100% (3/3) in OXC-induced SCR (AXC-SJS) cases. Locharenkul *et al.* reported four cases of SCR induced by PHT (PHT-SJS) in Thailand who were all positive for *HLA-B*1502*, which further confirmed the association between SJS/TEN and the *HLA-B*1502* allele in Southeast Asian countries. The frequency of the *HLA-B*1502* allele shows significant regional variations: 7.1% in South China, 1.9% in North China, 4.3% in Taiwan, 7.2% in Hong Kong, 6.1% in Thailand, 8.4% in Malaysia, 0.1% in Japan, 0.4% in South Korea, and lower or almost zero in European countries such as Germany and France. The results in European populations were also different from those in Southeast Asian countries. One study in Europe revealed that among the 12 cases of CBZ-SJS/TEN, 8 were Caucasian and did not carry the *HLA-B*1502* allele, whereas the other 4 were positive for *HLA-B*1502* and of Asian origin (China, Vietnam, and Cambodia). Thus, the frequency of *HLA-B*1502* is low in Japan and in

European Caucasians, and consequently, the incidence of CBZ-SJS/TEN is low. Conversely, the frequency of *HLA-B*1502* is relatively high in Southeast Asian countries and regions (Taiwan, Hong Kong, Malaysia, Singapore, Thailand, and others)and the incidence of CBZ-SJS/TEN is also high, which further proves the strong association between CBZ-SJS/TEN incidence and *HLA-B*1502*. Therefore, the U.S.A FDA has recommended that in Han Chinese and Southeast Asian populations, *HLA-B*1502* screening should be performed before prescribing CBZ, and individuals who are positive for *HLA-B*1502* should be cautious when taking CBZ in order to reduce CBZ-SJS/TEN incidence.

*3.1.1. Relationship between the HLA-B*1502 allele and SJS/TEN due to other AEDs*

Due to the structural similarity and clinical cross-reactivity of AAEDs, several subsequent studies have been conducted regarding the correlation between other AAEDs and the *HLA-B*1502* allele. In studies conducted in Hong Kong, Taiwan, and Mainland China, no association was found between *HLA-B*1502* and LTG-SJS/TEN in the Han Chinese population, a weak association was seen with PHT-SJS/TEN relative to CBZ-SJS/TEN, and all three OXC-SJS cases were positive for *HLA-B*1502*. However, due to the small number of cases, the correlation between SJS/TEN caused by other AAEDs and *HLA-B*1502* remains to be determined using a larger sample size.

*3.1.2. Mechanism of the association between HLA-B*1502-positive patients and AAEDs-SJS/TEN*

Currently, the mechanism of severe cutaneous adverse reactions (SCAR) induced by AAEDs is unclear. Most scientists believe that provocation of the media results in severe symptoms within 2–3 days. In addition, a large number of infiltrating inflammatory cells are found in patient lesions, and increased dosage of CBZ significantly shortened the time for inflammatory cells to appear, which aggravated the symptoms. Therefore, the mechanistic origin likely lies in activation of the immune system. Cytotoxic T lymphocytes cause skin lesions in SJS/TEN patients with a common indicator of keratinocyte apoptosis induced by cytotoxic T-cells, and T-cells in the blister fluid of patients are mainlyCD8+ T-cells, implicating CD8+ T-cell-mediated cytotoxicity. Drugs such as CBZ and its metabolites are small chemicals, insufficient to induce immune responses, and thus the hapten hypothesis was proposed; that a specific drug or its metabolite covalently interacts with a protein or a polypeptide as a hapten, and is processed by cells and presented to the MHC molecules, resulting in HLA-specific T-cell activation. Another hypothesis is the p-i concept(direct pharmacological interaction between drug and immune receptor), i.e., the drug can be directly and non-covalently associated withT-cell receptors that match MHC molecules. Both hypotheses indicate that skin adverse reactions are triggered through interactions with specific MHC molecules, T-cell receptors, and drug-modified antigens. In 2007, Yang *et al.* studied HLA-B*1502-bound peptides and found that CBZ or its metabolites non-covalently interacted with HLA-B*1502-bound peptides, which resulted in cytotoxic T-cell-mediated apoptosis in SJS/TEN patients. This result favored the p-i concept. However, current studies have not been able to explain the mechanism of SJS/TEN incidence in *HLA-B*1502*-negative patients, which requires further investigation.

3.1.3. Correlation of cADRs occurrence and other HLA loci

*HLA-B*1502* is associated with CBZ-SJS/TEN and is also polymorphic among ethnic groups. Japanese scientists performed a study on 15 CBZ-induced cADRs patients (10 MPE and 5 SJS) and found that the *HLA-B*1518, HLA-B*5901,* and *HLA-C*0704* alleles were highly significantly associated with SCR risk, and that the haplotype *HLA-A*2402-B*5901-C*0102* was significantly associated with SCR risk. This study revealed that individuals with these alleles may have an increased CBZ-cADRs incidence rate and that that *HLA-B*5901* locus is a risk locus for CBZ-SJS in the Japanese population. Another study in Japan indicated that *HLA-B*5801* locus positivity was significantly associated with CBZ-SJS. A study in Europe also discovered an association with *HLA-A*3101,* with a frequency of approximately 2–5% in Northern Europe and that this gene locus was significantly associated with HSS (P = 3.5 × 10-8) and MPE (P = 1.1 × 10-6), and a risk factor for HSS, MPE, and SJS/TEN. People of Northern European descent carrying the *HLA-A*3101* allele had an increased CBZ-HHS incidence (from 5.0% to 26.0%); conversely, those lacking this allele had a decreased incidence rate (from 5% to 3.8%). A recent report showed that several cases of CBZ-SJS/TEN in *HLA-B*1502*-negative children in Han Chinese were found to be associated with *HLA-A*2402*.Therefore, *HLA-B*1502*-negative patients should also be closely observed after taking CBZ.

Scientists in Taiwan have also found that *HLA-B*1301, Cw*0801,* and *DRB1*1602* were associated with PHT-SJS/TEN. A study in Europe indicated that in addition to the *HLA-B* locus, *HLA-Cw*0718, DQB1*0609, A*6801,* and *DQB1*1301* were borderline-associated with LTG-SJS/TEN, and *HLA-B*5801* and *B*38* were weakly associated with LTG-SJS/TEN. However, the sample sizes in these studies were small; thus, further investigations are necessary to determine if the above genes are risk factors for LTG-SJS/TEN or PHT-SJS/TEN.

4. Summary

In summary, cADRs incidence resulting from AEDs varies among different regions, and the associations with related gene loci are not consistent. *HLA-B*1502*-positivity is more frequent in Han Chinese and Southeast Asian populations than in populations from Japan and European countries, and is strongly associated with CBZ-SJS/TEN. *HLA-B*1502* screening is important in choosing to use AEDs in the clinic; however, close observation is equally necessary for *HLA-B*1502*-negative patients to avoid CBZ-SJS/TEN. Because of the high mortality rate of SJS/TEN, *HLA-B*1502*-positive patients should avoid using CBZ, and instead chose to use levetiracetam, sodium valproate, topiramate, or other non-AAEDs. In individuals of Northern European ancestry, CBZ-SJS/TEN incidence is not associated with *HLA-B*1502,* but it is associated with *HLA-A*3101,* carriers of which have a significantly increased risk of cADRs. In Japan, *HLA-B*5901* and *HLA-B*5801* loci are risk factors for CBZ-SJS/TEN. Further studies will likely discover more AEDs-cADRs-associated gene loci, which will enrich the field of pharmacogenetics to provide more evidence for the clinical use of AEDs, reduce the incidence of cADRs, improve AEDs efficacy, and significantly reduce the risk of adverse drug reactions such as cADRs.

Acknowledgements

Supported by grants from the State Key Development Program for Basic Research of China (No.2003CB515509 and 2009CB522401) and from National Natural Scientific Foundation of China(No.81070450 and 30470751) to Dr. X.-Y.Z.

Author details

Yuying Sun and Yongzhi Xi*

*Address all correspondence to: xiyz@yahoo.com

Department of Immunology and National Center for Biomedicine Analysis, Beijing Hospital Affiliated to Academy of Medical Sciences, Beijing, PRC

References

[1] Ling ZY, Sun Y, Jiang JF. New development about safe questions of carbamazepine in epileptic. China Mod Med, 2010, 17(13): 13-14.

[2] Beswick TC, Cohen JB. Dose-related levetiracetam-induced reticulated drug eruption. J Drugs Dermatol, 2010, 9(4): 409-410.

[3] Ouyan H, Liu GG. A review over adverse drug reaction of anti-epileptic drugs. J Pediatr Pharm, 2005, 11(4): 57-59.

[4] Lonjou C, Borot N, Sekula P, et al. A European study of HLA-B in Stevens-Johnson syndrome and toxic epidermal necrolysis related to five high-risk drugs. Pharmacogenet Genomics, 2008, 18(2) :99-107.

[5] Gao MM, Shi YW, Yu MJ, et al. Association between cutaneous adverse reactions to antiepileptic drugs and HLA-B* 1502 allele. Chin J Neuromed, 2009, 8(5): 493-496.

[6] Horton R, Wilming L, Rand V, et al. Gene map of the extended human MHC. Nat Rev Genet. 2004, 5(12): 889-899.

[7] Chung WH, Hung SI, Hong HS, et al. Medical genetics: a marker for Stevens-Johnson syndrome. Nature. 2004, 428(6982):486.

[8] Hung SI, Chung WH, Jee SH, et al. Genetic susceptibility to carbamazepine-induced cutaneous adverse drug reactions. Pharmacogenet Genomics. 2006, 16(4): 297-306.

[9] Man CB, Kwan P, Baum L, et al. Association between HLA-B*1502 allele and antiepileptic drug-induced cutaneous reactions in Han Chinese. Epilepsia. 2007, 48(5): 1015-8.

[10] Wang GQ, Zhou YQ, Zhou LM, et al. Association between HLA-B*1502 Allele and carbamazepine-induced cutaneous adverse reactions in han people f China mainland. J Sun Yat sen Univ Med Sci, 2010, 31(6):828-832.

[11] Mehta TY, Prajapati LM, Mittal B, et al. Association of HLA-B*1502 allele and carbamazepine-induced Stevens-Johnson syndrome among Indians.Indian J Dermatol Venereol Leprol. 2009, 75(6): 579-582.

[12] Ding WY, Lee CK, Choon SE. Cutaneous adverse drug reactions seen in a tertiary hospital in Johor, Malaysia. Int J Dermatol. 2010, 49(7):834-841.

[13] Locharernkul C, Loplumlert J Limotai C, et al. Carbamazepine and phenytoin induced Stevens-Johnson syndrome is associated with HLA-B*1502 allele in Thai population. Epilepsia. 2008, 49(12):2087-2091.

[14] Lonjou C, Thomas L, Borot N, et al. A marker for Stevens-Johnson syndrome ...: ethnicity matters. Pharmacogenomics J. 2006, 6(4):265-268.

[15] Kaniwa N, Saito Y, Aihara M, et al. HLA-B locus in Japanese patients with anti-epileptics and allopurinol-related Stevens-Johnson syndrome andtoxic epidermal necrolysis. Pharmacogenomics. 2008, 9(11) :1617-1622.

[16] Kaniwa N, Hasegawa R. Exploratory studies on genetic biomarkers related to serious drug adverse reactions. Kokuritsu Iyakuhin Shokuhin Eisei Kenkyusho Hokoku. 2009, (127):1-14.

[17] Ikeda H, Takahashi Y, Yamazaki E, et al. HLA class I markers in Japanese patients with carbama- zepine-induced cutaneous adverse reactions. Epilepsia. 2010, 51(2): 297-300.

[18] Hung SI, Chung WH, Liu ZS, et al. Common risk allele in aromatic antiepileptic-drug induced Stevens-Johnson syndrome and toxic epidermal necrolysis in Han Chinese. Pharmacogenomics, 2010, 11(3): 349-356.

[19] Kazeem GR, Cox C, Aponte J, et al. High-resolution HLA genotyping and severe cutaneous adverse reactions in lamotrigine treated patients. Pharmacogenet Genomics, 2009, 19(9): 661-665.

[20] Lin LC, Lai PC, Yang SF, et al. Oxcarbazepine-induced Stevens-Johnson syndrome: a case report. Kaohsiung J Med Sci, 2009, 25(2): 82-86.

[21] Kuwbara S. Guillain-Barré syndrome: epidemiology, pathophysiology and management. Drugs, 2004, 64(6):597-610.

[22] Nassif A, Bensussan A, Borothee G, et al. Drugs pecific cytotoxic T-cells in the skin lesions of a patient with toxic epidermal necrolysis. J Invest Dermatol, 2002, 118(4): 728-733.

[23] Nassif A, Bensussan A, Boumsell L, et al. Toxic epidermal necrolysis: effector cells are drug-specific cytotoxic T cells. J Allergy Clin Immunol. 2004, 114(5):1209-1215.

[24] Pichler WJ. Pharmacological interactionof drugs with antigen specific immunereceptors: the pi concept. Curr Opin Allergy Clin Immunol, 2002, 2(4): 301-305.

[25] Wu Y, Sanderson JP, Farrell J, et al. Activation of T cells by carbamazepine and carbamazepine metabolites. J Allergy Clin Immunol. 2006, 118(1): 233-241.

[26] Wu Y, Farrell J, Pirmohamed M, et al. Generation and characterization of antigen-specific CD4+, CD8+,and CD4+CD8+ T-cell clones from patients with carbamazepine hypersensitivity. J Allergy Clin Immunol. 2007, 119(4):973-981.

[27] Yang CW,Hung SI,Juo CG, et al. HLA-B*1502-bound peptides:implications for the pathogenesis of carbamazepine-induced Stevens-Johnsonsyndrome. J Allergy Clin Immunol. 2007, 120(4):870-877.

[28] Chung WH, Hung SI, Chen YT. Genetic predisposition of life-threatening antiepileptic-induced skin reactions. Expert Opin Drug Saf, 2010, 9(1) :15-21.

[29] Toledano R, Gil-Nagel A. Adverse effects of antiepileptic drugs. Semin Neurol, 2008, 28(3):317-327.

[30] Arif H, Buchsbaum R, Weintraub D, et al. Comparison and predictors of rash associated with 15 antiepileptic drugs. Neurology, 2007, 68(20): 1701-1709.

[31] Mockenhaupt M, Messenheimer J, Tennis P, et al. Risk of Stevens-Johnson syndrome and toxic epidermal necrolysis in new users of antiepileptics. Neurology, 2005, 64(7): 1134-1138.

[32] Mockenhaupt M, Viboud C, Dunant A, et al. Stevens-Johnson syndrome and toxic epidermal necrolysis assessment of medication risks with emphasis on recently marketed drugs. The EuroSCAR-study. J Invest Dermatol, 2008 128(1): 35-44.

[33] Tassaneeyakul W, Tiamkao S, Jantararoungtong T, et al. Association between HLA-B*1502 and carbamazepine-induced severe cutaneous adverse drug reactions in a Thai population. Epilepsia, 2010, 51(5): 926-930.

[34] Chang CC, Too CL, Murad S, et al. Association of HLA-B*1502 allele with carbamazepine-induced toxic epidermal necrolysis and Stevens-Johnson syndrome in the multi-ethnic Malaysian population. Int J Dermatol, 2011, 50(2): 221-224.

[35] Shi YW, Min FL, Liu XR, et al. Hla-B alleles and lamotrigine-induced cutaneous adverse drug reactions in the Han Chinese population. Basic Clin Pharmacol Toxicol, 2011, 109, 1: 42-46.

http://dx.doi.org/10.5772/57513

[36] Min FL, Shi YW, Liu XR, et al. HLA-B*1502 genotyping in two Chinese patients with phenytoin-induced Stevens-Johnson syndrome. Epilepsy Behav, 2011, 20(2): 390-391.

[37] Alfirevic A, Jorgensen AL, Williamson PR, et al. HLA-B locus in Caucasian patients with carbamazepine hypersensitivity. Pharmacogenomics, 2006, 7(6): 813-818.

[38] Ozeki T, Mushiroda T, Yowang A, et al. Genome-wide association study identifies HLA-A*3101 allele as a genetic risk factor for carbamazepine-induced cutaneous adverse drug reactions in Japanese population. Hum Mol Genet, 2011, 20(5): 1034-1041.

[39] Liao WP, Shi YW, Min FL. HLA-B*1502 screening and toxic effects of carbamazepine. N Engl J Med, 2011, 365(7): 672-673.

[40] Shi YW, Min FL, Qin B, et al. Association between HLA and Stevens-Johnson syndrome induced by Carbamazepine in Southern Han Chinese genetic markers besides B*1502. Basic Clin Pharmacol Toxicol. 2012, 111(1):58-64. 7843.

[41] Hung SI, Chung WH, Jee SH, et al. Genetic susceptibility to carbamazepine-induced cutaneous adverse drug reactions. Pharmacogenet Genomics, 2006, 16(4): 297-306.

[42] An DM, Wu XT, Hu FY, et al. Association study of lamotrigine-induced cutaneous adverse reactions and HLA-B*1502 in a Han Chinese population. Epilepsy Res, 2010, 92(2-3): 226-230.

[43] Hu FY, Wu XT, An DM, et al. Pilot association study of oxcarbazepine-induced mild cutaneous adverse reactions with HLA-B*1502 allele in Chinese Han population. Seizure, 2011, 20(2): 160-162.

[44] Chen P, Lin JJ, Lu CS, et al. Carbamazepine-induced toxic effects and HLA-B 1502 screening in Taiwan. N Engl J Med, 2011, 364(12): 1126-1133.

Section 3

HLA-Associated Important Infectious Diseases

Chapter 10

HLA and Infectious Diseases

Daniela Maira Cardozo,
Amanda Vansan Marangon, Ana Maria Sell,
Jeane Eliete Laguila Visentainer and
Carmino Antonio de Souza

Additional information is available at the end of the chapter

http://dx.doi.org/10.5772/57496

1. Introduction

The Human Leukocyte Antigen (HLA) system is the Major Histocompatibility Complex (MHC) in humans, and all knowledge on this system is of great interest to the field of medical sciences. HLA has become an important tool for understanding the pathogenesis of various infectious diseases; the alleles or HLA haplotypes inherited by an individual can predict several risk and protective factors related to infections caused by various agents.

The list of infectious diseases associated with the HLA system is constantly increasing and the level of association is quite variable. New classification methods and frequent nomenclature updates have facilitated the understanding of the role of polymorphisms in this system and the association with various diseases.

The purpose of this chapter is to show the genetic variability of HLA genes and its influence in the immunopathogenesis of diseases caused by different classes of pathogens. The first part of the chapter encompasses aspects of the structure and function of MHC genes and the role of the molecules encoded by these genes. Subsequently, we present some infectious diseases associated with the HLA system that have been highlighted in the global overview.

2. Structure and function of the HLA

MHC is divided into three main regions and has over 200 genes, most of which have functions related to immunity, and are contained within 4.2 Mbp of DNA on the short arm of chromosome 6 at 6p21.3 [1]. In the HLA Class I region, near to the telomere, are located the HLA-A, -B and -C classic genes and -E, -F and -G non-classic genes, among other genes and pseudogenes. The HLA Class II region, near to centromere, contains HLA-DR, -DQ and –DP genes. Sub-region DR includes DRA gene which codes for the low-polymorphic alpha-chain and can combine with any beta chains codifying for DRB genes [2]. The Class III region, located between class I and II region contains the C2, C4A, C4B and B genes, that code for complement proteins and tumor necrosis factor (TNF) [1,2].

HLA molecules are polymorphic membrane glycoproteins found on the surface of nearly all cells. Multiple genetic loci within MHC encode these proteins, and one individual expresses simultaneously several polymorphic forms from a large pool of alleles in the population. The overall structure of the HLA class I and class II molecules is similar, with most of the polymorphisms located in the peptide binding groove, where there is the antigens recognized [3].

Class I molecules are composed of one heavy chain (45kD) encoded within the MHC and a light chain called β2-microglobulin (12kD) whose gene is on chromosome 15. Class II molecules consist of one α (34kD) and one β chain (30kD) both coding within MHC [1]

The class I heavy chain has three domains of which the membrane-distal first (α1) and the second (α2) are the polymorphic ones. These polymorphic domains concentrate three regions: positions 62 to 83; 92 to 121; and 135 to 157. These areas are called hypervariable regions. The two polymorphic domains are encoded by exons 2 and 3 of the class I gene. The diversity in these domains is of great importance as this is where the two domains that form the antigen binding cleft (ABC) or peptide binding groove (PBG) of MHC class I molecule are located [4,5]. The sides of the antigen-binding cleft are formed by α helices, whereas the floor of the cleft is comprised of eight anti-parallel beta sheets. The antigenic peptides of eight to ten amino acids (typically nonamers) bind to the cleft with low specificity but high stability. The α_3 domain contains a conserved seven amino acid loop (positions 223 to 229), which serves as a binding site for CD8 [3,6-8].

Class II molecules comprised of two transmembrane glycoproteins: α and β chains, are restricted to the cells of the immune system (e.g. B cells, dendritic cells), but may also be induced on other cells during immune response. The PBG of class II molecules has open ends which allow the peptide to extend beyond the groove at both ends, and therefore to be longer (12-24 amino acids). The peptide is presented to CD4 T-cells [1]. Both α and β chains are usually polymorphic in class II molecules. In these chains, the α1 and β1 domains are of the PBG and therefore diversity is found mainly in these domains, which are encoded by the exon 2 of their class II A or B genes and the hypervariable regions tend to be found in the groove walls [7].

T cell activation occurs following recognition of peptide / MHC complexes on an antigen-presenting cell (APC). T cell activation can be viewed as a series of intertwined steps, ultimately resulting in the ability to secrete cytokines, replicate, and perform various effector functions. During antigen presentation, the antigen receptors of T cells (TCR) recognize both the antigen peptide and the MHC molecules, with the peptide being responsible for the fine specificity of antigen recognition and MHC residues contributes for the restriction of the T cells (CD4 and

CD8). During antigen presentation, CD4 and CD8 are intimately associated with the TCR and bind to the MHC molecule [9].

3. Haplotype, linkage disequilibrium and HLA genes expression

HLA genes are transmitted for Mendel segregation and allelic variant is expressed in a codominant mode. The set of HLA alleles present in each chromosome of the pair is denominated haplotype. The probability of a sibling having the same HLA haplotype as the other is 25%, different haplotypes is 25% and 50% are share only one haplotype [2].

Moreover, there is a fact that occurs in HLA genes called linkage disequilibrium which denotes that certain alleles occur together with a greater frequency than would be expected by chance (non-random gametic association). Variations in the expected combinations of alleles in the population, more often or less often than would be expected from a random formation of haplotypes from alleles, could be related to linkage disequilibrium [1]. For example, a determined population has a gene frequency of 14% for *HLA-A*01* and 9% for *HLA-B*08*, therefore the expected frequency for this haplotype would be 1.26% (0.14 x 0.09), the actual frequency is however, 8.8% in this population, a higher frequency than expected, characterizing a positive linkage disequilibrium [2].

4. HLA and infection diseases

The frequency and the presence of HLA alleles vary among different populations. Studies suggest that the alleles that can confer resistance to certain pathogens are prevalent in areas with endemic diseases. Furthermore, genomic analysis in families has helped to map and identify the loci related to a number of diseases. Moreover, a number of diseases have been mapped and had their related loci identified thanks to the genomic analysis of families.

4.1. Bacterial diseases

4.1.1. Tuberculosis and leprosy

Leprosy and tuberculosis (TB) have afflicted humanity since time immemorial, and a number of factors converge to a timely discussion on mycobacterial disease. These factors include the re-emergence of human tuberculosis in epidemic proportions on a global scale, and the special position of leprosy among communicable diseases, the frequency of disabilities, and the social and economic consequences of these diseases.

The immunological mechanism involved in the breakdown of host resistance in these individuals remains unclear. A better understanding of the mechanisms that lead to the protective immunity of the host is fundamental in order to develop novel therapies and vaccines.

Cell-mediated immunity is thought to be the major component of host defense against mycobacterium; consequently, the induction of optimal Th1 response is protective immunity against mycobacterial infection.

Whereas exposure to and infection by *M. leprae* are necessary to acquire the disease, heritable factors are equally important in determining who will eventually develop clinical signs of leprosy. Numerous studies that have recently been reviewed support the major role of host genetic factors in the large variability of the host response to bacillus infection.

The extensive polymorphism of the class II genes and molecules results in genetically controlled interindividual differences in antigen-specific immune responsiveness, which in turn may lead to differential susceptibility to or expression of disease. The induction of cytolytic CD4+ Th1-like cells during mycobacterial infections has been extensively documented [10,11]. Thus, under inflammatory conditions it would be conceivable for T cells to access Schwann cells and recognize the HLA/peptide complexes presented by the Schwann cell.

4.1.2. HLA and leprosy

Leprosy is a chronic infection disease caused by *Mycobacterium leprae* (*M. leprae*) (Hansen, 1874), an intracellular parasite of macrophages, with high infectivity and low pathogenicity, which primarily affects the peripheral nerves and the skin [12]. The contact with *M. leprae* occurs mainly through the superior aerial views, but may also occur through the skin and maternal milk. A long period of exposure to the microorganism, between 2 and 5 years, is needed to promote the infection [13].

A global increase in both prevalence and new case detection has been observed as compared to 2011. The prevalence of leprosy in 2012 was 181,941 (0.34), compared to 189,018 (0.33) at the end of the first quarter of 2013, and approximately, 232,857 new cases reported (4.00/100,000 population), in the population were detected during the year of 2012 [14]. Currently, the major prevalence is in the Southeast Asiatic, South American, and African continents.

In 1966, Ridley and Jopling, based on clinical, histological, and immunological criteria, classified the spectra of leprosy into 5 groups: tuberculoid (TT), borderline-tuberculoid (BT), borderline-borderline (BB), borderline-lepromatous (BL) and lepromatous (LL). The Madrid classification was presented to subdivide leprosy patients into four different types (lepromatous, tuberculoid, borderline, and indeterminate), and since the year of 1998, the World Health Organization has recommended a new classification based on the number of skin lesions: paucibacillary (PB) for patients who have up to five skin lesions (lower bacterial load) and multibacillary (MB) for patients who have six or more skin lesions (higher bacterial load) [15].

The major signals of this disease are hypostatical cutaneous lesions, dilation of peripheral nerves, and the presence of acid-resistant bacillus in the skin lesions [16]. The undetermined form is an initial stage where the clinical and histopathological courses are uncertain. In the TT form, the lesions are maculates or infiltrated and can reappear or develop from undetermined macula, whereas in the LL form there are multiple lesions with numerous bacillus detected by skin biopsies [17].

Leprosy has been considered a multifactorial disease; the expression of clinical manifestations reflects the relation between the host and the parasite. The infection evolution depends on to the specific response on behalf of the host to the parasite. There is a good relationship observed *in vitro* and *in vivo* between the immunity mediated by cells (CMI) against antigens of *M. leprae* and the course of the disease. In the located and non-severe form TT, an efficient CMI to *M. leprae* develops with low levels of antibodies. On the other side of the leprosy spectrum are polar LL patients, who have a high humoral immune response and a low cellular response. Most patients, however, are between these two poles and are classified as borderline leprosy cases [18].

The susceptibility to *M. leprae* infection is complex and influenced by several host, parasite, and environmental factors. In 1929, Hopkins and Denny postulated that genetic variability was the basis of family and racial differences regarding the expression and incidence of the disease. Many epidemiologic studies that aimed to identify susceptibility genes have indicated that genetic characteristics of the host play a role in the variability of the clinical response to M. *tuberculosis* and *M. leprae* infection [19].

HLA has been studied in several distinctive illnesses, including infectious diseases. HLA alleles codify class I and II crucial molecules for CMI cell interaction. The HLA system participates effectively in the immune response by promoting the interaction between pathogen epitopes and the host cell T repertory. Consequently, depending on host HLA, different host responses can occur against the same antigen.

Previous investigations demonstrated different class I HLA variants associated to TT and LL forms of leprosy, in several populations. In India, the most important country in number of infected individuals with the bacillus, an important association with leprosy was reported for HLA-B40 antigen and HLA-A2-B40, HLA-A11-B40, and HLA-A24-B40 haplotypes [20]. Further studies in India replicated these findings; HLA-A11 [21] and HLA-B60 (split of B40) [22] antigens were associated to the LL form. Subsequently, with the advent of molecular genotyping, HLA class I alleles were determined in Indian multibacillary leprosy patients, resulting in a positive association with *HLA-A*02:06, A*11:02, B*18:01, B*51:10, C*04:07,* and *C*07:03* alleles, and a negative association with *C*04:11* [23]. Moreover, the *A*11-B*40* haplotype was confirmed in multibacillary leprosy patients compared to controls [24].

Recent studies have shown a positive association between LD and *HLA-A*11, HLA-B*38,* and *HLA-C*12,* as well as a negative association with *HLA-C*16.* When groups were stratified, *HLA-B*35* and *HLA-C*04* were shown to be protective against lepromatous leprosy, whereas *HLA-C*07* was shown to be a susceptibility variant [25]. Furthermore, the allele *HLA-C*15:05* has been related to the LD phenotype in certain populations from India and Vietnam [26].

However, the main restriction determinants for *M. leprae* seem to reside on DR or DQ molecules. The HLA-DR2 molecule [26-28], later identified as *DRB1*15* and *DRB1*16* variants, is primarily associated with leprosy or different clinical forms [29-33]. Risk for leprosy associated with *DRB1*10* has been described in Turkish, Vietnamese, and Brazilian populations [30,34], whereas *HLA-DRB1*14* has been associated with the TT group in a population from north-eastern Brazil [33] and with leprosy *per se* in the Argentinean population [35].

HLA molecules with the highest affinity to peptide produce the greatest T cell proliferation and IFN-γ response [36], and the peptide presentation by low affinity class II molecules may result in muted cell-mediated immunity [36]. Alternatively, peptide presentation by specific class II molecules may result in activation of suppressor/regulatory T-cells [37]. A protective effect against leprosy has been described for *DRB1*04* in Brazilian, Korean, Japanese, Vietnamese, Argentinean, and Taiwanese populations [30,38-40].

In addition to the studies that have been performed to investigate the molecular mechanisms of mycobacterium antigens restricted to HLA, certain Class II HLA genes have been suggested, as the selection of determined groups of antigen peptides and specific T helper cells, can contribute to the development of leprosy polar [41] and also tuberculoses [42].

4.1.3. HLA and tuberculosis

Tuberculosis, or TB, is a chronic disease caused by *Mycobacterium tuberculosis*, considered a major public health problem worldwide. The infection most commonly affects the lungs (Pulmonary Tuberculosis). One-third of the world's population has been in contact with the pathogen, but approximately 90% of the infected persons do not present clinical symptoms [43].

According to the World Health Organization [14], in 2011, there were an estimated 8.7 million new cases of TB (13% co-infected with HIV) and 1.4 million people died from TB, including almost one million deaths among HIV-negative individuals and 430,000 among people who were HIV-positive. Among the TB high-burden countries (approximately, 80% of all new TB cases arising each year), the highest rates of case detection in 2011 were estimated to be in Brazil, China, Kenya, the Russian Federation, and the United Republic of Tanzania.

A great challenge in immunology is to understand the complexities, mechanisms, and consequences of host interactions with microbial pathogens. The innate immune response to intracellular bacteria involves mainly macrophages and natural killing cells (NK). Bacteria activate NK cells directly or stimulate macrophages to produce cytokines that activate NK cells, which results in a broad and fast antimicrobial response critical to the control of pathogen dispersion. Innate immunity can limit bacterium growth for some time, but in general, it does not succeed in eradicating infections, triggering the acquired immunity mainly through cell action.

Proteins are processed by APCs that interact with surface receptors of T-lymphocytes (T CD4+) as peptides associated with class II HLA molecules. Either the phagocyted bacteria are transported from the phagosome to the cytosol or they escape the phagosome and enter the cytoplasm of infected cells, and their degraded products are expressed on the cell surface associated with the HLA molecule, whose complex interacts with the specific cytotoxic T CD8+ receptors. Thus, the T cell eradicates the target cell. The activation of the macrophage can also result in tissue lesion in the form of late hypersensibility reaction to the protein antigens. Bacteria may resist death within the phagocytes for a long period, producing macrophage and lymphocyte cell infiltration around them and giving rise to granulomes [44,45].

A number of genes are thought to be important in the pathogenesis of TB [46,47]. HLA class I molecules are involved in antigen presentation to CD8 cytotoxic T-cell response stimulation. However, the participation of these molecules is controversial in tuberculosis. A meta-analysis study reported that subjects carrying HLA-B13 had a lower risk for thoracic TB, whereas other class I antigens could not be related to tuberculosis pathogenesis [48].

Earlier studies revealed that HLA-DR2/DR3, DR2/DR4 and DR2/DR5 are the major heterozygous combinations associated with susceptibility to TB [49]. These same authors have also identified the association of HLA-DRB1 alleles and cytokine secretion in response to live *M. tuberculosis* [50]. An increased IFN-γ response in *HLA-DRB1*03*-positive and a decreased IFN-γ response in *HLA-DRB1*15*-positive patients, an increased level of IL-12p40 in *DRB1*10* and IL-10 in *DRB1*12* positive and an increased level of IL-6 in *DRB1*04* positive patients were observed.

The HLA class II variant, DR2 encoded by *DRB1*15* and *DRB1*16,* is associated with TB in several populations [51,52]. In South Africans [53], a significant interaction between *HLA-DRB1*13:02* allele and susceptibility to TB was observed. A study in Poland [54] related a significant interaction between *HLA-DRB1*16* and *HLA-DRB1*14* and susceptibility to TB. Furthermore *HLA-DRB1*04* and *HLA-DQB1*02:01* were associated with TB in Chinese patients [55].

Hence, whether the presentation of mycobacterial epitopes by HLA molecules is beneficial or detrimental to mounting a protective response to tuberculosis and leprosy conditions has yet to be explored.

4.2. Viral diseases

4.2.1. HLA and dengue

Dengue is a resurging mosquito-borne disease that is often contracted by US travelers visiting Latin America, Asia, and the Caribbean. The clinical symptoms range from a simple febrile illness, called to Dengue Fever (DF), to hemorrhagic fever represented for Dengue Hemorrhagic Fever (DHF) or shock symptoms, called to Dengue Shock Sindrome (DSS) [56].

Nowadays, there are currently four known serotypes: DEN 1, 2, 3 and 4, which are strongly related. The viruses belong to the genus flavivirus, family *Flavaviridae* and are prevalent in tropical and sub-tropical regions around the world, predominantly in urban and semi-urban areas [57].

The pathophysiology of DF viral infections and factors that result in severe clinical disease are poorly understood. Cross-reactive memory T cells and antibodies have been suggested to contribute to the immunopathology by altering the cytokine profiles during secondary infection and are believed to be less effective in eliminating the newly infective virus serotype [58].

However, genetic factors appear to be important in the manifestation of DF as, even in endemic areas, only a small proportion of people develop DF or the most serious forms of the disease.

During infection by DF virus, a series of genes have their regulation mechanisms modified, among them, genes linked to high production of IFN-gamma, as well as MIP-1β, RANTES, MBL2, IL-8 and IL-10 [59,60]. Host genetic polymorphisms involved in innate immune responses have been shown to be correlated with resistance to DHF, such as a variant of the FcGRIIA [61], functional polymorphisms of MBL2 [62], and the polymorphisms the CD209 promoter [63].

Similarly, studies on MHC-encoded transporters associated with antigen processing (TAP) genes have also shown associations with DHF [64, 65]. In addition, the analyses of tumor necrosis factor (TNF) and lymphotoxin alpha (LTA) genes have revealed specific combinations of TNF, LTA, and HLA class I alleles that associate with DHF and production of LTA and TNF [66].

Several aspects of T cell functionality are altered in DHF patients, including proliferation, activation status, production of cytokines, and their survival [67–70]. All these functions are influenced by specific recognition, through TCRs, of the antigen associated with HLA molecules. Thus, polymorphisms of HLA genes may also play an important role in dengue severity. Several genetic variations in HLA class I alleles have been found to correlate with dengue severity in Southeast Asian populations.

Some studies have revealed positive associations, whereas others have reported negative associations between DF and HLA classes I and II alleles. In Mexico and Cuba, *HLA-B*35, DRB1*04, *07, *11,* and *DQB1*03:02* were associated to protection against classical DF [12,13]. Meanwhile in Mexico, Thailand, and Cuban the *HLA-A*02:03, *31, B*15, *51, *52, DQB1*01,* and **02:02* have been associated with susceptibility to the classical disease [71,72].

Results based on a study with 85 dengue fever cases, 29 dengue hemorrhagic fever and 110 health controls (HCs) on Western India population, revealed a significantly higher frequency of *HLA-A*33* in DF cases compared to HCs, the frequency of *HLA-A*02:11* was higher in DHF cases compared to DF cases. The frequency of *HLA-B*18* was significantly higher in dengue (DEN) cases. The frequency of *HLA-C*07* was significantly higher in DEN cases. Significance was observed even when the cases were categorized into DF and DHF [73].

The combined frequency of *HLA-C*07* with *HLA-DRB1*07/*15* genotype was significantly higher in DHF cases compared to DF and HCs. On the other hand, the frequency of combination of *HLA-C*07* without *HLA-DRB1*07* was significantly higher in DF cases compared to HCs. The results suggest that *HLA-A*33* may be associated with DF whereas *HLA-B*18* and *HLA-C*07* may be associated with symptomatic dengue requiring hospitalization. In the presence of *HLA-DRB1*07/*15* genotype, *HLA-C*07* is associated with increased risk of developing DHF whereas in the presence of other HLA-DRB1 alleles, *HLA-C*07* is associated with DF [73].

Our group had previously found a strong association between HLA-DQ1 and classical DF, during an epidemic that occurred in a Southern Brazilian population in 1995, characterized by the presence of DF virus serotype 1, however no association between DF and HLA class I antigens was detected [74].

http://dx.doi.org/10.5772/57496

The statistical analysis revealed however, an association between *HLA-A*01* and DHF in the Brazilian population, whereas analysis of *HLA-A*31* suggested a potential protective role in DHF that should be further investigated. This study provides evidence that HLA class I alleles might represent important risk factors for DHF in Brazilian patients. [75].

In addition, HLA class I and II have been associated to primary and the several forms of DF around the world [76]. The host HLA allele profile influenced the reactivity of DF-specific T cells, and may be responsible for the immunopathology of DF infection [77].

HLA Allele	Infection	Serotype	Case (n)	Control	Population	Reference
Susceptible						
*A*02:03*	2nd	DV-1	DF (49)	140	Thai	Stephens et al., 2002
*A*02:03*	2nd	DV-3	DF (26)	140	Thai	Stephens et al., 2002
*A*02:03*	2nd	all	DF (106)	140	Thai	Stephens et al., 2002
*B*52*	2nd	DV-2	DF (17)	140	Thai	Stephens et al., 2002
*B*52*	2nd	-	DF (106)	140	Thai	Stephens et al., 2002
*DQB1*01*	-	-	DF (23)	34	Mexican	Falcón-Lezama et. al., 2009
*DQB1*02:02*	-	-	DF (23)	34	Mexican	Falcón-Lezama et. al., 2009
DQ1	-	-	DF (64)	64	Brazilian	Polizel et. al., 2004
*A*24*, codon 70 histidine	-	-	DHF (59)	200	Vietnamese	Lan et. al., 2008
*A*24*, codon 70 histidine	-	-	DHF (117)	250	Vietnamese	Lan et. al., 2008
*A*02:07*	2nd	DV-1	DHF/DSS (32)	140	Thai	Stephens et al., 2002
*A*02:07*	2nd	DV-2	DHF/DSS (36)	140	Thai	Stephens et al., 2002
*A*02:07*	2nd	DV-1, DV-2	DHF/DSS (103)	140	Thai	Stephens et al., 2002
*A*02:07*	2nd	all	DHF/DSS (103)	140	Thai	Stephens et al., 2002
*A*03*	-	-	DHF/DSS (51)	95	Malay, Chinese, Indian	Appanna et. al., 2010
*B*13*	-	-	DHF/DSS (19)	95	Malay	Appanna et. al., 2010
*B*51*	2nd	all	DHF/DSS (103)	140	Thai	Stephens et al., 2002
*B*51*	2nd	DV-1	DHF/DSS (32)	140	Thai	Stephens et al., 2002
*B*53*	-	-	DHF/DSS (51)	95	Malay, Chinese, Indian	Appanna et. al., 2010

HLA Allele	Infection	Serotype	Case (n)	Control	Population	Reference
*A*24*			DHF/DSS (309)	251	Vietnamese	Fernández-Mestre et. al., 2004
*A*02*	2nd	-	DSS (41)	138	Thai	Chiewsilp et. al., 1981
*A*24*, codon 70 histidine	-	-	DSS (152)	250	Vietnamese	Lan et. al., 2008
*A*24*, codon 70 histidine	-	-	DSS (170)	200	Vietnamese	Lan et. al., 2008
*A*24*, codon 70 histidine			DSS (96)	200	Vietnamese	Lan et. al., 2008
B blank	2nd	-	DSS (41)	138	Thai	Chiewsilp et. al., 1981
*A*31*	-	DV-2	DF, DHF/DSS (120)	189	Cuban	Sierra et. al., 2007
*B*15*	-	DV-2	DF, DHF/DSS (120)	189	Cuban	Sierra et. al., 2007
*B*51*	2nd	DV-3	DF, DHF/DSS (51)	140	Thai	Stephens et al., 2002
Resistant						
*DRB1*11*	-	-	DF (47)	34	Mexican	La Fleur et. al., 2002
*DQB1*03:02*	-	-	DF (23)	34	Mexican	Falcón-Lezama et. al., 2009
*DRB1*09:01*	1st	-	DHF (59)	200	Vietnamese	Lan et. al., 2008
*A*33*	-	-	DHF/DSS (309)	251	Vietnamese	Fernández et. al., 2004
*B*18*	-	-	DHF/DSS (51)	95	Malay, (Chinese, Indian	Appanna et. al., 2010
*B*13*	2nd	-	DSS (41)	138	Thai	Chiewsilp et. al., 1981
*DRB1*09:01*	-	-	DSS (170)	200	Vietnamese	Lan et. al., 2008
*DRB1*09:01*	-	-	DSS (96)	200	Vietnamese	Lan et. al., 2008
*B*35*	-	-	DF, DHF/DSS (39)	34	Mexican	Falcón-Lezama et. al., 2009
*DRB1*04*	2nd	DV-2	DF, DHF/DSS (77)	189	Cuban	Sierra et. al., 2007
*DRB1*07*	-	DV-2	DF, DHF/DSS (120)	189	Cuban	Sierra et. al., 2007

Table 1. Cases vs. healthy controls Adaptated to [78].

4.2.2. HLA and hepatitis C

Hepatitis C virus (HCV) is one of the major causes of chronic liver inflammation worldwide [79,80]. HCV was first identified in 1989 [81] and has since then been the subject of intense research and clinical investigation due to the role this virus plays in causing liver disease and the ability of HCV to persist despite cellular immune defense.

The majority of the individuals infected by HCV are asymptomatic and only a small number will clear the virus whereas most individuals, approximately 50–85%, end up with persistent chronic viremia. Chronic disease can be evidenced by histopathological changes, which begin with an inflammation of the liver, often associated with fibrosis and which may progress towards cirrhosis, and in some cases, towards hepatocellular carcinoma [82,83]. An estimated 20% of chronic patients develop cirrhosis, especially 20 years after infection, and of these, 0 to 3% develop hepatocellular carcinoma [84,85].

The exact mechanisms responsible for liver damage during chronic hepatitis C have not yet been defined. The factors that influence the disease progression include viral genotype, age, gender, duration of the infection, concurrent infections and alcohol abuse; these factors taken individually, however, do not explain the reason that many patients spontaneously recover and escape from persistent infection whereas others progress towards end-stage liver disease [86-89].

In this context, these clinical features appear to be the result of the host's immune response, a complex interaction between the innate and adaptive immune response, involved in the control of viral replication. HLA class I and II play an important role in the immune response against viral infections because they are key proteins to antigen presentation by antigen presenting cells to T lymphocytes. Several studies have analyzed HLA class I and class II in patients with hepatitis C in different populations and there is strong evidence that some, mainly HLA class II, alleles are involved in the control of viral infection by HCV. Table 1 summarizes the various HLA class II specificities that have been associated with HCV infection [90-123].

The most consistent data seems to be related to *HLA-DRB1*11* associated with the asymptomatic disease in individuals hosting HCV in Italy (*DRB1*11:04* allele) [95], and has been associated with normal levels of alanine aminotransferase (ALT) in patients infected in France [105]. In another study in France, *HLA-DRB1*11* has been more frequently detected in patients without cirrhosis when compared to cirrhotic patients [103]. In Europe, *HLA-DRB1*11* has been observed to be less frequent in those individuals who had received transplants for HCV-induced end-stage liver disease compared to blood donors. In fact, *HLA-DRB1*11* seems to be a favorable prognosis factor not only in facilitating spontaneous HCV clearance [96,98,104,115,124,125], but also in increasing resistance against the development of more advanced stages of the chronic HCV infection [121].

Another allele group that has been correlated to self-limiting HCV is *DQB1*03* [101,104,114,124]. *HLA-DQB1*03* is found in linkage disequilibrium (LD) with *HLA-DRB1*11* and, alone or in conjunction with *DRB1*11*, has been strongly associated with spontaneous viral clearance [96,100,115,122] and with the avoidance of further liver damage in chronically infected hepatitis C virus patients. In a meta-analysis, individuals with *HLA-DRB1*11:01* and *DQB1*03:01* had a reduced risk of acquiring chronic HCV infection in 102% and 136%, respectively [126]. *HLA-DQB1*03* once again seems to influence treatment response, *HLA-*

*DQB1*03:01* has been associated with sustained viral response (SVR) treated with pegylated interferon-alpha and ribavirin [120]. In another study carried out with patients from Pakistan, an association between *DQB1*03* and improved antiviral defense in patients treated with inferferon-alpha plus ribavirin was detected [100].

Although some studies have been conducted to evaluate the influence of HLA class I in the course of hepatitis C disease and on the treatment response, the data is not yet consistent. The HLA-B35 antigen has been found more frequently in HCV carriers when compared to healthy individuals [111]. *HLA-B*18* has been observed more frequently in patients with advanced stages of fibrosis (F2-F4) [127]. In a study carried out in Spain, this specificity was also more frequently found in patients with hepatocellular carcinoma, suggesting a possible involvement in progression towards more severe forms of the disease and a more unfavorable prognosis [128]. African-American patients with *HLA-A*23* showed a higher susceptibility to develop chronic HCV infection [101].

Some HLA class I alleles have been described in treated patients: *HLA-C*07* has been associated with SVR in patients on interferon-alpha therapy in Croatia [129]. The HLA-B55, B62, Cw3 and Cw4 antigens have been associated with improved response to interferon-alpha treatment in Japanese's patients [130]. In Taiwan, the HLA- *A*11, B*51, C*15* and *DRB1*15* allele groups were related to a sustained response to interferon-alpha treatment, whereas *A*24* was linked to non-response to treatment [108]. In addition, *HLA-A*24* and *B*40* as well as haplotypes *B*40-DRB1*03, B*46-DRB1*09, C*01-DQB1*03* and *C*01-DRB1*09* were associated with SVR in Taiwan [131]. Furthermore, in Caucasian Americans, *HLA-A*02* was associated with SVR [132].

This lack of consensus in the literature may be result of the variations in the methodology of each study, such as different criteria or treatment response diagnoses, sample size, ethnic differences, mixing viral genotypes during analysis, and differences in treatment.

Associated HLA class II specificity	**Population/ Country**	**Outcome**	**Reference**
*DRB1*04:05* and *DQB1*04:01*	Japan	Viral persistence	Aikawa et al. (1996)
*DRB1*03:01*	Germany	Viral persistence	Hohler et al. (1997)
*DRB1*11* and *DQB1*03*	France	Viral clearance	Alric et al. (1997)
*DRB1*04:05* and *DQB1*04:01*	Japan	Viral persistence	Kuzushita et al. (1998)
*DRB1*07*	Caucasians/France	Nonresponders to IFN-a therapy	Alric et al. (1999)
*DQB1*06*	Caucasians/France	Sustained virological response	Alric et al. (1999)
*DRB1*10:01* and *DRB1*11:01*	Italy	Viral persistence	Asti et al. (1999)
*DRB1*11:04* and *DRB3*03*	Italy	Protection	Asti et al. (1999)
*DQB1*05:02*	Italy	Viral persistence	Mangia et al. (1999)

Associated HLA class II specificity	**Population/ Country**	**Outcome**	**Reference**
*DRB1*11:04* and *DQB1*03:01*	Italy	Viral	Mangia et al. (1999)
*DRB1*07:01,* and *DRB4*01:01*	European (UK)	Viral persistence	Thursz et al. (1999)
*DRB1*01*	Ireland	Spontaneous clearance	Fanning et al. (2000)
*DRB1*03:01* and *DQB1*02:01*	Thailand	Viral persistence	Vejbaesya et al. (2000)
*DRB1*11* and *DQB1*03*	Caucasians/UK	Viral clearance	Harcourt et al. (2001)
*DQB1*03:01*	Black/USA	Viral clearance	Thio et al. (2001)
*DRB1*01:01* and *DQB1*05:01*	Caucasians/USA	Viral clearance	Thio et al. (2001)
*DRB1*03:01* and *DQB1*02:01*	Caucasians/USA	Viral persistence	Thio et al. (2001)
*DRB1*13*	Poland	Viral persistence	Kryczka et al. (2001)
*DQB1*02:01*	France	Viral persistence	Hue et al. (2002)
*DRB1*11*	Turkey	Protection	Yenigun & Durupinar (2002)
*DRB1*11*	France	less severe liver disease	Renou et al. (2002)
DR14 and *DR17*	Italy	Viral persistence	Scotto et al. (2003)
*DQB1*05:03*	Japan	Viral persistence	Yoshizawa et al. (2003)
*DRB1*15*	Taiwan	Sustained virological response	Yu et al. (2003)
*DQB1*02:01*	Ireland	Viral persistence	McKiernan et al. (2004)
*DRB1*07*	China	Sustained virological response	Jiao & Wang (2005)
*DRB1*08:03, DQB1*06:01* and *DQB1*06:04*	Korea	Viral persistence	Yoon et al. (2005)
*DRB*40:01*	Taiwan	High viral load	Wang et al. (2005)
*DRB1*15*	Tunisia	Viral persistence	Ksiaa et al. (2007)
*DRB1*08*	Tunisia	Spontaneous clearance	Ksiaa et al. (2007)
*DRB1*03*	Brazil	Viral clearance	Cursino-Santos et al. (2007)
*DRB1*11, DQB1*03* and *DRB3*02*	USA	Viral clearance	Harris et al. (2008)
*DRB1*04* and *DQB1*02*	Egypt	Viral persistence	El-Chennawi et al. (2008)
*DQB1*06*	Egypt	Protection	El-Chennawi et al. (2008)
*DRB1*07*	Brazil	Viral persistence	Corghi et al. (2008)
*DRB1*08* and *DQB1*04*	Brazil	Protection	De Almeida et al. (2011)

Associated HLA class II specificity	Population/ Country	Outcome	Reference
*DRB1*11*	Brazil	Viral clearance	De Almeida et al. (2011)
*DRB1*11* and *DQB1*03*	Brazil	Protection	Cangussu et al. (2011)
*DQB1*03:01*	Spain	Sustained virological response	Rueda et al. (2011)
*DRB1*11*	Brazil	Protection	Marangon et al. (2012)
*DRB1*11-DQA1*05-DQB1*03*	Brazil	Protection	Marangon et al. (2012)
*DRB1*11*	Brazil	Sustained virological response	Marangon et al. (2012)
*DRB1*04*	Pakistan	Protection to HCV	Ali et al. (2013)
*DRB1*11* and *DQB1*03*	Pakistan	Viral clearance	Ali et al. (2013)
*DRB1*07* and *DQB1*02*	Pakistan	Viral persistence	Ali et al. (2013)
*DQB1*02, DQB1*06, DRB1*13* and *DRB1*15*	Egypt	Sustained virological response	Shaker et al. (2013)

Table 2. HLA class II specificities associated with hepatitis C infection

4.2.3. HLA and hepatitis B

Similar to HCV, Hepatitis B virus (HBV) is a hepatotrophic virus considered a serious public health problem. HBV infection is endemic in many parts of the world and more than 2 billion people are estimated to be infected with HBV [133-134].

The clinical features of the disease can vary from virus clearance to fulminating hepatitis. Some HBV carriers have an unapparent self-limiting hepatitis and others develop chronic hepatitis, which may lead to cirrhosis and in some cases to hepatocellular carcinoma [133-134].

Persistent HBV infection or HBV clearance is influenced by many factors such as level of viral replication, age at infection, gender, chronic alcohol abuse, co-infection with other hepatitis viruses, and genetic makeup, with most studies having identified susceptibility loci at HLA class II [133-134].

A meta-analysis demonstrated that *HLA-DR*03* and *HLA-DR*07* were associated with an increased risk of persistent HBV infection in 18 individual case-control studies including 9 Han Chinese cohorts, 3 Korean cohorts, 2 Iranian cohorts, and 1 cohort each of Caucasian, Gambian, Taiwanese, Thai, and Turkish subjects [135].

In Chinese Han populations, *HLA-DR*01* was associated with clearance of HBV infection, whereas in other ethnic groups there was no association between *HLA-DR*01* and HBV infection.

The haplotypes *HLA-DQA1*01:02-DQB1*03:03* and *HLADQA1*03:01-DQB1*06:01* were associated to persistent HBV infection, whereas *HLA-DQA1*01:02-DQB1*06:04* and *HLA-DQA1*01:01-DQB1*05:01* were protective to HBV infection [135].

A genome-wide association study identified a significant association of chronic hepatitis B in Asians with 11 SNPs in a region including HLA-DPA1 and HLA-DPB1 and subsequent analyses revealed risk haplotypes (*HLA-DPA1*02:02-DPB1*05:01* and *HLA-DPA1*02:02-DPB1*03:01*) and protective haplotypes (*HLADPA1* 01:03-DPB1*04:02* and *HLA-DPA1*01:03-DPB1*04:01*) for HBV infection [136].

HLA haplotype analysis indicated that *HLA-DQA1*01:02-DQB1*03:03* and *HLADQA1*03:01-DQB1*06:01* were risk types for persistent HBV infection, whereas *HLA-DQA1*01:02-DQB1*06:04* and *HLA-DQA1*01:01-DQB1*05:01* were protective types for HBV infection [137].

4.2.4. HLA and HIV

Human immunodeficiency virus (HIV) infection has indeed spread worldwide with over 30 million people living with HIV/AIDS. HIV infection represents a major challenge for physicians and scientists and is typically associated with an acute viral syndrome, with an asymptomatic period until the development of acquire immunodeficiency syndrome (AIDS). When left untreated the infection causes a decline in the CD4+ T cell number to less than 200 cells/ mm^3, resulting in immunodeficiency, opportunistic infections, and death [138].

A great number of disease-protective and disease-susceptible HLA alleles have been well characterized in HIV infection and the strongest associations seems to be related to HLA class I alleles (mainly HLA-A and B alleles) with differential rates of HIV disease outcome. Herein, we intend to review and discuss the HLA alleles related to HIV infection.

The virologic and immunologic outcomes in patients with HIV infection can be highly variable, with only a small number of individuals capable of controlling HIV replication without therapy [138]. Despite the mechanism involved in control and progress of HIV infection not yet being fully understood, the implication of some host immunogenetic factors, as the HLA molecules, in the course of disease has been well established.

Earlier studies revealed a relationship between *HLA-B*27* and *HLA-B*57* and the slow progression to AIDS [139]. Since then, a great number of studies have investigated the influence of HLA class I and class II alleles in both acute and chronic HIV infection and the strongest associations seem to be related to HLA class I alleles.

Regarding the association of HLA class I alleles and protection against HIV infection, the *HLA-B*44* and *B*57* have been described as favorable factors in both the acute and chronic phases of sub-Saharan Africans seroconverters [140]. In China, *HLA-A*03* has been described as a protective factor against HIV-1 infection and disease progression [141].

In another study, *HLA-A*32, A*74, B*14, B*45, B*53, B*57* have been associated with disease control in African Americans infected by HIV-1 subtype B [142].

A large multiethnic cohort with HIV-1 controllers and progressors found diverse alleles associated with virologic and immunologic control: *HLA B*57:01, B*27:05, B*14/C*08:02, B*52,* and *A*25* [143]. Furthermore, *HLA-B*13:02* [144,145] and *B*58:01* [146-148], have also been described as favorable prognostic factors.

Although all these alleles seem to be implicated in HIV infection the most consistent data are related to three HLA-B specificities: *HLA-B*57* (*HLA-B*57:01* in European population, **57:02* and **57:03* alleles mainly in African population) [140,143,147-152], *HLA B*27* (*HLA-B*27:05*) [139,143,145,150] and also *HLA-B*81* (*HLA-B*81:01*) [140,143,146,148]. These variants are strongly associated with viral load control and slow disease progression in different populations. In fact, the HLA-B molecules have impact on HIV infection as the majority of detectable HIV-specific CD8+T-cell responses described seems to be restricted by HLA-B alleles.

Regarding HIV susceptibility and rapid disease progression, *HLA-B*35* (*B*35:01, B*35:02* and *35:03*) seems to have the greatest impact on the disease: patients with these alleles seem to have less effective control of viral replication and progress towards AIDS more rapidly [143, 153].

Other unfavorable alleles have been described: *B*18/*18:01* [148,151], *B*45/*45:01* [140,148], *B*51:01* [148], *B*53:01* [143,153], *B*58:02* [140,146,148], *A*36:01* [140,148], and *B*07:02* [143], however with no actual consistency.

In addition, some HLA-C alleles have been described in association with HIV. *HLA-C*08* and *C*18* have been associated with viral load [142]. In 2010 and 2011 respectively, HIV escape mutants within cytolitic T lymphocytes (CTL) epitopes restricted of to two different HLA-C alleles were reported: *C*03* [154] and *HLA-C*12:02* [155]. In HLA-C associations, some HLA-C alleles tend to be in linkage disequilibrium (LD) with HLA-B alleles and the results could be due to the presence of these HLA-B alleles, such as *B*81:01-C*04:01*. To elucidate the genetic factors predisposing to AIDS progression, the first genomewide association study (GWAS) identified several new associations, all of them involving HLA genes: MICB, TNF, RDBP, BAT1-5, PSORS1C1, and HLA-C: This study underscores the potential for some HLA genes to control disease progression soon after infection [151].

4.2.5. HLA and papillomavirus infection

Infection by human papillomavirus (HPV) is a common sexually transmitted infectious disease and most sexually active women have been infected during their lifetime. HPV infections frequently occur in healthy individuals and the high carcinogenic risk (HR) HPV types are a major causal factor for cervical cancer (CC). Persistent infection with one among approximately 15 genotypes of carcinogenic HPV causes almost all cases of cervical cancer; type 16 and HPV-18 account for more than 70% of the cervical cancers detected worldwide [156,157].

A number of genetic risk factors have been identified, but their effects are generally weak. The most prominent among the known risk factors is the HLA complex, which plays a critical role in susceptibility to CC [3]. Since the first reported association of HLA-DQ3 with CC, a large number of studies of HLA association with cervical cancer have been published with variable results depending on the ethnic group [157,158].

A study with CC described that *DRB1*04:07-DQB1*03:02* and DRB1**15:01-DQB1*06:02* were clearly associated with susceptibility to HPV-16 positive invasive CC, high squamous intrae-

http://dx.doi.org/10.5772/57496

pithelial lesion (HSIL), and carcinoma in situ [159]. Studies with Honduran women showed *HLA-DQA1*03:01* in linkage disequilibrium with all HLA-DR4 subtypes in Mestizos, as an increased risk of developing high squamous intraepithelial lesion and CC [160]

Some DR-DQ haplotypes containing *DQB1*03:01* have been positively associated with CC susceptibility: *DRB1*11:01-DQB1*03:01* in Senegalese and US Caucasian Europeans, and *DRB1*04:01-DQB1*03:01* in US Caucasian Europeans and British females. *DRB1*11:02-DQB1*03:01* was also increased in Hispanics with carcinoma in situ or HSIL.

Protection has been mainly linked with the *HLA-DRB1*13* group: *DRB1*13:01* in patients from Costa Rica, and *DRB1*13:01-DQB1*06:03-DQA1*01:03* in Swedish, French and Dutch women with CC. A protective effect against CC progression was also claimed to be correlated with *DQB1*05, DQA1*01:01/04, DRB1*01:01* and *DRB1*13:02* in Brazilians. In Caucasians, *HLA-DRB1*13* and HPV-16/18-negative status, were independently associated with an increased probability of regression of low squamous intraepithelial lesion (LSIL), also suggesting a protective effect against CC progression [161-163].

Continuing trials pursue an explanation for the relationship between HLA and HPV infection. Silva (2013) showed that *HLA-DQB1*05:01* allele might be associated with susceptibility of HPV reinfection in Mexican women, allele frequency of *HLA-DRB1*14* was particularly reduced in patients with cancer when compared with the HPV–persistent group (p=0.04), suggesting that this allele is a possible protective factor for the development of cervical cancer.

A study analyzed the associations between HLA-G polymorphisms and HPV infection and squamous intraepithelial lesions (SIL) in Inuit women from Nunavik, northern Quebec. The group demonstrated that *HLA-G*01:01:01* was associated with an increased risk of period prevalent alpha groups 1 and 3 [164]. The *HLA-G*01:04:01* genotype was associated with a decreased risk of alpha group 3 infection period prevalence. No HLA-G alleles were significantly associated with HPV persistence. *HLA-G*01:01:02, G*01:04:01* and *G*01:06* were associated with HSIL, however the association did not reach statistical significance. In this trial, HPV genotypes were classified according to tissue-tropism groupings of alpha-papillomavirus species: alpha group 1 including low risk (LR) cervical species, group 2 including high risk (HR) cervical species, and group 3 including LR vaginal species.

One Korean study related the relationship between HLA and recurrent respiratory papillomatosis (RRP) and showed that the gene frequencies of *HLA-DRB1*11:01* and *DQB1*03:01* and the haplotype frequency of *DRB1*11:01-DQB1*03:01* were higher in RRP patients than in controls. *DRB1*11:01* and *DRB1*11:01-DQB1*03:01* haplotype were strongly associated with disease susceptibility to severe RRP in Koreans [165]. In Brazil, the *HLA-A*02-HLA-B*51* haplotype presented a reduced frequency in HPV patients compared to controls; and was associated with resistance against the disease [156].

In China population, HLA-DRB alleles were associated with cervical cancer and HPV infections [166]. For the assessment of these genotypes, 69 cervical cancer patients and 201 controls were examined. *HLA-DRB1*13* and *DRB1*03(17)* were associated with an increased risk of cervical cancer, and *DRB1*09:012* and *DRB1*12:01* were associated with a decreased risk. The risk associations of HPV infection were increased in women carrying *HLA-DRB1*09:012* and *DRB3(52)*01:01* alleles.

Among cervical cancer patients, the association risks differed between HPV positive and negative cases for several alleles; an increased risk of cervical cancer was observed in patients with *DRB3(52)*02/03* and *DRB1*3(17)* and a decreased risk was observed with *DRB1*09:012* and *DRB5(51)*01/02* [166].

4.3. Parasitic diseases

4.3.1. HLA and Chagas disease

Many genetic linkage and association studies have attempted to identify genetic variations that are involved in immunopathogenesis of Chagas disease. However, the causal genetic variants underlying susceptibility remain unknown due to parasite and host complexity [167]. Susceptibility or resistance to Chagas disease involves multiple genetic variants functioning jointly, each with small or moderate effects. To identify possible host genetic factors that may influence the clinical course of Chagas disease, the role of classic and non-classic MHC genes will be addressed.

Chagas disease is an infection caused by the protozoan *Trypanosoma cruzi,* described in 1907 by Carlos Chagas. The disease is endemic and is characterized by acute and chronic phases, which develop into the indeterminate, cardiac and/or gastrointestinal forms [168,169]. Ten million people are estimated to be infected with *T. cruzi* worldwide, mostly in Latin America (WHO, 2012) with a total estimated incidence of 800,000 new cases per year [170].

The mechanisms of the transmission of Chagas infection include transmission through insect vectors mainly, but blood transfusion, contaminated food, congenital and secondary transmissions mechanism may occur [171].The phases of infection include the early or acute phase, characterized by high parasitaemia or trypomastigote circulating forms in the blood for two to four months [170]. Mortality, during this period, ranges from 5% to 10% due to episodes of myocarditis and meningocefalite [172,173].

The clinical signs are a local inflammatory reaction with formation of strong swelling at the site of entry of the parasites (chagoma or Romaña sign), fever, splenomegaly and cardiac arrhythmia [174]. During the acute phase, the majority of the infected individuals develop a humoral and cellular immune response responsible for the decrease of parasites in the blood.

Following this phase, patients progress to the chronic asymptomatic stage which affects most individuals (50 to 60%): this condition characterizes the indeterminate clinical form (IND) of the disease, and may remain in effect for long periods of time [175]. Approximately 20% to 30% of the individuals develop cardiomyopathy, which reflects a progressively damaged myocardium due to extensive chronic inflammation and fibrosis and, in terminal phases, usually presents as dilated cardiomyopathy. Chronic Chagas cardiomyopathy (CCC) is the most relevant clinical manifestation leading to death from heart failure in endemic countries. Eight to 10% have the digestive form (DF), characterized by dilation of the oesophagus or colon (megaoesophagus and megacolon). Some patients have associated cardiac and digestive manifestations, known as the mixed or cardiodigestive form [176-178].

There is a consensus that during *T. cruzi* infection the host immune system induces complex processes to ensure the control of parasite growth. The immune response is crucial for protection against the disease; however, immunological imbalances can lead to heart and digestive tract lesions in chagasic patients. Several studies have evaluated the innate, cellular and humoral immune responses in chagasic patients in an attempt to correlate immunological findings with clinical forms of Chagas disease. However, in all clinical forms of Chagas disease the involvement of cell-mediated immunity is undoubtedly of major importance [179- 189].

The spectrum of expression of Chagas disease brings strong evidence of the influence of the genetic factors on the clinical course of the disease, and the polymorphic genes involved in the innate and specific immune response is being widely studied such as the molecules and genes in the region of the HLA.

The polymorphic HLA class I (A, B and C) and II (DR, DQ and DP) molecules determine the efficiency of presentation of the *T. cruzi* epitopes to $CD8^+$ and $CD4^+$ T-cells, respectively. The type of the presentation could affect the clinical course of diseases because patients may respond differently to the same antigen, depending on their HLA repertory [190]. Several HLA alleles and haplotypes have been reported to be associated with Chagas disease.

Regarding the association of HLA and Chagas disease, HLA-Dw22 was firstly associated to the susceptibility of developing the disease in Venezuelans [191]. A subsequent study compared class II allele frequencies between patients and controls and identified a decreased frequency of *DRB1*14* and *DQB1*03:03* in patients, suggesting protective effects unrelated to chronic infection in this population [192]. A study in southeastern Brazil showed that *HLA-A*30* confers susceptibility to Chagas disease, whereas *HLA-DQB1*06* confers protection, regardless of the clinical form of the disease [193] and, in a South Brazilians population, HLA-DR2 antigens were related to susceptibility to chronic Chagas disease [194]. HLA-DR4 and HLA-B39 were associated with the infection by the *T. cruzi* in the Mexican population [195] and *HLA-DRB1*04:09* and *DRB1*15:03* in Argentineans [196,197]. In the latter study, *DRB1*11:03* allele was associated with disease resistance [197]. The haplotype *HLA-DRB1*14-DQB1*03:01* was involved in resistance to *T. cruzi* infection in the rural mestizo population of Southern Peru [198] and the *HLA-DRB1*01-B*14-MICA*011* haplotype was associated with resistance against chronic Chagas disease in Bolivian individuals [199].

As to the association of HLA and the clinical form of CCC, the first publication related HLA-B40 antigen, in the presence of Cw3, with a resistance to cardiac manifestations in Chilean patients [200], which was later confirmed [201]. However, *HLA-C*03* was associated with susceptibility to cardiomiopathy in the Venezuelan *T. cruzi* serologically positive individuals [202]. An increase of HLA-A31, B39, DR8, HLA-DR16 and *DRB1*15:03* and *HLA-DPB1*04:01* alleles and a decrease of HLA-A68, DR4, DR5, DQ1, DQ3 and *DRB1*15:01* were observed in several Latin American mestizos from different countries with CCC [192,195,203,204]. *DPB1*04:01-HLA-DPB1*23:01* and *DPB1*04:01-DPB1*39:01* haplotypes were susceptibility factors in this clinical form [204].

The studies conducted with the mixed or cardiodigestive form revealed that *DRB1*01, DRB1*08* and *DQB1*05:01* was more frequent in patients conferring susceptibility to the disease [192], as occurs with the *HLA-DPB1*04:01* allele in homozygous or in combination with *HLA-DPB1*23:01* or *DPB1*39:01* [204]. Contrarily, a decreased frequency of *DRB1*15:01* was found in patients with arrhythmia and congestive heart failure, conferring resistance against these disorders [192,204]. Recently, resistance conferred by *HLA-DRB1*01* and *HLA-B*14:02* was associated with the patients suffering from megacolon, as well as in those with ECG alterations and/or megacolon when they were compared with a group of patients with indeterminate symptoms [199].

Another study showed that contrarily, the polymorphism of HLA-DR and -DQ molecules did not influence the susceptibility to different clinical forms of Chagas' disease or the progression to severe Chagas' cardiomyopathy [205].

The polymorphism of MICA may be involved in the susceptibility to various diseases; however this association has been suggested to be secondary, due to the strong linkage disequilibrium with HLA-B alleles. *MICA*011*, which was closely linked to *HLA-B*14* and *DRB1*01*, might stimulate Tγδ cells in the gut mucosa, a phenomenon that could be related to megacolon [206]. In Chagas disease the same *HLA-DRB1*01-B*14-MICA*011* haplotype was associated with resistance against the chronic form [199]. *MICA-A5* and *HLA-B35* synergistically enhanced susceptibility to CCC [207].

These different results between the HLA allele and haplotypes and Chagas disease could be the result of the variability of HLA allele's distribution in different ethnic groups, the selection of the patients and the clinical form, and the biological variability of the parasite, among other factors. Nevertheless, genetic factors related to the HLA system reflect an important role in susceptibility or protection to Chagas disease and its clinical forms.

4.3.2. HLA and malaria

Malaria is an infectious disease caused by intracellular protozoan of the genus *Plasmodium*. Genes located in the HLA complex appear to protect populations in endemic areas against the severe forms caused by *Plasmodium falciparum* and *Plasmodium vivax.*

The antibody response generated during malaria infections is of particular interest, since the production of specific IgG antibodies is required for acquisition of clinical immunity. However, variations in antibody responses could result from genetic polymorphism s of the HLA class II genes. Given the increasing focus on the development of subunit vaccines, studies of the influence of class II alleles on the immune response in ethnically diverse populations is important, prior to the implementation of vaccine trials. Junior et al.(2012) showed that *HLA-DRB1*04* alleles were associated with a high frequency of antibody responses to five out of nine recombinant proteins tested in Rondonia State, Brazil [208].

The Fulani of West Africa have been shown to be less susceptible to malaria and to mount a stronger immune response to malaria than sympatric ethnic groups. *HLA-DRB1*04* and - *DQB1*02* have been shown to be implicated in the development of several autoimmune diseases, to be present at high frequency in the Fulani, suggesting their potential involvement in the enhanced immune reactivity observed in this population [209].

Trials have been performed seeking to determine the associations between HLA-A, B, and DRB1 group of alleles and severe malaria in northern Ghana. *HLA-DRB1*04* was analyzed in 4,032 subjects from a severe malaria case-control study, 790 severe malaria cases, 1,611 mild malaria controls, and 1631 asymptomatic controls. The presence of *HLA-DRB1*04* was associated with severe malaria. The frequency of *DRB1*04* was similar in the two major ethnic groups in the study population, Kassem (4.4%) and Nankam (4.7%), and the OR for the association between *DRB1*04* and severe malaria was similar in both ethnic groups. These findings were consistent with results from Gabon suggesting that *DRB1*04* to be a risk factor for severe malaria [210].

To test for associations between HLA alleles and the severity of malaria in a Thai population, polymorphisms of HLA-B and HLA-DRB1 genes were investigated in 472 adult patients in northwest Thailand with *Plasmodium falciparum* malaria. In the study, malaria patients were classified into three groups: mild malaria, non-cerebral severe malaria, and cerebral malaria. The results revealed that the allele frequencies of *HLA-B*46, B*56,* and *DRB1*10:01* were statistically different between non-cerebral severe malaria and cerebral malaria, between mild malaria and cerebral malaria (P = 0.032), and between mild malaria and non-cerebral malaria [211].

Individuals from Mumbai, an area of low and seasonal *Plasmodium falciparum* transmission, were investigated for HLA associations. A cohort of 171 severe *P. falciparum* malaria patients were compared with that of 101 normal gender, age, and ethnically matched control samples. Significant differences were observed between patients with malaria and controls in the following HLA: A3, B27, B49, *DRB1*04,* and *DRB1*08:09,* which were increased, whereas A19, A34, B18, B37, and *DQB1*02:03* were decreased. HLA B49 and *DRB1*08:09* were found to be positively associated with the complicated severe malaria patients. HLA-A19, B5 and B13 were protective in patients with high parasite index (> 2%). These observations revealed the importance of ethnic background, which has to be taken into consideration when developing an ideal malaria vaccine. Furthermore, when compared to HLA associations of other world populations the study indicated the relative importance of different HLA alleles that may vary in different populations [212].

5. Concluding remarks

Many genetic linkage and association studies have attempted to identify HLA variations that are involved in immunopathogenesis of infection diseases. However, in the infection diseases multiple genetic variants functioning jointly, each with small or moderate effects, may protect against diseases, or could contribute to aggression and tissue damage. Different results between the alleles and haplotypes HLA and infection diseases could be caused by: variability of HLA alleles distribution in different ethnic groups; the typing test (serological or molecular techniques); the methods of statistical analyses (chi-square test, logistic or linear regression) and interpretation (*p* or *pc* values that apply the Bonferroni correction for multiple comparations); the selection of the patients and the clinical form; the numbers of individuals; linkage disequilibrium that vary among populations; and biological variability of the parasite.

The characterisation of the susceptibility genes and their variants has important implications, not only for a better understanding of disease pathogenesis, but for the control and development of new therapeutic strategies for infectious diseases. Using the basic knowledge acquired in the studies of the influence of genetics upon the immune response against parasite in different populations, one can look for proteins that induce the immunological phenotype needed for protection. At present, vaccination is an effective preventive measurement for these disorders, and researches for peptides with the best-predicted binding affinities for HLA molecules are an alternative. Overall, this type of analysis could potentially define high-risk patient groups, and result in effective therapeutic strategies for infectious disorders.

Author details

Daniela Maira Cardozo[1], Amanda Vansan Marangon[1], Ana Maria Sell[2], Jeane Eliete Laguila Visentainer[2] and Carmino Antonio de Souza[1]

1 Immunogenetics Laboratory, Hematology and Hemotherapy Center-University of Campinas/Hemocentro-Unicamp, Instituto Nacional de Ciência e Tecnologia do Sangue, Campinas, São Paulo, Brazil

2 Immunogenetics Laboratory, Department of Healthy Basic Science, Maringá State University, UEM, Maringá, Paraná, Brazil

References

[1] Jawdat D, Al Saleh S, Sutton P, Al Anazi H, Shubaili A, Uyar FA, et al. HLA-C Polymorphisms in two cohorts of donors of bone marrow transplantation. Saudi J Kidney Dis Transpl. 2012;23:467-70. http://www.sjkdt.org/article.asp?issn=1319-2442; year=2012; volume=23; issue=3;spage=467;epage=470 ;aulast=Jawdat (accessed 13 August 2012).

[2] Voltarelli JC, Pasquini R, Ortega ETT, Transplante de Células-Tronco Hematopoiéticas. Ed. Atheneu 2010.

[3] Bjorkman PJ, Saper MA, Samraoui B, Bennett WS, Strominger JL, Wiley DC. Structure of the human class I histocompatibility antigen, HLA-A2. J Immunol 2005;174:6-9. http://www.jimmunol.org/content/174/1/6.long (accessed 13 August 2012).

[4] Steinmetz M, Hood L. Genes of the major histocompatibility complex in mouse and man. Science 1983; 222: 727-33. http://www.sciencemag.org/content/222/4625/727.long (accessed 14 August 2012)

[5] Le Bouteiller P. HLA class I chromosomal region, genes, and products: facts and questions. Critical Reviews in Immunology1994;14:89-129. http://www.ncbi.nlm.nih.gov/pubmed?term=HLA%20class%20I%20chromosomal%20region%2C%20genes%2C%20and%20products%3A%2 (accessed 16 August 2012).

[6] Bjorkman PJ, Saper MA, Samraoui B, Bennett WS, Strominger JL, Wiley DC. The foreign antigen binding site and T cell recognition regions of class I histocompatibility antigens. Nature 1987;329:512-8. http://www.nature.com/nature/journal/v329/n6139/abs/329512a0.html (accessed 18 August 2012).

[7] Rammensee HG, Friede T, Stevanovic S. MHC ligands and peptide motifs: first listing. Immunogenetics 1995;41:178-28. http://www.ncbi.nlm.nih.gov/pubmed?term=MHC%20ligands%20and%20peptide%20motifs%3A%20first%20listing (accessed 29 August 2012).

[8] Salter RD, Benjamin RJ, Wesley PK, et al. A binding site for the T-cell co-receptor CD8 on the alpha 3 domain of HLA-A2. Nature 1990;345:41-6. http://www.nature.com/nature/journal/v345/n6270/abs/345041a0.html (accessed 30 August 2012).

[9] Croft M, Dubey C. Accessory molecule and costimulation requirements for CD4 T cell response. Crit Rev Immunol.1997;17:89-118. http://www.ncbi.nlm.nih.gov/pubmed?term=Accessory%20molecule%20and%20costimulation%20requirements%20for%20CD4%20T%20cell%20response (accessed 02 September 2012).

[10] Kaleab BR, Kiessling JD, van Embden JE, Thole DS, Kumararatne P, Pisa A, Wondimu and Ottenhoff THM. Induction of antigen-specific CD41 HLA-DR-restricted cytotoxic T lymphocytes as well as nonspecific nonrestricted killer cells by the recombinant mycobacterial 65-kDa heat-shock protein. Eur. J. Immunol. 1990;20:369.

[11] Mutis T, Cornelisse YE and Ottenhoff THM. Mycobacteria induce CD41 T cells that are cytotoxic and display Th1-like cytokine secretion profile: heterogeneity in cytotoxic activity and cytokine secretion levels. Eur. J. Immunol. 1993;23:2189.

[12] Hunter SW, Gaylord H, Brennan PJ. Structure and antigenicity of the phosphorylated lipopolysaccharide antigens from the leprosy and tubercle bacilli. J Biol Chem. 1986;26: 12345-51.

[13] Meyers WM. Leprosy. Dermatol Clin. 1992;10:73-96.

[14] World Health Organization, "Global leprosy: update on the 2012 situation," Weekly Epidemiological Record. 2013, 88:365-380.

[15] WHO Expert Committee on leprosy. 17th report. Geneva, World Health Organization; 1998. (Technical Report Series, 874).

[16] Brandsma JW, Heerkens YF, Lakerveld-Heyl K, Mischner-Van Ravensberg CD. The international classification of impairments, disabilities and handicaps in leprosy-control projects. Lepr Rev. 1992;63:337-44.

[17] Schurr E, Morgan K, Gros P, Skamene E. Genetics of leprosy. Am J Trop Med Hyg. 1991;44:4-11. http://www.ajtmh.org/content/44/4_Part_2/4.long (accessed 23 October 2013).

[18] Spierings E, De Boer T, Zulianello L, Ottenhoff TH. Novel mechanisms in the immunopathogenesis of leprosy nerve damage: the role of Schwann cells, T cells and Mycobacterium leprae. Immunol Cell Biol. 2000;78:349-55. http://www.nature.com/icb/journal/v78/n4/full/icb200047a.html (accessed 02 October 2013).

[19] Marquet S and Schurr E. Genetics of susceptibility to infections disease: tuberculosis and leprosy as example. Drug Metab Dispos. 2001;29:479-83. http://dmd.aspetjournals.org/content/29/4/479.long (accessed 03 September 2013).

[20] Bale UM, Mehta MM, Contractor NM. HLA antigens in leprosy patients. Tissue Antigens. 1982;20:141–143. http://www.ncbi.nlm.nih.gov/pubmed/?term=Bale+1982+leprosys (accessed 03 October 2013).

[21] Agrewala JN, Ghei SK, Sudhakar KS, Girdhar BK, Sengupta U. HLA antigens and erythema nodosum leprosum (ENL). Tissue Antigens. 1989;33:486–487.

[22] Rani R, Zaheer SA, Mukherjee R. Do human leukocyte antigens have a role to play in differential manifestation of multibacillary leprosy: a study on multibacillary leprosy patients from North India. Tissue Antigens. 1992;40:124–127.

[23] Shankarkumar U, Ghosh K, Badakere S, Mohanty D. Novel HLA class I alleles. Associated with Indian leprosy patients. Journal of Biomedicine and Biotechnology. 2003;3:208–211. http://www.ncbi.nlm.nih.gov/pmc/articles/PMC400212/ (accessed 02 October 2013).

[24] Shankarkumar U. HLA associations in leprosy patients from Mumbai, India. Leprosy Review. 2004;75:79–85. http://www.ncbi.nlm.nih.gov/pmc/articles/PMC400212/ (Accessed 29 September 2013).

[25] Franceschi DSA, Tsuneto LT, Mazini PS et al., Class-I human leukocyte alleles in leprosy patients from southern Brazil. Revista da Sociedade Brasileira de Medicina Tropical. 2011;44:616–620.

[26] Alter A, Huong NT, Singh M et al., Human leukocyte antigen class I region single-nucleotide polymorphisms are associated with leprosy susceptibility in Vietnam and India. The Journal of Infectious Diseases. 2011;203:1274–1281.

[27] Mehra NK, Verduijn W, Taneja V, Drabbels J, Singh SP, Giphart MJ. Analysis of HLA-DR2-associated polymorphisms by oligonucleotide hybridization in an Asian Indian population. Hum Immunol. 1991;32:246-53.

[28] Visentainer JEL, Tsuneto LT, Serra MF, Peixoto PRF and Petzl-Erler ML. Association of leprosy with HLA-DR2 in a Southern Brazilian population. Brazilian Journal of Medical and Biological Research. 1997;30:51–59.

[29] Singh M, Balamurugan A, Katoch K, Sharma SK and Mehra NK. Immunogenetics of mycobacterial infections in the North Indian population. Tissue Antigens. 2007;69:228–230.

[30] Vanderborght PR, Pacheco AG, Moraes ME et al. HLADRB1*04 and DRB1*10 are associated with resistance and susceptibility, respectively, in Brazilian and Vietnamese leprosy patients. Genes and Immunity. 2007;8:320–324.

[31] da Silva SA, Mazini PS, Reis PG, et al. HLA-DR and HLADQ alleles in patients from the south of Brazil: markers for leprosy susceptibility and resistance. BMC Infectious Diseases. 2009;9:134–140. http://www.ncbi.nlm.nih.gov/pmc/articles/PMC2746224/ (Accessed 30 September 2013).

[32] Zhang F, Liu H, Chen S, et al. Evidence for an association of HLA-DRB1*15 and DRB1*09 with leprosy and the impact of DRB1*09 on disease onset in a Chinese Han population. BMC Medical Genetics. 2009;10:133. http://www.ncbi.nlm.nih.gov/pmc/articles/PMC2797507/ (Accessed 12 October 2013).

[33] Correa RDG, Aquino DM, Caldas ADJ, et al. Association analysis of human leukocyte antigen class II, (DRB1) alleles with leprosy in individuals from São Luís, state of Maranhão, Brazil. Memórias Instituto Oswaldo Cruz. 2012;107:150–155. http://www.scielo.br/scielo.php?script=sci_arttext&pid=S0074-02762012000900022&lng=en&nrm=iso&tlng=en (accessed 12 October 2013).

[34] Koçak M, Balci M, Pençe B and Kundakç N. Associations between human leukocyte antigens and leprosy in the Turkish population. Clinical and Experimental Dermatology. 2002;27:235–239. http://onlinelibrary.wiley.com/doi/10.1046/j.1365-2230.2002.01004.x/full (Accessed 23 October 2013).

[35] Borrás SG, Cotorruelo C, Racca L, et al. Association of leprosy withHLA-DRB1 in an Argentinean population. Annals of Clinical Biochemistry. 2008;45:96–98. http://acb.sagepub.com/content/45/1/96.long (Accessed 12 October 2013).

[36] Agrewala JN and Wilkinson RJ. Influence of HLA-DR on the phenotype of CD4+ T lymphocytes specific for an epitope of the 16-kDa alpha-crystallin antigen of Mycobacterium tuberculosis. European Journal of Immunology. 1999;29:1753–1761. http://onlinelibrary.wiley.com/doi/10.1002/(SICI)1521-4141(199906)29:06%3C1753::AID-IMMU1753%3E3.0.CO;2-B/pdf (Accessed 23 September 2013).

[37] Mutis T, Cornelisse YE, Datema G, van den Elsen PG, Ottenhoff THM and de Vries RRP. Definition of a human suppressor T-cell epitope. Proceedings of the National Academy of Sciences of the United States of America. 1994;91:9456–9460. http://www.ncbi.nlm.nih.gov/pmc/articles/PMC44831/ (Accessed 12 September 2013).

[38] Joko S, Numaga J, Kawashima H, Namisato M and Maeda H. Human leukocyte antigens in forms of leprosy among Japanese patients. International Journal of Leprosy and Other Mycobacterial Diseases. 2000;68:49–56. http://www.ncbi.nlm.nih.gov/pubmed/10834069 (Accessed 10 September 2013).

[39] Motta PMF, Cech N, Fontan C, et al. Role of HLA-DR and HLA-DQ alleles in multibacillary leprosy and paucibacillary leprosy in the province of Chaco (Argentina). Enfermedades Infecciosas y Microbiologia Clinica. 2007;25:627–631. http://www.ncbi.nlm.nih.gov/pubmed/18053473 (Accessed 02 September 2013).

[40] Hsieh NK, Chu CC, Lee NS, Lee HL and Lin M. Association of HLA- DRB1*0405 with resistance to multibacillary leprosy in Taiwanese. Human Immunology. 2010;71:712–716. http://www.sciencedirect.com/science/article/pii/S0198885910000790 (Accessed 11 October 2013).

[41] Goldfeld AE, Delgado JC, Thim S, Bozon MV, Uglialoro AM, Turbay D, Cohen C, Yunis EJ. Association of an HLA-DQ allele with clinical tuberculosis. JAMA. 1998;279:226-8. http://jama.jamanetwork.com/article.aspx?articleid=187149 (Accessed 30 September 2013).

[42] Zerva L, Cizman B, Mehra NK, Alahari SK, Murali R, Zmijewski CM, Kamoun M, Monos DS. Arginine at positions 13 or 70-71 in pocket 4 of HLA-DRB1 alleles is associated with susceptibility to tuberculoid leprosy. J Exp Med. 1996;183:829-36. http://www.ncbi.nlm.nih.gov/pmc/articles/PMC2192353/ (Accessed 14 October 2013).

[43] Dye, C, Williams, BG, Espinal, MA, Raviglione, MC. Erasing the world's slow stain: strategies to beat multidrug-resistant tuberculosis. Science. 2002. 295:2042-2046. DOI: 10.1126/science.1063814.

[44] Frigui W, Bottai D, Majlessi L, Monot M, Josselin E, Brodin P, Garnier T, Gicquel B, Martin C, Leclerc C, Cole ST, Brosch R. Control of M. tuberculosis ESAT-6 secretion and specific T cell recognition by PhoP. PLoS Pathog. 2008;8:e33. http://www.ncbi.nlm.nih.gov/pmc/articles/PMC2242835/ (accessed 10 October 2013).

[45] Urdahl KB, Shafiani S, Ernst JD. Initiation and regulation of T-cell responses in tuberculosis. Mucosal Immunol. 2011; 4(3):288-93. http://www.ncbi.nlm.nih.gov/pmc/articles/PMC3206635/ (accessed 10 September 2013).

[46] Hoal EG. Human genetic susceptibility to tuberculosis and other mycobacterial diseases. IUBMB Life. 2002;53:225–229. http://onlinelibrary.wiley.com/doi/10.1080/15216540212644/abstract (accessed 10 September 2013).

[47] Malik S and Schurr E. Genetic susceptibility to tuberculosis. Clinical Chemistry and Laboratory Medicine. 2002;40:863–868. DOI: 10.1515/CCLM.2002.153.

[48] Kettaneh L, Seng KP, Tiev C, Tolédano B, Fabre JC. Human leukocyte antigens and susceptibility to tuberculosis: a meta-analysis of case-control studies. Int J Tuberc

Lung Dis. 2006;10:717–725. http://www.ncbi.nlm.nih.gov/pubmed/16848331 (accessed 03 September 2013).

[49] Selvaraj P, Reetha AM, Uma H, et al. Influence of HLA-DR and -DQ phenotypes on tuberculin reactive status in pulmonary tuberculosis. Tuber Lung Dis 1996;77:369–73.

[50] P. Selvaraj D, Nisha Rajeswari MS, Jawahar PRN. Influence of HLA-DRB1 alleles on Th1 and Th2 cytokine response to Mycobacterium tuberculosis antigens in pulmonary tuberculosis. Tuberculosis. 2007;87:544–550. http://www.tuberculosisjournal.com/article/S1472-9792(07)00089-3/abstract (accessed 10 September 2013).

[51] Dubaniewicz A, Lewko B, Moszkowska G, Zamorska B, Stepinski J. Molecular subtypes of the HLA-DR antigens in pulmonary tuberculosis. International Journal of Infectious Diseases. 2000;4:129–133. http://www.ncbi.nlm.nih.gov/pubmed/11179915 (accessed 10 September 2013).

[52] Rojas-Alvarado MDL, Diaz-Mendoza ML, Said-Fernandez S, Caballero-Olın G, Cerda-Flores RM. Association of pulmonary tuberculosis with HLA systemantigens in Northeastern Mexico. Gaceta Medica de Mexico. 2008;144:233–238.

[53] Lombard Z, Dalton D, Venter PA, Williams RC and Bornman L. Association of HLA-DR, -DQ, and vitamin D receptor alleles and haplotypes with tuberculosis in the Venda of South Africa. Human Immunology. 2006;67:643–654. http://www.sciencedirect.com/science/article/pii/S0198885906001078 (accessed 15 October 2013).

[54] Dubaniewicz A. and Moszkowska G. Analysis of occurrence of DRB and DQ alleles in sarcoidosis and tuberculosis from Northern Poland. Pneumonologia i Alergologia Polska. 2007;75:13–21. http://www.ncbi.nlm.nih.gov/pubmed/17541908 (accessed 03 September 2013).

[55] Wu F, Zhang W, Zhang L, Wu J, Li C, Meng X, Wang X, He P, Zhang J. NRAMP1, VDR, HLA-DRB1, and HLA-DQB1 Gene Polymorphisms in Susceptibility to Tuberculosis among the Chinese Kazakh Population: A Case-Control Study. BioMed Research International. 2013;2013:1-8. http://www.ncbi.nlm.nih.gov/pmc/articles/PMC3758880/ (accessed 04 September 2013).

[56] Mangold KA, Reynolds SL. A review of dengue fever: resurging tropical disease. Pediatric Emergency Care. 2013;29:665-669. http://www.ncbi.nlm.nih.gov/pubmed/23640151 (accessed 17 September 2013).

[57] Ministério da Saúde. "Tabulação de dados. Dengue - Notificações registradas no sistema de informação de agravos de notificação," - SinanNet, 2011. [cited 2011 September 08]. Available from: dtr2004.saude.gov.br/sinanweb/index.php.

[58] Appanna R, Ponnampalavanar S, Chai See LL and Sekaran SD. Susceptible and protective HLA class I alleles against Dengue Fever and Dengue Hemorrhagic Fever patients in a Malaysian population. Plos One. 2010;5:e13029. http://www.ncbi.nlm.nih.gov/pmc/articles/PMC2946915/ (accessed 14 September 2013).

[59] Dong T, Moran E, Vinh Chau N, et al. High proinflammatory cytokine secretion and loss of high avidity cross-reactive cytotoxic hemorrhagic fever and virus load in a dengue-2 outbreak. Clinical Immunology. 2007;131:404-409. http://www.ncbi.nlm.nih.gov/pmc/articles/PMC2092391/ (accessed 14 September 2013).

[60] Ubol S, Masrinoul P, Chaijaruwanich J, et al. Differences in global gene expression in peripheral blood mononuclear cells indicate a significant role of the innate responses in progression of Dengue Fever but not Dengue Hemorrhagic Fever. Jornal Infectious. Diseases. 2008;197:1459-1467. http://jid.oxfordjournals.org/content/197/10/1459.long (accessed 14 September 2013).

[61] Cardozo DM, Guelsin GA, Clementino SL, et al. Extração de DNA a partir de sangue humano coagulado para aplicação nas técnicas de genotipagem de antígenos leucocitários humanos e de receptores semelhantes à imunoglobulina. Revista Sociedade Brasileira Medicinal Tropical. 2009;42:651-656. http://www.scielo.br/scielo.php?script=sci_arttext&pid=S0037-86822009000600008&lng=en&nrm=iso&tlng=en (accessed 14 September 2013).

[62] Alves-Silva M, da Silva Santos PE, Guimarães et al. The ancestry of Brazilian mtDNA lineages. American Journal of Human Genetics. 2000;67:444-461. http://www.ncbi.nlm.nih.gov/pmc/articles/PMC1287189/ (accessed 12 September 2013).

[63] Carvalho-Silva JDR, Santos FR, Rocha J, and Pena SD. The phylogeography of Brazilian Y-chromosome lineages. American Journal of Human Genetics 2001;68:281-286. http://www.ncbi.nlm.nih.gov/pmc/articles/PMC1234928/ (accessed 10 October 2013).

[64] Nishimura Y, Kamikawaji N, Fujisawa K. et al. Genetic control of immune response and disease susceptibility by HLA-DQ gene. Research Immunology. 1991;142:559-566. http://www.ncbi.nlm.nih.gov/pubmed/1684444 (accessed 01 September 2013).

[65] Huang X, Ling H, Mao W, et al. Association of HLA-A, B, DRB1 alleles and haplotypes with HIV-1 infection in Chongqing, China. BMC Infectious Diseases. 2009;9:201-209. http://www.ncbi.nlm.nih.gov/pmc/articles/PMC2797796/ (accessed 10 September 2013).

[66] Hu J, Li L, Pang L, et al. HLA-DRB1*1501 and HLA-DQB1*0301 alleles are positively associated with HPV16 infection–related Kazakh esophageal squamous cell carcinoma in Xinjiang China. Cancer Immunology Immunotherapy. 2012;61:2135-2141. http://link.springer.com/article/10.1007%2Fs00262-012-1281-x (accessed 10 September 2013).

[67] Martín JL, Brathwaite O, Zambrano B, et al. The Epidemiology of Dengue in the Americas Over the Last Three Decades: A Worrisome Reality. The American Journal of Tropical Medicine and Hygiene. 2010;82:128-135. http://www.ncbi.nlm.nih.gov/pmc/articles/PMC2803522/ (accessed 10 September 2013).

[68] Marangon AV, Moliterno RA, Sell AM, et al. Influence of HLA alleles in response to treatment with pegylated interferon-alpha and ribavirin in patients with chronic hep-

atitis C. International Journal of Immunogenetics. 2012;39:296-302. http://onlinelibrary.wiley.com/doi/10.1111/j.1744-313X.2012.01088.x/abstract (accessed 10 September 2013).

[69] Alagarasu K, Mulay AP, Singh R, Gavade VB, Shah PS, Cecilia D. Association of HLA-DRB1 and TNF genotypes with dengue hemorrhagic fever. Human Immunology. 2013;74:610-617. http://www.sciencedirect.com/science/article/pii/S0198885913000384 (accessed 01 October 2013).

[70] Falcón-Lezama JA, Ramosa C, Zuñigab J, et al. HLA class I and II polymorphisms in Mexican Mestizo patients with dengue fever. Acta Tropica. 2009;112:193-197. http://www.sciencedirect.com/science/article/pii/S0001706X09002058 (accessed 01 September 2013).

[71] LaFleur C, Granados J, Alarcon GV, et al. HLA-DR Antigen Frequencies in Mexican Patients with Dengue virus infection: HLA-DR4 as a Possible Genetic Resistance Factor for Dengue Hemorrhagic Fever. Human Immunology. 2002;63:1039-1044. http://www.sciencedirect.com/science/article/pii/S0198885902006821 (accessed 10 September 2013).

[72] Sierra B, Alegre R, Pérez AB, et al. HLA-A, B, C, and DRB1 allele frequencies in Cuba individuals with antecedents of dengue 2 disease: Advantages of the Cuban population for HLA studies of dengue infection. Human Immunology. 2007;68:531-540. http://www.sciencedirect.com/science/article/pii/S019888590700050X (accessed 11 September 2013).

[73] Alagarasu K, Mulay AP, Sarikhani M, Rashmika D, Shah PS, Cecilia D. Profile of human leukocyte antigen class I alleles in patients with dengue infection from Western India. Hum Immunol. 2013;20:198-8859.

[74] Stephens HAF, Klaythong R, Sirikong M, et al. HLA-A and B allele associations with secondary dengue virus infections correlate with disease severity and the infecting viral serotype in ethnic Thais. Tissue Antigens. 2002;60:309-318. http://www.sciencedirect.com/science/article/pii/S0198885913002292 (accessed 12 September 2013).

[75] Monteiro SP, Brasil PE, Cabello GM, Souza RV, Brasil P, Georg I, Cabello PH, De Castro L. HLA-A*01 allele: a risk factor for dengue haemorrhagic fever in Brazil's population. Mem Inst Oswaldo Cruz. 2012;107:224-30. http://dx.doi.org/10.1590/S0074-02762012000200012 (accessed 12 September 2013).

[76] Santos BA, Segat L, Dhalia R, et al. MBL2 Gene polymorphisms protect against development of thrombocytopenia associated with sever dengue phenotype. Human Immunology. 2008;69:122-128. http://dx.doi.org/10.1016/j.humimm.2008.01.005 (accessed 12 September 2013).

[77] Zivna I, Green S, Vaughn DW, et al. T Cell responses to an HLA-B*07-restricted epitope on the dengue NS3 protein correlate with disease severity. Journal Immunology.

2002;168:5959-5965. http://www.jimmunol.org/content/168/11/5959.long (accessed 13 September 2013).

[78] Lan NTP and Hirayama K. Host genetic susceptibility to severe dengue infection. Tropical Medicine and Health. 2011;39:73-81. http://www.ncbi.nlm.nih.gov/pmc/articles/PMC3317601/ (accessed 14 September 2013).

[79] Berenguer M, Lopez-Labrador FX, Wright TL. Hepatitis C and liver transplantation. J Hepatol. 2001;35:666–78. http://www.sciencedirect.com/science/article/pii/S221074011100146X (accessed 20 September 2013).

[80] Thomson BJ, Finch RG. Hepatitis C virus infection. Clin Microbiol Infect. 2005;11:86–94. http://onlinelibrary.wiley.com/doi/10.1111/j.1469-0691.2004.01061.x/abstract (accessed 20 October 2013).

[81] Trepo C, Vierling J, Zeytin FN, Gerlich WH. The First Flaviviridae Symposium. Intervirol. 1997;40:279–88. http://www.ncbi.nlm.nih.gov/pubmed/9612731 (accessed 10 September 2013).

[82] Villano SA, Vlahov D, Nelson KE, Cohn S, Thomas DL. Persistence of viremia and the importance of long-term follow-up after acute hepatitis C infection. Hepatology. 1999;29:908-914. http://www.ncbi.nlm.nih.gov/pubmed/10051497 (accessed 13 September 2013).

[83] Thomas DL, Seef LB. Natural history of hepatitis C. Clin Liver Dis 2005;9:383– 398. http://dx.doi.org/10.1016/j.cld.2005.05.003

[84] Goodman ZD, Ishak KG. Histopathology of hepatitis C virus infection. Semin Liver Dis 1995;15: 70 – 81. DOI: 10.1055/s-2007-1007264.

[85] NIH Consensus Statement On Management Of Hepatitis C, NIH Consens State Sci Statements 2002;19:1–46.

[86] Freeman AJ, Dore GJ, Law MG, et al. Estimating progression to cirrhosis in chronic hepatitis C virus infection. Hepatology 2001;34:809-816. DOI: 10/S0270-9139(01)33319-0.

[87] Kobayashi M, Tanaka E, Sodeyama T, Urushihara A, Matsumoto A, Kiyosawa K. The natural course of chronic hepatitis C: a comparison between patients with genotypes 1 and 2 hepatitis C viruses. Hepatology 1996;23:695–699. DOI: 10/S0270-9139(96)00112-7.

[88] Mallat A, Hezode C, Lotersztajn S. Environmental factors as disease accelerators during chronic hepatitis C. J Hepatol 2008;48:657–665. http://www.journal-of-hepatology.eu/article/S0168-8278(08)00049-4/abstract (accessed 14 October 2013).

[89] Poynard T, Bedossa P, Opolon P. Natural History Of Liver Fibrosis Progression In Patients With Chronic Hepatitis C. The Obsvirc, Metavir, Clinivir, and Dosvirc groups. Lancet. 1997;349:825-832. doi:10.1016/S0140-6736(96)07642-8.

[90] Aikawa T, Kojima M, Onishi H, Tamura R, Fukuda S, Suzuki T, Tsuda F, Okamoto H, Miyakawa Y. & other authors. HLA DRB1 and DQB1 alleles and haplotypes influencing the progression of hepatitis C. J Med Virol. 1996;49,274–278.

[91] Hohler T, Gerken G, Notghi A, Knolle P, Lubjuhn R, Taheri H, Schneider P. M., Meyer zum Buschenfelde KH & Rittner C. MHC class II genes influence the susceptibility to chronic active hepatitis C. J Hepatol. 1997;27,259–264. http://www.journal-of-hepatology.eu/article/S0168-8278(97)80169-9/abstract (accessed 29 September 2013).

[92] Alric, M. Fort, J. Izopet et al. Genes of the major histocompatibility complex class II influence the outcome of hepatitis C virus infection. Gastroenterology. 1997;113:1675–1681. http://www.gastrojournal.org/article/S0016-5085(97)00536-2/abstract?referrer=http://www.ncbi.nlm.nih.gov/pubmed/9352872 (accessed 10 September 2013).

[93] Kuzushita N, Hayashi N, Moribe T,Katayama K, Kanto T, Nakatani S, Kaneshige K, Tatsumi T, Ito A, Mochizuki K, Sasaki Y, Kasahara A, Hori M. Influence of HLA haplotypes on the clinical courses of individuals infected with hepatitis C virus. Hepatol. 1998;27:240–244. DOI: 10/S0270913998000354.

[94] Alric L, Izopet J, Fort M, Vinel JP, Fontenelle P, Orfila C, Payen JL, Sandres K, Desmorat H, Charlet JP, Duffaut M, Abbal M. Study of the association between major histocompatibility complex class II genes and the response to interferon alpha in patients with chronic hepatitis C infection. Hum Immunol. 1999;60:516-23. http://dx.doi.org/10.1016/S0198-8859(99)00021-X (accessed 10 September 2013).

[95] Asti M, Martinetti M, Zavaglia C, Cuccia MC, Gusberti L, Tinelli C, Cividini A, Bruno S, Salvaneschi L, Ideo G, Mondelli MU, Silini ME. Human leukocyte antigen class II and III alleles and severity of Hepatitis C Virus-Related chronic liver disease. Hepatol. 1999;1272–1279. DOI: 10/S0270913999001937.

[96] Renou C, Halfon P, Pol S, et al. Histological Features And HLA Class II Alleles In Hepatitis C Virus Chronically Infected Patients With Persistently Normal Alanine Aminotransferase Levels. Gut. 2002;51:585–590. http://www.ncbi.nlm.nih.gov/pmc/articles/PMC1773404/ (accessed 10 September 2013).

[97] Thursz M, Yallop R, Goldin R et al. Influence of MHC class II genotype on outcome of infection with hepatitis C virus. Lancet 1999; 354: 2119–2124.

[98] Fanning LJ, Levis J, Kenny-Walsh E, Wynne F, Whelton M, Shanahan F. 2000. Viral Clearance In Hepatitis C (1b) Infection: Relationship With Human Leukocyte Antigen Class II In a Homogeneous Population. Hepatol 31:1334–1337.

[99] Vejbaesya S, Songsivilai S, Tanwandee T, Rachaibun S, Chantangpol R, Dharakul T. HLA association with hepatitis C virus infection. Hum Immunol 2000; 61: 348-353.

[100] Harcourt G, Hellier S, Bunce M, Satsangi J, Collier J, Chapman R, Phillips R & Klenerman P. Effect of HLA Class II genotype on T Helper lymphocyte responses and

viral control in Hepatitis C virus infection. J Viral Hepatitis. 2001;8,174-9. DOI: 10.1046/j.1365-2893.2001.00289.x. (accessed 22 October 2013).

[101] Thio CL, Thomas DL, Goedert JL, et al. Racial differences in HLA class II associations with hepatitis C virus outcomes. J Infect Dis 2001; 184: 16-21. http://jid.oxfordjournals.org/content/184/1/16.long (accessed 22 October 2013).

[102] Kryczka W, Brojer E, Kalinska A, et al. DRB1 alleles in relation to severity of liver disease in patients with chronic hepatitis C. Med Sci Monit 2001;7(Suppl 1):217–220.

[103] Hue S, Cacoub P, Renou C, et al. Human leukocyte antigen class ii alleles may contribute to the severity of hepatitis C virus–related liver disease. J Infect Dis. 2002;186:106–9. http://jid.oxfordjournals.org/content/186/1/106.long (accessed 15 September 2013).

[104] Yenigun A, Belma Durupinar. Decreased frequency of the HLA-DRB1*11 allele in patients with chronic hepatitis C virus infection. J Virol. 2002;76:1787–9. http://www.ncbi.nlm.nih.gov/pmc/articles/PMC135873/ (accessed 23 September 2013).

[105] Renou C, Halfon P, Pol S, et al. Histological Features And HLA Class II Alleles In Hepatitis C Virus Chronically Infected Patients With Persistently Normal Alanine Aminotransferase Levels. Gut. 2002;51:585–90. http://www.ncbi.nlm.nih.gov/pmc/articles/PMC1773404/ (accessed 10 September 2013).

[106] Scotto G, Fazio V, D'Allessandro G, et al. Association between HLA class II antigens and hepatitis C virus infection. J Biol Regul Homeost Agents 2003;17(4):316–321.

[107] Yoshizawa K, Ota M, Saito S, et al. Long-term follow-up of hepatitis C virus infection: HLA class II loci influences the natural history of the disease. Tissue Antigens 2003;61(2):159–165.

[108] Yu ML, Dai CY, Chen SC, Chiu CC, Lee LP, Lin ZY, Hsieh MY, Wang LY, Chuang WL & Chang WY. Human leukocyte antigen class I and II alleles and response to interferon-alpha treatment, in Taiwanese patients with chronic hepatitis C virus infection. J Infect Dis. 2003;188:62-5. http://jid.oxfordjournals.org/content/188/1/62.long (accessed 13 September 2013).

[109] Mckiernan SM, Hagan R, Curry M, MCDonald JSA, Nolan N, Crowley J, Hegarty J, Lawlor E, Kelleher, D. The MHC is a major determinant of viral status, but not fibrotic stage, in individuals infected with Hepatitis C. Gastroenterology. 2000; 118:1124-1130.

[110] Jiao J, & Wang JB. Hepatitis C virus genotypes, HLADRB alleles and their response to interferon-alfa and ribavirin in patients with chronic hepatitis C. Hepatobiliary and Pancreatic Diseases International. 2005; 4:80-83.

[111] Yoon SK, Han JY, Pyo C-W, et al. Association between human leukocytes antigen alleles and chronic hepatitis C virus infection in the Korean population. Liver Int. 2005;25:1122–7. DOI: 10.1111/j.1478-3231.2005.01105.x.

[112] Wang LY, Lin HH, Lee TD, Wu YF, Hu CT, Cheng ML, Lo SY. Human leukocyte antigen phenotypes and hepatitis C viral load. J Clin Virol 2005; 32: 144-150.

[113] Ksiaa L, Ayed-Jendoubi S, Sfar I, Gorgi Y, Najjar HAT, Abdallah TB, Ayed K. Viral Immunology. June 2007, 20(2): 312-9. doi:10.1089/vim.2006.0060.

[114] Cursino-Santos JR, Donadi EA, Martinelli AL, Louzada-Junior P, Martinez-Rossi NM. Evolution of hepatitis C virus infection under host factor influence in an ethnically complex population. Liver Int. 2007;27(10):1371-8. http://onlinelibrary.wiley.com/doi/10.1111/j.1478-3231.2007.01600.x/abstract (accessed 10September 2013).

[115] Harris RA, Sugimoto K, Kaplan DE, Ikeda F, Kamoun F, Chang KM. Human leukocyte antigen class II associations with hepatitis c virus clearance and virus-specific CD4 T cell response among caucasians and african americans. Hepatology. 2008;48:70-9. http://www.ncbi.nlm.nih.gov/pmc/articles/PMC2749605/ (accessed 12 September 2013).

[116] El-Chennawi FA, Auf FA, Metwally SS, Mosaad YM, El-Wahab MA, Tawhid ZE. HLA-Class II Alleles in Egyptian Patients with Hepatocellular Carcinoma Immunological Investigations, 2008 37:661–74. doi:10.1080/08820130802111605(accessed 12 September 2013).

[117] Corghi DB, Gonc¸ales NSL, Marques SBD, Junior FLG. Distribution of the human leukocyte antigen class II alleles in brazilian patients with chronic hepatitis C virus infection. Braz J Med Biol Res 2008;41:884–889.

[118] De Almeida BS, Silva GMF, Silva PM, Perez RM, Figueiredo FAF,Porto LC. Ethnicity and route of HCV infection can influence the associations of HLA with viral clearance in an ethnically heterogeneous population Journal of Viral Hepatitis, 2011, 18, 692–9 doi:10.1111/j.1365-2893.2010.01429.x. (accessed 12 September 2013).

[119] Cangussu LOF,Teixeira R,Campos EF, Rampim GF, Mingoti SA, Martins-Filho OAM. Gerbase-DeLima. HLA Class II Alleles and Chronic Hepatitis C Virus Infection Clinical Immunology.282-7 doi: 10.1111/j.1365-3083.2011.02568.x

[120] De Rueda PM, Lo pez-Nevot MA, Saenz-Lopez P, Casado J, Martın-casares A, Palomares P. et al. Importance of host genetic factors HLA and IL28B as predictors of response to pegylates interferon and ribavirin. American Journal of Gastroenterology. 2011;106:1246-54. http://www.nature.com/ajg/journal/v106/n7/full/ajg201182a.html (accessed 23 September 2013).

[121] Marangon AV, Silva GF, de Moraes CF, Grotto RM, Pardini MI, de Pauli DS, Visentainer JE, Sell AM, Moliterno RA. Protective effect of HLA-DRB1 11 and predisposition of HLA-C 04 in the development of severe liver damage in Brazilian patients with chronic hepatitis C virus infection. Scand J Immunol. 2012;76:440-7. http://onlinelibrary.wiley.com/doi/10.1111/j.1365-3083.2012.02755.x/abstract (accessed 22 September 2013).

[122] Ali L, Mansoor A, Ahmad N, Siddiqi S, Mazhar K, Muazzam AG, Qamar R, KhanKM. Patient HLA-DRB1* and -DQB1* allele and haplotype association with hepatitis C virus persistence and clearance. J Gen Virol. 2010;91:1931-8. http://vir.sgmjournals.org/content/91/8/1931.long (accessed 12 October 2013).

[123] Shaker O, Bassiony H, Raziky ME, El-Kamary SS, Esmat G, El-Ghor S, Mohamed MM. Human Leukocyte Antigen Class II Alleles (DQB1 and DRB1) as Predictors for Response to InterferonTherapy in HCV Genotype 4 Hindawi Publishing Corporation Mediators of Inflammation. 2013, Article ID 392746, 10 pageshttp://dx.doi.org/10.1155/2013/392746.

[124] Yee LJ. Host genetic determinants in Hepatitis C virus infection. Genes Immun. 2004; 5, 237-45. http://www.nature.com/gene/journal/v5/n4/full/6364090a.html (accessed 23 September 2013).

[125] Tillmann HL, Chen D-F, Trautwein C, Kliem V, Grundey A, Berning-Haag A, Boker K, Kubicka S, Pastucha L, Stangel W, & Manns M. Low frequency of HLA-DRB1*11 in hepatitis C virus induced end stage liver disease. Gut. 2001;48,714-8 http://www.ncbi.nlm.nih.gov/pmc/articles/PMC1728277/ (accessed 15 September 2013).

[126] Hong X, Yu RB, Sun NX, Wang B, Xu YC, Wu GL. Human leukocyte antigen class II DQB1*0301, DRB1*1101 alleles and spontaneous clearance of hepatitis C virus infection: a meta-analysis. World J Gastroenterol. 2005;11:7302-7. http://www.wjgnet.com/1007-9327/full/v11/i46/7302.htm (accessed 12 September 2013).

[127] Patel K, Norris S, Lebeck L, et al. HLA class I allelic diversity and progression of fibrosis in patients with chronic hepatitis C. Hepatology. 2006;2:241-6. http://onlinelibrary.wiley.com/doi/10.1002/hep.21040/abstract (accessed 10 September 2013).

[128] López-Vázquez A, Rodrigo L, Mina-Blanco A, et al. Extended human leukocyte antigen haplotype EH18.1 influences progression to hepatocellular carcinoma in patients with hepatitis C virus infection. J Infect Dis. 2004;189:957–63. http://jid.oxfordjournals.org/content/189/6/957.long (accessed 12 September 2013).

[129] Ivić I, Bradarić N, Puizina-Ivić N, Ledina D, Lukšić B, & Martinić R. Hla-Cw7 Allele as Predictor of favorable therapeutic response to Interferon-α in Patients with Chronic Hepatitis C. Croat Med J. 2007;48:807-13. http://www.ncbi.nlm.nih.gov/pmc/articles/PMC2213809/ (accessed 12 September 2013).

[130] Miyaguchi S, Saito H, Ebinuma H, Morizane T & Ishii H. Possible association between HLA antigens and the response to interferon in Japanese patients with chronic hepatitis C. Tissue Antigens. 1997; 49, 605-611.

[131] Dai C-Y, Chuang W-L, Hsieh M-Y, Huang JF, Lin Y-Y, Chu P-Y, Hou NJ, Lin ZY, Chen SC, Hsieh MY, Wang LY & Yu ML. Human leukocyte antigen alleles and the response to pegylated interferon/ribavirin therapy in chronic hepatitis C patients. Antiviral Res. 2010;85:396-402. http://www.sciencedirect.com/science/article/pii/S016635420900535X (accessed 16 September 2013).

[132] Rhodes SL, Erlich H, Im KA, Wang J, Li J, Bugawan T, Jeffers L, Tong X, Su X, Rosen HR, Yee LJ, Liang TJ, Yang H. Associations between the human MHC and sustained virologic response in the treatment of chronic hepatitis C virus infection. Genes Immun 2008; 9, 328-33. http://www.ncbi.nlm.nih.gov/pmc/articles/PMC2696808/ (accessed 12 September 2013).

[133] McMahon BJ.Chronic hepatitis B virus infection.Med Clin North Am. 2014;98(1): 39-54. doi: 10.1016/j.mcna.2013.08.004.(accessed 12 September 2013).

[134] Lai CL, Ratziu V, Yuen MF, Poynard T. Viral hepatitis B. Lancet 2003; 362: 2089-94.

[135] Tamori A, Kawada N. HLA class II associated with outcomes of hepatitis B and C infections. World J Gastroenterol. 2013;19:5395-401. http://www.ncbi.nlm.nih.gov/pmc/articles/PMC3761092/ (accessed 12 September 2013).

[136] Nishida N, Sawai H, Matsuura K, Sugiyama M, Ahn SH, Park JY, et al. Genome-wide association study confirming association of HLA-DP with protection against chronic hepatitis B and viral clearance in Japanese and Korean. PLoS One. 2012;7(6):e39175. doi: 10.1371/journal.pone.0039175 accessed 12 September 2013).

[137] Mbarek H, Ochi H, Urabe Y, Kumar V, Kubo M, Hosono N, Takahashi A, Kamatani Y, Miki D, Abe H, Tsunoda T, Kamatani N, Chayama K, Nakamura Y, Matsuda K. A genomewide association study of chronic hepatitis B identified novel risk locus in a Japanese population. Hum Mol Genet 2011; 20: 3884-92. http://hmg.oxfordjournals.org/content/20/19/3884.long (accessed 12 October 2013).

[138] Buchbinder SP, Katz MH, Hessol NA, O'Malley PM, Holmberg SD. Long-term HIV-1 infection without immunologic progression. AIDS. 1994;8:1123– 8. http://www.ncbi.nlm.nih.gov/pubmed/7986410 (accessed 12 September 2013).

[139] Kaslow RA, Carrington M, Apple R, Park L, Munoz A, Saah AJ, et al. Influence of combinations of human major histocompatibility complex genes on the course of HIV-1 infection. Nat. Med. 1996;2:405–411.

[140] Tang J, Cormier E, Gilmour J, Price MA, Prentice HA, Song W, Kamali A, Karita E, Lakhi S, Sanders EJ, Anzala O, Amornkul PN, Allen S, Hunter E, Kaslow RA. Human leukocyte antigen variants B*44 and B*57 are consistently favorable during two distinct phases of primary HIV-1 infection in sub-Saharan Africans with several viral subtypes. J.Virol. 2011;85:8894–902. http://www.ncbi.nlm.nih.gov/pmc/articles/PMC3165830/ (accessed 12 September 2013).

[141] Zhang W, Wang L, Hong K, Liu Y, Su B, Xu C, Xu J, Ruan Y, Shao Y, Zheng D. Frequency of HLA-A*03 associates with HIV-1 infection in a Chinese cohort. Sci China Life Sci. 2013.1404-9. http://link.springer.com/article/10.1007%2Fs11427-013-4555-4 (accessed 21 September 2013).

[142] Lazaryan A, Song W, Lobashevsky E, Tang J, Shrestha S, Zhang K, McNicholl JM, Gardner LI, Wilson CM, Klein RS, Rompalo A, Mayer K, Sobel J, Kaslow RA. The influence of human leukocyte antigen class I alleles and their population frequencies

on human immunodeficiency virus type 1 control among African Americans. Hum. Immunol. 2011;72:312–8. http://www.ncbi.nlm.nih.gov/pmc/articles/PMC3778654/ (accessed 20 September 2013).

[143] Pereyra F, Jia X, McLaren PJ, Telenti A, de Bakker PI, Walker BD, Ripke S, Brumme CJ, Pulit SL, Carrington M, et al. International HIV Controllers Study. The major genetic determinants of HIV-1 control affect HLA class I peptide presentation. Science. 2010;330:1551–7. http://www.ncbi.nlm.nih.gov/pmc/articles/PMC3235490/ (accessed 10 September 2013).

[144] Honeyborne I, Prendergast A, Pereyra F, Leslie A, Crawford H, Payne R, Reddy S, Bishop K, Moodley E, Nair K, et al. Control of human immunodeficiency virus type 1 is associated with HLA-B*13 and targeting of multiple gag-specific CD8+ T-cell epitopes. J. Virol. 2007;81:3667–3672. http://www.ncbi.nlm.nih.gov/pmc/articles/PMC1866034/ (accessed 10 September 2013).

[145] Fellay J, Ge D, Shianna KV, Colombo S, Ledergerber B, Cirulli ET, Urban TJ, Zhang K, Gumbs CE, Smith JP, et al; NIAID Center for HIV/AIDS Vaccine Immunology (CHAVI). Common genetic variation and the control of HIV-1 in humans. PLoS Genet. 2009;5:e1000791. http://www.ncbi.nlm.nih.gov/pmc/articles/PMC2791220/ (accessed 10 September 2013).

[146] Kiepiela P, Leslie AJ, Honeyborne I, Ramduth D, Thobakgale C, Chetty S, Rathnavalu P, Moore C, Pfafferott KJ, Hilton L, et al. Dominant influence of HLA-B in mediating the potential co-volution of HIV and HLA. Nature. 2004;432:769–75. http://www.nature.com/nature/journal/v432/n7018/full/nature03113.html (accessed 10 September 2013).

[147] Lazaryan A, Lobashevsky E, Mulenga J, Karita E, Allen S, Tang J, and Kaslow RA. Human leukocyte antigen B58 supertype and human immunodeficiency virus type 1 infection in native Africans. J. Virol. 2006;80:6056–60. http://www.ncbi.nlm.nih.gov/pmc/articles/PMC1472610/ (Accessed 01 October 2013).

[148] Carlson JM, Listgarten J, Pfeifer N, Tan V, Kadie C, Walker BD, Ndung'u T, Shapiro R, Frater J, Brumme ZL, et al.. Widespread impact of HLA restriction on immune control and escape pathways of HIV-1. J. Virol. 2012;86:5230–43. http://www.ncbi.nlm.nih.gov/pmc/articles/PMC3347390/ (accessed 20 October 2013).

[149] Migueles SA, Sabbaghian MS, Shupert WL, Bettinotti MP, Marincola FM, Martino L, Hallahan CW, Selig SM, Schwartz D, Sullivan J, and Connors M. HLA B*5701 is highly associated with restriction of virus replication in a subgroup of HIV-infected long term nonprogressors. Proc. Natl. Acad. Sci. 2000;97:2709–14. http://www.ncbi.nlm.nih.gov/pmc/articles/PMC15994/ (accessed 14 September 2013).

[150] O'Brien SJ, Gao X, and Carrington M. HLA and AIDS: a cautionary tale. Trends Mol.Med. 2001;7: 379–81. doi:10.1016/S1471-4914(01)02131-1.

[151] Leslie A, Matthews PC, Listgarten J, Carlson JM, Kadie C, Ndung'u T, Brander C, Coovadia H, Walker BD, Heckerman D, and Goulder, PJ. Additive contribution of

HLA class I alleles in the immune control of HIV-1 infection. J. Virol. 2010;84:9879–88. http://www.ncbi.nlm.nih.gov/pmc/articles/PMC2937780/ (accessed 20 September 2013).

[152] Lécuroux C, Sáez-Cirión A, Girault I, Versmisse P, Boufassa F, Avettand-Fenoël V, Rouzioux C, Meyer L, Pancino G, Lambotte O, Sinet M, Venet A. Both HLA-B*57 and plasma HIV RNA levels 1 contribute to the HIV-specific CD8+T cell response in HIV controllers. J. Virol. 2013; doi:10.1128/JVI.02098-13.

[153] Gao X, Nelson GW, Karacki P, Martin MP, Phair J, Kaslow R, Goedert, J.J., Buchbinder, S., Hoots, K., Vlahov, D, et al. Effect of a single amino acid change in MHC class I molecules on the rate of progression to AIDS. N.Engl. J. Med. 2001;344:1668–75. http://www.nejm.org/doi/full/10.1056/NEJM200105313442203 (accessed 10 October2013).

[154] Honeyborne I, Codoner FM, Leslie A et al. HLA-Cw*03-restricted CD8+ T-cell responses targeting the HIV-1 gag major homology region drive virus immune escape and fitness constraints compensated for by intracodon variation. J Virol. 2010;84:11279–88. http://www.ncbi.nlm.nih.gov/pmc/articles/PMC2953179/ (accessed 20 September 2013).

[155] Honda K, Zheng N, Murakoshi H et al. Selection of escape mutant by HLC-C-restricted HIV-1 Pol-specific cytotoxic T lymphocytes carrying strong ability to suppress HIV-1 replication. Eur J Immunol. 2011;41:97–106. DOI: 10.1002/eji.201040841.

[156] Marangon AV, Guelsin GAS, Visentainer JEL, Borelli SD, Watanabe MAE, Consolaro MEL, KRC Ferracioli, Rudnick CCC and Sell AM. The Association of the Immune Response Genes to Human Papillomavirus-Related Cervical Disease in a Brazilian Population. Biomed Res Int. 2013;2013:1-11. http://www.ncbi.nlm.nih.gov/pmc/articles/PMC3722781/ (accessed 23 September 2013).

[157] Silva SB, Granados J, Gorodezky C, Aláez C, Aguilar HF, Flores RMC, González GG,LDV Chapa, Casas JM, Guerrero JFG and Saldaña HAB. HLA-DRB1 Class II antigen level alleles are associated with persistent HPV infection in Mexican women; a pilot study. Infectious Agents and Cancer. 2013;8:31. http://www.ncbi.nlm.nih.gov/pmc/articles/PMC3766142/ (accessed 30 September 2013).

[158] Peng S, Trimble C, Wu L, Pardoll D, Roden R, Hung CF, Wu TC. HLA-DQB1*02-restricted HPV-16 E7 peptide-specific CD4+ T-cell immune responses correlate with regression of HPV-16-associated high-grade squamous intraepithelial lesions. Clin Cancer Res 2007, 13(8):2479–87, Wank R, Thomssen C: High risk of squamous cell carcinoma of the cervix for women with HLA-DQw3. Nature. 1991;352:723–5. http://www.ncbi.nlm.nih.gov/pmc/articles/PMC3181117/ (accessed 10 September 2013).

[159] Apple RJ, Becker TM, Wheeler CM, Erlich HA. Comparison of human leukocyte antigen DR-DQ disease associations found with cervical dysplasia and invasive cervical

carcinoma. J Natl Cancer Inst. 1995;87:427–36. http://jnci.oxfordjournals.org/content/87/6/427.long (Accessed 10 September 2013).

[160] Ferrera A, Olivo A, Alaez C, Melchers WJ, Gorodezky C. HLA DOA1 and DOB1 loci in Honduran women with cervical dysplasia and invasive cervical carcinoma and their relationship to human papillomavirus infection. Hum Biol. 1999;71:367–379. http://digitalcommons.wayne.edu/humbiol/vol71/iss3/5/ (accessed 03 October 2013).

[161] Lin P, Koutsky LA, Critchlow CW, Apple RJ, Hawes SE, Hughes JP, Touré P, Dembele A, Kiviat NB. HLA class II DR-DQ and increased risk of cervical cancer among Senegalese women. Cancer Epidemiol Biomarkers Prev. 2001;10:1037–45. http://cebp.aacrjournals.org/content/10/10/1037.long (accessed 24 October 2013).

[162] Madeleine MM, Brumback B, Cushing-Haugen KL, Schwartz SM, Daling JR, Smith AG, Nelson JL, Porter P, Shera KA, McDougall JK, Galloway DA. Human leukocyte antigen class II and cervical cancer risk: a population-based study. J Infect Dis. 2002;186:1565–74. http://jid.oxfordjournals.org/content/186/11/1565.long (accessed 20 September 2013).

[163] Cuzick J, Terry G, Ho L, Monaghan J, Lopes A, Clarkson P, Duncan I. Association between high-risk HPV types, HLA DRB1* and DQB1* alleles and cervical cancer in British women. Br J Cancer. 2000;82:1348–52. http://www.ncbi.nlm.nih.gov/pmc/articles/PMC2374489/ (accessed 27 October 2013).

[164] Metcalfe S, Roger M, Faucher MC, Coutlée F, Franco EL, Brassard P. The association between human leukocyte antigen (HLA)-G polymorphisms and human papilloma virus (HPV) infection in Inuit women of northern Quebec. Hum Immunol. 2013;74(12):1610-1615.

[165] Song EY, Shin S, Park KU, Park MH, Sung MW, Kim KH, Kwon TK. Associations of HLA-DRB1 and -DQB1 alleles with severe recurrent respiratory papillomatosis in Korean patients. Hum Immunol. 2013;74:961-4. http://www.sciencedirect.com/science/article/pii/S0198885913001067 (accessed 23 September 2013).

[166] Zhao M, Qiu L, Tao N, Zhang L, Wu X, She Q, Zeng F, Wang Y, Wei S, Wu X. HLA DRB allele polymorphisms and risk of cervical cancer associated with human papillomavirus infection: a population study in China. Eur J Gynaecol Oncol. 2013;34:54-9.

[167] Macedo AM, Pena SDJ. Genetic Variability of Trypanosoma cruzi: implications for the pathogenesis of Chagas disease. Parasitol Today. 1998;14:119-124.

[168] Chagas C. Nova tripanozomiaze humana. Estudos sobre a morfologia e o ciclo evolutivo do Schizotrypanum cruzi n. gen., n. sp. Agente etiológico de uma nova entidade mórbida para o homem. Mem Inst Oswaldo Cruz. 1909;1:59-218. http://www.sciencedirect.com/science/article/pii/S0001706X05002500 (accessed 25 October 2013).

[169] Köberle F. 50 Years of Chagas' disease. Munch Med Wochenschr 1957;99 1193-1198.

[170] Moncayo A, Ortiz Yanine MI. An update Chagas disease (human American trypanosomiasais). Ann Trop Med Parasitol. 2006;100:663-677. http://dx.doi.org/10.1179/136485906X112248.

[171] Coura JR. Chagas disease: what is known and what is needed - a background article.Mem Inst Oswaldo Cruz 2007;102:113-122. http://dx.doi.org/10.1590/S0074-02762007000900018.

[172] Silva LJ. A evolução da doença de Chagas no Estado de São Paulo. São Paulo: Editora Hucitec; 1999. http://dx.doi.org/10.1590/S0102-311X2003000400019.

[173] Dutra WO, Gollob KJ. Current concepts in immunoregulation and pathology of human Chagas disease. Curr Opin Infec Dis. 2008;21:287-292. http://www.ncbi.nlm.nih.gov/pmc/articles/PMC3322114/ (accessed 23 September 2013).

[174] Barrett MP, Burchmore RJ, Stich A, et al. The trypanosomiases Lancet 2003;362:1469-480. doi:10.1016/S0140-6736(03)14694-6.

[175] Brener Z. Pathogenesis and immunopathology of chronic Chagas disease. Mem Inst Oswaldo Cruz 1987;82: 205-213.

[176] Moncayo A, Silveira AC. Current epidemiological trends for Chagas disease in Latin America and future challenges in epidemiology, surveillance and health policy. Mem Inst Oswaldo Cruz 2009;104:31-40. http://dx.doi.org/10.1590/S0074-02762009000900005.

[177] Coura JR, Vinãs PA. Chagas disease: a new worldwide challenge. Nature 2010;465:S6-S7. http://www.nature.com/nature/journal/v465/n7301_supp/full/nature09221.html (accessed 23 September 2013).

[178] Moolani Y, Bukhman G, Hotez PJ. Neglected Tropical Diseases as Hidden Causes of Cardiovascular Disease. PLoS Negl Trop Dis. 2012;6:e1499.

[179] Dias E, Laranja FS, Miranda A, et al. Chagas disease. A clinical, epidemiologic and pathologic study. Circulation 1956;14:1035-1060. http://www.ncbi.nlm.nih.gov/pmc/articles/PMC3383757/ (accessed 20 October 2013).

[180] Dutra WO, Martins-Filho OA, Cançado JR. Activated T and B lymphocytes in peripheral blood of patients with Chagas disease. Int Immunol. 1994;6:499-506.

[181] Dutra WO, Martins-Filho OA, Cançado JR. et al. Chagasic patients lack CD28 expression on many of their circulating T lymphocytes. Scand J Immunol. 1996;43:88-93.

[182] Tarleton RL. Trypanosoma cruzi- induced suppression of IL-12 production. II. Evidence for a role for suppressor cells. J Immunol. 1988;140:2769-2773. http://www.jimmunol.org/content/140/8/2769.long (accessed 10 September 2013).

[183] Tarleton RL, Grusky MJ, Postan M, et al. Trypanosoma cruzi infection in MHC-deficient mice: further evidence for the role of both class I- and class II-restricted T cells

in immune resistance and disease. Int Immunol. 1996;8:13-22. http://intimm.oxfordjournals.org/content/8/1/13.long (accessed 10 October 2013).

[184] Clark RK, Kuhn RE. Trypanosoma cruzi does not induce apoptosis in murine fibroblasts. Parasitology. 1999;118:167–75.

[185] Corrêa-Oliveira R, Gomes JAS, Lemos EM, et al. The Role of the Immune Response on the Development of Severe Clinical Forms of Human Chagas Disease. Mem Inst Oswaldo Cruz. 1999; 94:253-255. http://dx.doi.org/10.1590/S0074-02761999000700042.

[186] Dutra WO, Colley DG, Pinto-Dias JC, et al. Self and nonself stimulatory molecules induce preferential expansion of CD5C B cells or activated T cells chagasic patients, respectively. Scand J Immunol. 2000;51:91–97. http://onlinelibrary.wiley.com/doi/10.1046/j.1365-3083.2000.00648.x/abstract (accessed 20 September 2013).

[187] d'Avila Reis D, Lemos EM, Silva GC, et al. Phenotypic characterization of the inflammatory cells in chagasic megaoesophagus. Trans R Soc Trop Med Hyg. 2001;95:177–178.

[188] Cardoso GM, Morato MJ, Gomes JA. Comparative analysis of cell phenotypes in different severe clinical forms of Chagas' disease. Front Biosci. 2006;11:1158–1163.http://www.bioscience.org/2006/v11/af/1870/fulltext.htm (accessed 13 September 2013).

[189] da Silveira AB, Adad SJ, Correa-Oliveira R, et al. Morphometric study of eosinophils, mast cells, macrophages and fibrosis in the colon of chronic chagasic patients with and without megacolon. Parasitology 2007;134:789-796. DOI: http://dx.doi.org/10.1017/S0031182007002296.

[190] Mack DG, Jonhson JJ, Roberts F, et al. HLA-classe II genes modify outcome of Toxoplasma gondii infection. Int J Parasitol. 1999;29:1351-1358. http://www.sciencedirect.com/science/article/pii/S0020751999001526 (accessed 20 September 2013).

[191] Acquatella H, Catalioti F, Gómez JR, et al. Asociación entre HLA-DB9 y Enfermedad de Chagas. In Rodríguez-Lemoine V, editor. Genética: VI Congreso Latinoamericano de Genética. Venezuela: Ars. Gráfica S.A; 1984

[192] Fernandez-Mestre MT, Layrisse Z, Montagnani S, et al. Influence of the HLA class II polymorphism in chronic Chagas' disease. Parasite Immunol. 1998;20:197-203.

[193] Deghaide NH, Dantas RO, Donadi EA. HLA Class I and II Profiles of Patients Presenting with Chagas' Disease. Dig Dis Sci. 1998;43:246-252.

[194] Dalalio MMO, Visentainer JEL, Moliterno RA, et al. Association of HLA-DR2 with chronic Chagasic cardiopathy in a population at Paraná Northeast region, Brazil. Acta Scientiarum. 2002;24:727-730.

[195] Cruz-Robles D, Reyes PA, Monteón-Padilla VM, et al. MHC Class I and Class II Genes in Mexican Patients With Chagas Disease. Hum Immunol. 2004;65:60–65.

http://www.sciencedirect.com/science/article/pii/S0198885903006360 (accessed 23 October 2013).

[196] García Borrás S, Diez C, Cotorruelo C, et al. HLA class II DRB1 polymorphism in Argentinians undergoing chronic Trypanosoma cruzi infection. Ann Clin Biochem. 2006;43:214-216. http://acb.sagepub.com/content/43/3/214.long (accessed 03 October 2013).

[197] García-Borrás S, Racca L, Cotorruelo C, et al. Distribution of HLA-DRB1 alleles in Argentinean patients with Chagas' disease cardiomyopathy. Imunol Invest. 2009;38:268-275.

[198] Nieto A, Beraún Y, Collado MD, et al. HLA haplotypes are associated with differential susceptibility to Trypanosoma cruzi infection. Tissue Antigens. 2000;55:195-198. http://onlinelibrary.wiley.com/doi/10.1034/j.1399-0039.2000.550301.x/abstract (accessed 20 September 2013).

[199] del Puerto F, Nishizawa JE, Kikuchi M, et al. Protective Human Leucocyte Antigen Haplotype, HLA-DRB1*01-B*14, against Chronic Chagas Disease in Bolivia PLoS Negl Trop Dis. 2012;6:e1587. http://www.ncbi.nlm.nih.gov/pmc/articles/PMC3308929/ (accessed 20 October 2013).

[200] Llop E, Rothhammer F, Acuña M, et al. HLA antigens in cardiomyopathic Chilean chagasics. Am J Hum Genet.1988;43:770-773. http://www.ncbi.nlm.nih.gov/pmc/articles/PMC1715553/ (accessed 04 October 2013).

[201] Llop E, Rothhammer F, Acuña M, et al. HLA antigens in Chagas cardiomyopathy:new evidence based on a case control study. Rev Med Chil. 1991;119:633-636.

[202] Layrisse Z, Fernandez MT, Montagnani S, et al. HLA-C(*)03 is a risk factor for cardiomyopathy in Chagas disease. Hum Immunol. 2000;61:925-92.

[203] Sierp GM, Albert ED. Analysis of the HLA data of the 5th Latin American Histocompatibility Workshop. In: Gorodezky C, Sierp G, Albert E (ed) Immunogenetics Laboratory. Munich; 1992.

[204] Colorado IA, Acquatella H, Catalioti F, et al. HLA class II DRB1, DQB1, DPB1 polymorphism and cardiomyopathy due to Trypanosoma cruzi chronic infection. Hum Immunol. 2000;61:320-325. http://www.sciencedirect.com/science/article/pii/S0198885999001779 (accessed 02 October 2013).

[205] Faé KC, Drigo SA, Cunha-Neto E, et al. HLA and beta-myosin heavy chain do not influence susceptibility to Chagas disease cardiomyopathy. Microbes Infect. 2000;2:745-751. http://www.sciencedirect.com/science/article/pii/S1286457900005013 (accessed 03 October 2013).

[206] Groh V, Steinle A, Bauer S, et al. Recognition of stress-induced MHC molecules by intestinal epithelial gammadelta T cells. Science 1998;279:1737–1740.

[207] Aida K, Juarez S, Kikuchi M, et al. HLA-B35 and MICA-A5 synergistically enhanced susceptibility to Chagas Heart disease. MHC 2000;7:63-70.

[208] Lima-Junior JC, Rodrigues-da-Silva RN, Banic DM, Jiang J, Singh B, Fabrício-Silva GM, Porto LC, Meyer EV, Moreno A, Rodrigues MM, Barnwell JW, Galinski MR, de Oliveira-Ferreira J. Influence of HLA-DRB1 and HLA-DQB1 alleles on IgG antibody response to the P. vivax MSP-1, MSP-3α and MSP-9 in individuals from Brazilian endemic area. PLoS One. 2012;7(5). http://www.ncbi.nlm.nih.gov/pmc/articles/PMC3359319/ (accessed 30 September 2013).

[209] Lulli P, Mangano VD, Onori A, Batini C, Luoni G, Sirima BS, Nebie I, Chessa L, Petrarca V, Modiano D. HLA-DRB1 and -DQB1 loci in three west African ethnic groups: genetic relationship with sub-Saharan African and European populations. Hum Immunol. 2009 Nov;70:903-9. http://www.sciencedirect.com/science/article/pii/S0198885909002006 (accessed 03 October 2013).

[210] Osafo-Addo AD, Koram KA, Oduro AR, Wilson M, Hodgson A, Rogers WO. HLA-DRB1*04 allele is associated with severe malaria in northern Ghana. Am J Trop Med Hyg. 2008 Feb;78:251-5. http://www.ajtmh.org/content/78/2/251.long (accessed 03 September 2013).

[211] Hananantachai H, Patarapotikul J, Ohashi J, Naka I, Looareesuwan S, Tokunaga K.Polymorphisms of the HLA-B and HLA-DRB1 genes in Thai malaria patients. Jpn J Infect Dis. 2005 Feb;58:25-8. http://www0.nih.go.jp/JJID/58/25.html (accessed 04 September 2013).

[212] Shankarkumar U, Devaraj JP, Ghosh K, Karnad D, Anand K, Mohanty D. HLA associations in P. falciparum malaria patients from Mumbai, western India. Indian J Malariol. 2002 Sep-Dec; 39:76-82.

Chapter 11

Association Between HLA Gene Polymorphism And The Genetic Susceptibility Of HIV Infection

Fang Yuan and Yongzhi Xi

Additional information is available at the end of the chapter

http://dx.doi.org/10.5772/57538

1. Introduction

Human leukocyte antigen (HLA) complex, which refers to a group of closely linked genes on the short arm of the sixth human chromosome, is considered the most polymorphic genetic marker that has so far been reported in the human. HLA plays a significant role in the immune response, particularly in antiviral immunity. Although HLA and genetic predisposition to various autoimmune diseases have been separately studied for the past 40 years, the evaluation of the correlation between the two was initiated only within the last 10 years. In recent years, research on HLA polymorphisms and susceptibility to various infectious diseases has attracted significant attention owing to the critical role of HLA in diseases such as SARS and hepatitis B. In particular, HLA polymorphism, HIV, and genetic predisposition to AIDS have emerged as research areas of immense clinical significance.

Human immunodeficiency virus (HIV) infection is able to perturb and alter gene expression through several mechanisms that can, lastly, cause acquired immunodeficiency syndrome (AIDS) Figure 1. Meanwhile, associations between disease parameters and the genetic makeup of the host and virus may be crucial in determining the outcome of HIV-1 infection.

According to Joint United Nations Programme on HIV/AIDS, there were approximately 40 million HIV-infected people worldwide at the end of 2004. Limiting the susceptibility to HIV, predicting the course of AIDS, and reversing it are some of the challenging tasks that need to be addressed urgently. Existing data demonstrates that the susceptibility to HIV differs among individuals, and significant differences exist in the disease progression in HIV-infected persons. In general, it takes less than 10 years from the time of HIV infection to the manifestation of typical AIDS symptoms. However, a small subset of HIV-infected people (0.8%) are

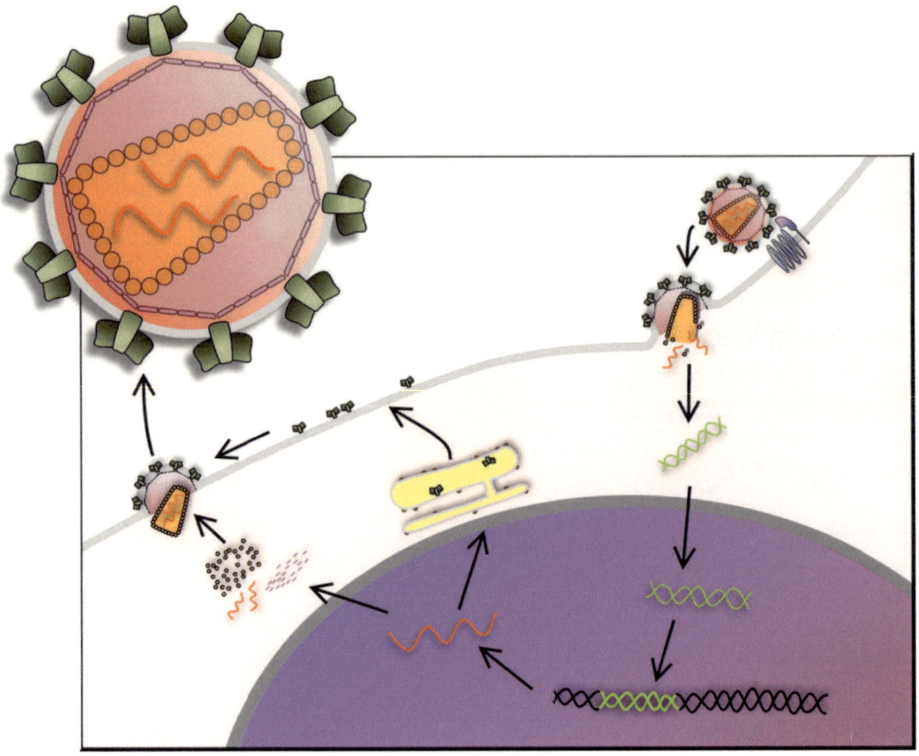

Figure 1. HIV virus is formed by a diploid single strand RNA genome enclosed in a truncated cone capsid with a phospholipidic bilayer envelope, containing the proteins that allow the virus entry into the cells. The HIV-1 infection is mediated by interaction between the proteins of the viral envelope, leukocyte receptor, and coreceptor. This interaction causes the membranes fusion and the uncoating of the virion core. The viral RNA is reverse transcribed in DNA which enters in the nucleus where the integrase enzyme catalyzes the insertion of the viral genome into the genome of the host cell. The expression of integrated viral genome is controlled by the RNA-binding proteins tat and rev. A set of RNAs are transported from the nucleus to the cytoplasm, where they can be translated or packaged. The new core proteins localize near the cell membrane, while the envelope mRNA is translated at the endoplasmic reticulum (ER) and subsequently the envelope proteins are placed on the cell membrane. Finally, the capsid proteins are assembled with the viral genomic RNA, and an immature virion begins to bud from cell surface.

asymptomatic for over 10 years. According to a number of studies, the HLA complex is considered as the most noteworthy genetic marker that is closely related to AIDS progression and highlights the differences in genetic susceptibility of HIV-infected individuals.

2. HLA polymorphism and genetic predisposition to HIV

1. Epidemiological survey: Worldwide epidemiological surveys indicate that there is a close relationship between HIV/AIDS and HLA. Although global research reports at different times have demonstrated the involvement of HLA in the differential susceptibility to HIV, the individual HLA locus has not been validated to correlate with HIV infection or AIDS progression. For example, some reports indicate a correlation between HIV susceptibility

and HLA-B*35 in ethnic groups of Han. However, findings of research on Caucasian individuals did not agree with this notion. HLA-B*07, found among people of African descent, is considered to correlate with the susceptibility to HIV, but the similar correlation has not been reported among people of other ethnic groups. Research on other ethnic groups indicates that HLA-B*18 and the HLA-A2 either influence HIV-1 infectivity or act as protective genes that inhibit the incidence of AIDS. The homozygous HLA-G 14-bp nsertion/deletion genotype is associated with higher viral load, lower CD4 cell count, and increased mortality compared with HLA-G 14-bp carriers.

Considering the limitation of the small population evaluated, polymorphisms outside the peptide binding region of the HLA class I molecule can play a key role in HIV progression through interaction with other immune-relevant receptors. Some results identify co-operative effects between HLA Class I alleles in the control of HIV-1 in an extended Southern African cohort, and underline complementarity and breadth of the CD8+ T cell targeting as one potential mechanism for this effect. HLA-A-restricted Gag-specific responses can impose selection pressure on HIV. Vaidya et al analyzed the associations between HLA-B alleles and HIV-1 viral replication during acute infection and VLSP in untreated subjects. The results show that the effect of HLA-B*57 on viral control is more pronounced during the later stages of primary HIV-1 infection, while HLA-B*97 is more broadly associated with HIV-1 viral load during primary infection. In HIC (HIV controllers, a unique group of infected individuals who are able to control HIV naturally), HLA-B*57 and the amount of ultrasensitive viral load seem to play a role in the HIV-specific CD8+ T cell responses. Some results provide support for the role of HLA-B*51-restricted CTLs and functional avidity in the control of early HIV-1 infection. HALS (HIV/Highly active antiretroviral therapy-associated lipodystrophy syndrome) is associated with combined low-expression TS (thymidylate synthase) and MTHFR (methylene-tetrahydrofolate reductase) associated with high activity polymorphisms but not with HLA-B*40:01 carriage in Caucasian patients with long-term exposure to stavudine. For details, see Table 1.

Richard et al characterized the differential cell surface expression levels of all common HLA-C allotypes and tested directly for effects of HLA-C expression on outcomes of HIV infection in 5243 individuals. They found that HIV peptides presented by higher expressed HLA-C alleles were more likely to elicit CTL responses than peptides presented by low expression HLA-C allotypes, such that higher HLA-C expression was correlated with increased likelihood of cytotoxic T lymphocyte responses and frequency of viral escape mutation. It is also pointed out that HLA-C and HLA-E collaborate to keep the HIV-1 virus at bay. HLA-C can present antigens to CTL, and it is able to inhibit NK cell lysis, but for some reason it is normally expressed on the cell surface at levels approximately 10-fold less than most HLA-A and HLA-B allotypes. The mechanisms that regulate HLA-C expression and the link between this molecule and HIV infection are not yet completely understood. Maybe a new miRNA targeting sequences identified on HLA-C gene and the low level of affinity between β2M and the HLA-C heavy chains can explain for this low level of expression.

Cohorts used in study	HLA locus or haplotype or supertype	
	Susceptible to HIV or AIDS FP	Non-susceptible to HIV or AIDS SP
Han Ethnicity	B*35	-
Zambian	A*02-Cw*16, A*23-B*14, A*23-Cw*07(FP)	B*57, B*39, A*30-Cw*03(SP)
European	A1-Cw7-B8-DR3, A24(FP)	-
Yi Ethnicity	B*07, B*35, B*46	B*55, B*44, B*78
Kenya	A*29, Cw*07, Cw*08 (HT)	B*18(LT)
Kenya	A*2301	A2/6802 supertype(LT)
Argentina	A*24, B*18, B*39	B*44, B*55
African-American	DQB1*0201	DQB1*0303
Caucasian	DQB1*0603, DRB1*04	DQB1*0303
European	A*29, B*22, DR*11(FP)	B*14, Cw*08(SP)
Caucasian	Heterozygous HLA locus, Type I	B*35, Cw*04
American	B*54, B*55, B*56	-
American	-	B*18(LT)
Male Caucasian Homosexuals	B*35	A2 supertype
Zimbabwean	HLA-G 14-bp insertion/deletion	
European-American	HLA-C low expression	HLA-C high expression

FP, fast progression; SP, slow progression; HT, high transmission; LT, low transmission

Table 1. HLA genes, haplotype, and supertype related to HIV-1 susceptibility and AIDS progression

2. *In vitro* study on HLA and HIV infection susceptibility: It is difficult to extrapolate the common characteristics from the results of epidemiological surveys owing to the abundance of inherent variation. Some researchers try to analyze HLA and HIV infection susceptibility by using *in vitro* approaches, and speculate the relationship between HLA polymorphism and HIV infection susceptibility or AIDS progression. *In vitro* studies can better control significant influencing factors such as the type, developmental stage and culturing conditions of cells, type of HIV strain, density of infection, and mechanisms, as well as minimize the variable factors that will have an effect on statistical findings. Second, *in vitro* experiments facilitate the consistent evaluation of critical factors as well as the application of uniform testing standards.

Jabri and his colleagues used two strains of HIV-1 and HIV-2 to infect peripheral blood cells with different HLA antigenic specificities, and reported that no single HLA antigen was capable of preventing both types of HIV infection. For example, HLA-B52 showed susceptibility to HIV-1 viral strains, whereas it was not susceptible to HIV-2 viral strains. HLA-B58 showed susceptibility to HIV-2 viral strains, but it was not susceptible to HIV-1 viral strains. HLA-B44 influenced the immune function only against certain HIV-1/2 strains. It is still therefore still ambiguous whether different HLA phenotypes influence the susceptibility to and *in vivo* effects of HIV infection, which needs to be verified by experiments with larger sample sizes.

HLA-G variant expression has a considerable impact on the control of HIV replication, an effect that seems to be mediated primarily by the protein specificity of CD4(+) T cell responses to HIV Gag and Nef. Numerous studies have been conducted, aimed at observing the expression of the molecule HLA-G in the early stage of infection by HIV and its progression. In 2004, Derrien and colleagues demonstrated that during HIV-1 infection the HLA-G1 isoform was down regulated by a Vpu dependent mechanism, which recognizes a double lysine residues in 4 and 5 positions of the C terminus. The HLA-G1 isoform has the major ability to present viral peptides to CD8+ T lymphocytes; therefore, the recognition of HIV-1 infected cells by CD8+ T lymphocytes could depend on the expression of HLA-G1.More results show that HLA-G Treg plays an important role for balancing by stander immune activation and anti-viral immune activity in HIV-1 infection and suggest that the loss of these cells during advanced HIV-1 infection may contribute to immune dysregulation and HIV-1 disease progression. The connection between miRNA, HLA-G expression, and HIV-1 also needs to be further explored because it can reveal novel information about HIV-1 control of the immune system.

3. Statistical analysis of the correlation between HLA gene polymorphism and HIV infection or AIDS susceptibility: Previously published research findings have been analyzed to evaluate the diversity in the correlation of HLA with HIV/AIDS susceptibility. Meta-analysis was anticipated to identify the common features. Research articles that satisfy the selection criteria were retrieved and the original data in the documents were processed and analyzed, wherein B35, B62, DR5, and DR11 were identified as genes that facilitate HIV-1 susceptibility and/or occurrence of AIDS, while A10, B18, B27, B5, and DR1 were identified as protective genes against HIV-1 infection and/or occurrence of AIDS. Since meta-analysis is an observational study, variations are likely to be introduced in each step of the analysis, and the results need to be validated by testing in laboratories with a large sample size.

3. Possible mechanisms that HLA influence HIV infection susceptibility or AIDS progression

1. Infection receptors: HIV combines with the CD4 molecule and other coreceptors to invade T cells during infection. HIV susceptibility is affected when the above-mentioned receptors have natural defects or mutations. So far, it has been verified that receptors of

chemotactic factors (CCR35 and CXCR4) are coreceptors for HIV-1. When HIV-1 infects target cells, the viruses that combine with CD4 molecules combine with coreceptors in order to enter the target cells. In high-risk populations with close contact to infected individuals but no infection, approximately one-third of the CCR5 alleles undergo deletion mutation; for instance, deletion of 32 bases of CCR5 genes (referred to as CCR5Δ32 mutation), which results in a natural immunity of the organism against HIV-1 infection at the gene level. The mutation and polymorphism changes of alleles not only influence the ability of HIV-1 to infect the target cells, but also change the onset and progression of AIDS. It is possible that HLA participates in HIV invading process through similar means, and affects AIDS progression. However, there are no validated reports on HLA's direct participation in HIV-1 infection by acting as the receptor, so far. Therefore, the susceptibility theory, which suggests that HLA acts as a receptor, needs to be subjected to further scientific scrutiny.

2. HLA molecules selection pressure: The antigen-binding groove of HLA molecules combine with a specific epitope of the HIV protein (For example, gap 120), inducing the generation of helper T cells and cytotoxic T cells. In particular, CD8+ cytotoxic T lymphocytes can kill infected $CD4^+$ T lymphocyte in a direct manner, which can influence virus replication, transmission, and AIDS progression. HLA molecules can employ different epitopes for the same molecule, and stimulate generation of CTLs featuring different quantities as well as specific properties, which has been confirmed in previous studies. Therefore, this can better explain the differences in AIDS progress when individuals with certain HLA phenotypes infected with HIV.

During viral infection, some viruses undergo degradation by cellular proteasome complex, and the cytosolic antigenic peptides are carried into the ER. In this organelle, the peptides are captured by HLA I molecules and then exposed on the cell surface, triggering the cytotoxic activity of the circulating CD8+ T lymphocytes, as described previously. The HIV has devised different ways to evade the immune response including a Nef-dependent mechanism that downregulates the HLA I expression, thus avoiding the recognition of the infected cells by CD8+ T lymphocytes (Fig2). Selectively, Nef alters the expression of HLA-A and -B by recognition of a sequence (Y320SQAASS) present on the cytoplasmic tail of these HLA molecules accelerating their endocytosis from the plasma membrane and blocking the transport of newly synthesized MHC class I molecules to the cell surface. Nef maintains the expression of HLA-C -G and -E unchanged, in order to inhibit the innate response of the natural killer cells (NK). Furthermore, the gp41 protein of the viral envelope upregulates the synthesis of IL-10 by monocytes; in turn, as mentioned before, this cytokine increases the expression of HLA-G molecules to control immune response and facilitate infection.

Meanwhile, under the influence of CTLs that are induced by HLA, mutation of HIV can occur. For example, TW10 peptide fragment (TAILQEQIAW) of gap protein in the HIV-1 virus, has a specific mutation on the residue 242 in the individuals with HLA-B57 or B58 and can revert to the wild type after the viruses detach from HLA-B57 or B58 molecules. This HIV mutation can cause functional loss of specific CTL, and enable HIV to adapt to the HLA environment

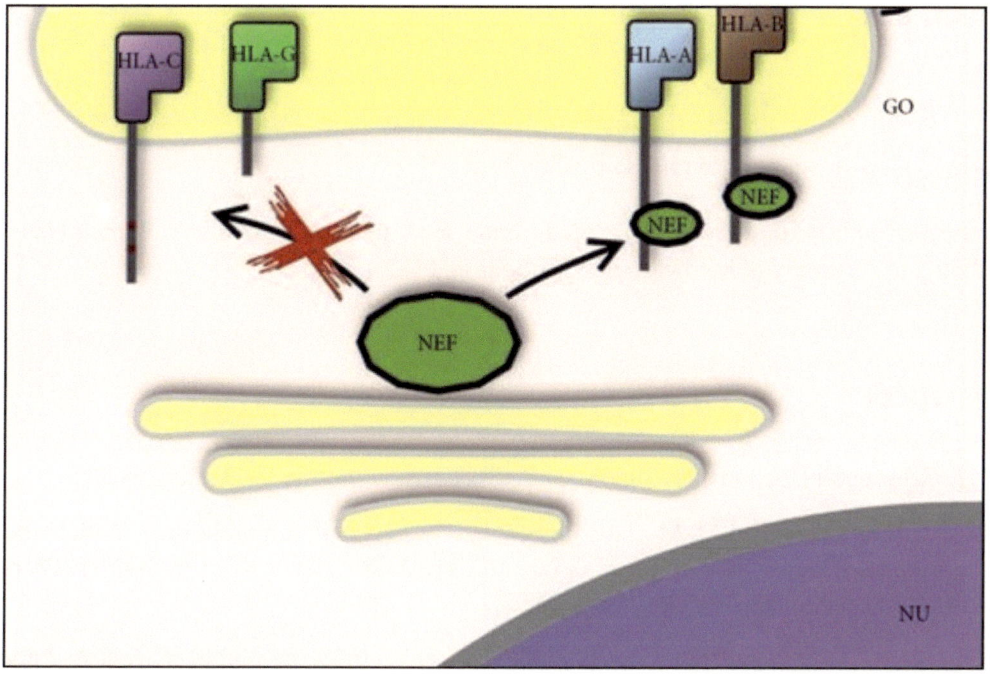

Figure 2. The HIV has devised different ways to evade the immune response, including a Nef-dependent mechanism that downregulates the HLA I expression, thus avoiding the recognition of the infected cells by CD8+ T lymphocytes. Selectively, Nef alters the expression of HLA-A and -B by recognition of a sequence (Y320SQAASS) present on the cytoplasmic tail of these HLA molecules accelerating their endocytosis from the plasma membrane and blocking the transport of newly synthesized MHC class I molecules to the cell surface. Nef maintains the expression of HLA-C, -G, and -E unchanged, in order to inhibit the innate response of the natural killer cells (NK). NU: nucleus; GO: golgi apparatu

and overcome the immune responses, resulting in HIV susceptibility of specific HLA types as well as a rapid progression of AIDS. Children of mothers with AIDS who have similar HLA genes are at a higher risk of being infected with HIV, and they tend to progress to AIDS in a shorter time. The possible reason for this is that the HIV of the mother might have adapted to the HLA environment in the host, and the virus replication increases when HLA similarity is high between the mother and child, which in turn makes it is easier for HIV to propagate and lead to a faster progression of AIDS. But sometimes specific mutation of HIV can also lead to a decrease in its virulence, enabling a reduced susceptibility of individuals towards HIV and a slower progression of AIDS.

Acknowledgements

Supported by grants from the State Key Development Program for Basic Research of China (No.2003CB515509 and 2009CB522401) and from National Natural Scientific Foundation of China(No.81070450 and 30470751) to Dr. X.-Y.Z.

Author details

Fang Yuan and Yongzhi Xi*

*Address all correspondence to: xiyz@yahoo.com

Department of Immunology and National Center for Biomedicine Analysis, Beijing Hospital Affiliated to Academy of Medical Sciences, Beijing, PRC

References

[1] Grimwood J. Schmutz J. Genomics: six is seventh. Nature, 2003, 425:775-776.

[2] Lefrere JJ, Mariotti M, Morand-Joubert L, et al. Plasma human immunodeficiency virus RNA below 40 Copies/ml is rare in untreated persons even in the first years of infection. J Infect Dis, 1999, 180: 526-529.

[3] Tang J, Tang S, Lobashevsky E, et al. Favorable and unfavorable HLA class I alleles and haplotypes in Zambians predominantly infected with clade C human immunodeficiency virus type 1. J Virol, 2002, 76: 8276-8284.

[4] Xu MY, Hong KX, Deng XL , et al. Association of HLA-B alleles with human immunodeficiency virus type 1 infection in the Yi ethnic group in Sichuan province. Biomed Environ Sci, 2004, 17: 203-208.

[5] MacDonald KS, Matukas L, Embree JE, et al. Human leucocyte antigen supertypes and immune susceptibility to HIV-1, implications for vaccine design. Immunol Lett, 2001, 79: 151-157.

[6] Roe DL, Lewis RE, Cruse JM. Association of HLA-DQ and -DR alleles with protection from or infection with HIV-1. Exp Mol Pathol, 2000, 68: 21-28.

[7] Carrington M, Nelson GW, Martin MP, et al. HLA and HIV-1: heterozygote advantage and B*35-Cw*04 disadvantage. Science, 1999, 283: 1748-1752.

[8] Dorak MT, Tang J, Tang S, et al. Influence of human leukocyte antigen-B22 alleles on the course of human immunodeficiency virus type 1 infection in 3 cohorts of white men. J Infect Dis, 2003, 188: 856-863.

[9] Farquhar C, Rowland-Jones S, Mbori-Ngacha D, et al. Human leukocyte antigen (HLA) B*18 and protection against mother-to-child HIV type 1 transmission. AIDS Res Hum Retroviruses, 2004, 20: 692-697.

[10] Liu C, Carrington M, Kaslow RA, et al. Association of polymorphisms in human leukocyte antigen class I and transporter associated with antigen processing genes with

resistance to human immunodeficiency virus type 1 infection. J Infect Dis, 2003, 187: 1404-1410.

[11] Al Jabri AA. HLA and in vitro susceptibility to HIV infection. Mol Immunol, 2002, 38: 959-967.

[12] Liu H, Hwangbo Y, Hotle S, et al. Analysis of genetic polymorphisms in CCR5, CCR2, stromal cell-derived factor-1, RANTES, and dendritic cell-specific intercellular adhesion molecule-3-grabbing nonintegrin in seronegative individuals repeatedly exposed to HIV-1. J Infect Dis, 2004, 190: 1055-1058.

[13] Jansen CA, Kostense S, Vandenberghe K, et al. High responsiveness of HLA-B57-restricted Gag-specific CD8+ T cells in vitro may contribute to the protective effect of HLA-B57 in HIV-infection. Eur J Immunol, 2005, 35: 150-158.

[14] Walker BD, Korber BT. Immune control of HIV: the obstacles of HLA and viral diversity. Nat Immunol, 2001, 2: 437-475.

[15] Leslie AJ, Pfafferott KJ, Chetty P, et al. HIV evolution: CTL escape mutation and reversion after transmission. Nat Med, 2004, 10: 282-289.

[16] Kuhn L, Abrams EJ, Palumbo P, et al. Maternal versus paternal inheritance of HLA class I alleles among HIV-infected children: consequences for clinical disease progression. AIDS, 2004, 18: 1281-1289.

[17] Grifoni A, Montesano C, Palma P. et al. Role of HLA-B α-3 domain amino acid position 194 in HIV disease progression. Mol Immunol. 2013, 53(4):410-3.

[18] Matthews PC, Listgarten J, Carlson JM, et al. Co-operative additive effects between HLA alleles in control of HIV-1. PLoS One. 2012, 7(10):e47799.

[19] Kloverpris HN, Stryhn A, Harndahl M, et al. HLA-A*68:02-restricted Gag-specific cytotoxic T lymphocyte responses can drive selection pressure on HIV but are subdominant and ineffective. AIDS. 2013, 27(11):1717-23.

[20] Vaidya SA, Streeck H, Beckwith N, et al. Temporal effect of HLA-B*57 on viral control during primary HIV-1 infection. Retrovirology. 2013, 10(1):139.

[21] Lecuroux C, Saez A, Girault I, et al. Both HLA-B*57 and plasma HIV RNA levels contribute to the HIV-specific CD8+ T cell response in HIV controllers. J Virol. 2013.

[22] Yager N, Robinson N, Brown H, et al. Longitudinal analysis of an HLA-B*51-restricted epitope in integrase reveals immune escape in early HIV-1 infection. AIDS. 2013, 27(3):313-23.

[23] Ranasinghe S, Cutler S, Davis I, et al. Association of HLA-DRB1-restricted CD4 T cell responses with HIV immune control. Nat Med. 2013, 19(7):930-3.

[24] Levitz L, Koita OA, Sangare K, et al. Conservation of HIV-1 T cell epitopes across time and clades: validation of immunogenic HLA-A2 epitopes selected for the GAIA HIV vaccine. Vaccine. 2012, 30(52):7547-60.

[25] Li C, Toth I, Schulze ZW, et al. Functional characterization of HLA-G regulatory T cells in HIV-1 infection. PLoS Pathog. 2013, 9(1):e1003140.

[26] Lenfant F, Pizzato N, Liang S, C. et al. Induction of HLA-G-restricted human cytomegalovirus pp65 (UL83)-specific cytotoxic T lymphocytes in HLA-G transgenic mice. the Journal of General Virology, 2003, 84(2):307-317.

[27] Apps R, Qi Y, Carlson JM, et al. Influence of HLA-C expression level on HIV control. Science. 2013, 340(6128):87-91.

[28] Buranapraditkun S, Hempel U, Pitakpolrat P, et al. A novel immunodominant CD8+ T cell response restricted by a common HLA-C allele targets a conserved region of Gag HIV-1 BioMed Research International 11 clade CRF01AE infected thais. PLoS ONE. 2011, 6(8):23603.

[29] Fellay J, Shianna KV, .Ge D, et al. A whole-genome association study of major determinants for host control of HIV-1. Science, 2007, 317(5840):944–947.

[30] Trachtenberg E, Bhattacharya T, Ladner M, et al. The HLA-B/-C haplotype block contains major determinants for host control of HIV. Genes and Immunity, 2009, 10(8): 673-677.

[31] Segat L, Catamo E, Fabris A, et al. HLA-G*0105N allele is associated with augmented risk for HIV infection in white female patients. AIDS, 2010, 24(12):1961-1964.

[32] Larsen MH, Zinyama R, Kallestrup P, et al. HLA-G 3′ untranslated region 14-base pair deletion: association with poor survival in an HIV-1-infected zimbabwean population. The Journal of Infectious Diseases, 2013, 207(6): 903-906.

[33] Kulkarni S, Savan R, Qi Y, et al, Differential microRNA regulation of HLA-C expression and its association with HIV control. Nature, 2011, 472(7344):495-498.

[34] Gall SL, Buseyne F, Trocha A, Walke BD, et al. Distinct trafficking pathways mediate Nef induced and clathrin-dependent major histocompatibility complex class I down-regulation. Journal of Virology, 2000 74(19): 9256-9266.

[35] Kasper MR and Collins KL. Nef-mediated disruption of HLA-A2 transport to the cell surface in T cells. Journal of Virology, 2003 77(5):3041-3049.

[36] Pizzato N, Derrien M, and Lenfant F. The short cytoplasmic tail of HLA-G determines its resistance to HIV-1 Nef-mediated cell surface down regulation. Human Immunology, 2004, 65(11):1389–1396.

[37] Nattermann J, Nischalke HD, Hofmeister V et al, HIV-1 infection leads to increased HLA-E expression resulting in impaired function of natural killer cells. Antiviral Therapy, 2005, 10(1):95-107.

Chapter 12

Association Between HLA Gene Polymorphism and the Genetic Susceptibility of SARS Infection

Yuying Sun and Yongzhi Xi

Additional information is available at the end of the chapter

http://dx.doi.org/10.5772/57561

1. Introduction

Theoretically, any infectious disease with an infection source, transmission route, and susceptible population is able to infect any population. However, studies of human development history, especially those of infectious disease history, have clearly shown that ethnic and regional differences in susceptibility to some infectious diseases actually exist, even if their infection sources and transmission routes are the same. In terms of the 40 types of new infectious diseases that have occurred worldwide in the past 40 years, the epidemiology of some infectious diseases (including severe acute respiratory syndrome (SARS)) has been dominated by regional/territorial or ethnic oriented infections. Examples, along with the year of first occurrence, include:Ebola hemorrhagic fever caused by Ebola virus (1977), Legionnaires' disease caused by *Legionella pneumophila* (1977), hemorrhagic fever with renal syndrome caused by hantavirus (1977), T cell lymphoma leukemia caused by human T-lymphotropic virus type I (1980), hemorrhagic colitis caused by E. coli O157:H7 (1982), hairy cell leukemia caused by human T-lymphotropic virus type II (1982), and the British BSE (bovine spongiform encephalopathy) that created worldwide shock. Along with the effects of infection sources and transmission routes, the contributions of racial or genetic factors to these regional/territorial diseases are still under discussion. Clearly, these infectious diseases occurred more frequently and with greater severity in certain regions and ethnicities. The SARS outbreak in 2002-2003 spread mainly in Asia, especially in China; the most susceptible populations were mainland and overseas Chinese. These observations lead us to consider the important theoretical and practical topic of the relationship between SARS genetic predisposition and individual clinical onset. However, the sudden disappearance of SARS also left us with many revelations.

2. The correlation of disease genetic predisposition and MHC gene polymorphism

It is well known that the investigation of genetic predisposition is an important topic in modern medicine. It helps to clarify not only the fundamental reasons for patients' individual differences but also the pathogenesis of many diseases. Better understanding of genetic predisposition can provide prevention and treatment strategies for the corresponding diseases, an especially important consideration for individualized disease prevention and treatment. Modern medical studies have shown that disease is a specific life process formed by interactions of environmental factors (external) and the human body (internal). Genetic factors are the major basis of an organism's reactivity, including defensive immunity, the functional states of the nervous and endocrine systems, nutritional status, psychological factors, age, gender, etc. Among these numerous factors, genetic factors predominate because, besides external factors, immune responses and neuropsychological and endocrine functions are constrained by genetic factors. Even nutrition status is not based only on the quality and quantity of the exogenous nutrient supply. It is also influenced by digestion, absorption, and utilization functions controlled by genetic factors. Gender and age (an organism's reactive characteristics at different ages) are even more determined by genetic factors. Therefore, organism reactivities determined by genetic factors have been collectively called genetic predisposition. Numerous studies have demonstrated that many severe diseases, such as cancer, atherosclerosis, coronary heart disease, diabetes, schizophrenia, and high blood pressure, have significant genetic predispositions. In addition, some infectious diseases caused by bacteria and viruses have significant individual genetic predispositions. The human immune and genetic system most closely related to genetic predisposition to disease is the major histocompatibility complex (MHC).

Human MHC is also named as human leucocyte antigens (HLA) system, which codes for the most polymorphic antigen system that is known. The correlation of HLA and human diseases has been studied for nearly 40 years. The rapid development of advanced technologies in modern molecular biology and their wide applications to HLA studies have effectively promoted studies of HLA mechanisms and their associations with disease, leading to significantly increased accuracy of disease association analysis. Many alleles have been identified as being primarily associated with certain aspects of diseases. For example, in autoimmune diseases, Hodgkin's disease and HLA-A1 have relative risk (RR) of 32. 0; congenital adrenal hyperplasia and HLA-B47 have relative risk of 15. 4; ankylosing arthritis and HLA-B27 have relative risk of 87. 4; Reiter's syndrome and HLA-B27 have relative risk of 37. 0; acute anterior uveitis and HLA-B27 have relative risk of 10. 4; psoriasis and HLA-Cw6 have relative risk of 13. 3, etc. In infectious diseases, Hepatitis B virus associated glomerulonephritis and HLA-DQB1*03 have relative risk of 12. 90; infection and development of AIDS are highly correlated with HLA-A29, HLA-B35, and B57; infection and development of flu are closely correlated with HLA-A2 antigen; hepatitis B is separately correlated with HLA-B13, B8, DR7, DR13; and infection and development of hepatitis C are closely correlated with HLA-DRB1*0402, DRB1*12 and DQB1*0301. Therefore, correlation studies of HLA and different diseases can help the identification and classification of diseases. The studies could also be treated as auxiliary diagnostic tools. While conducting such studies, researches could further clarify the relationships between diseases and genetic inheritance, provide genetic consulting services to specific families, detect HLA-linked disease genes, and, most importantly, provide early predictions and preventions of these diseases.

3. The correlation of SARS genetic predisposition and HLA gene polymorphism

SARS virus is a recently discovered infectious pathogen that can cause severe human diseases, and, to date, we know little about it. Knowledge of its occurrence and development pattern remains limited, and studies of its pathogenesis, treatment, and prevention strategies remain limited. Considering that SARS displays significant regional/territorial and ethnic and individual specificity, and that the SARS-associated antigen epitopes are almost all related to HLA antigen recognition, as inferred by known SARS gene and protein sequences, we hypothesize that there is a close correlation between the occurrence of a SARS epidemic and the HLA system.

3.1. Speculations regarding susceptible genes based on SARS coronavirus (SARS-CoV) structure

Previous studies demonstrated that although SARS-CoV and other known coronaviruses have less than 40%-50% homology in amino acid sequence, their structures and functions are similar to those of other known coronaviruses. The antisera of transmissible gastro-enteritis virus (TGEV), murine hepatitis virus (MHV), Feline infectious peritonitis virus (FIPV), and 229E human coronavirus can inhibit the growth of cultured SARS viruses. In the known OC43 and 229E coronavirus strains, HLA-A3. 1was shown by some studies to be the receptor of OC43 and aminopeptidase N (APN), also known as metalloproteinases or CD13, and the co-receptor of human coronavirus 229E and cats/pigs coronavirus. A recent study using molecular 3D structure simulation showed that CD13 also interacted with the S protein of SARS virus. Carcinoembryonic antigen (CEA) is the S protein receptor of human/rats coronavirus. The invasion, infection, and disease caused by OC43 must be accompanied by the presence and expression of HLA-A3. 1. The invasion, infection, and disease caused by coronavirus 229E must be accompanied by the presence and expression of aminopeptidase N. On the other hand, carcinoembryonic antigen may be the required co-receptor for many coronavirus infections. Theoretically, HLA-A3.1 is the susceptible gene of SARS coronavirus, and individuals without this susceptible gene are not easily affected or have resistance to the disease.

3.2. Population genetics studies of HLA gene polymorphism and SARS genetic predisposition

SARS is a highly contagious disease with high disease incidence and mortality rate. The limited diffusion mode based on East and Southeast Asian countries has indicated the existence of susceptible genes in these populations. This has been corroborated in numerous clinical case-control studies, but some other studies yielded opposite results. In the 2 months immediately following the last outbreak of SARS in Taiwan, Taiwan scholars recruited 658 employees from hospitals who had just experienced their initial or the most severe SARS infections to help the investigation of related infectious and genetic factors of SARS-CoV. They used an enzyme immunoassay to test the infections of SARS-CoV and then employed western blot analysis, antibody neutralization, and commercial SARS tests for verification. Risk evaluations were prepared through questionnaires and sequence-specific oligonucleotide probe analysis of the human leukocyte antigen (HLA) allele. The study showed that 3% (20/658) of the participants were positive. A female nurse with a subclinical case was identified. Identified risk factors of SARS-CoV infection included working in the same building, such as hospital emergency rooms and infection wards, direct nursing for SARS patients, and carrying the HLA-Cw*0801 allele. The SARS-CoV infection ratio of homozygous and heterozygous Cw*0801 carriers was 4. 4:1 (95% confidence interval, 1. 5-12. 9; *P*=0. 007). However, in September 2006, 3 years after the SARS outbreak in Taiwan, 130 diagnosed SARS patients were studied to evaluate the correlation of their SARS antibody levels and HLA types. Western blot analysis illustrated that 6. 9%of the participants still had anti-spike and antinuclear antibodies. HLA-SARS case-control studies revealed that HLA-Cw*1502 and DRB1*0301 genes might be the resistance factors of SARS infection (*P*<0. 05).

Another study in the Taiwan population also proved the correlation between HLA and SARS. The researchers used PCR-sequence specific oligonucleotides probe (SSOP) to study the genotyping of HLA type I and type II alleles. The study population included 37 suspected SARS cases (28 fever patients were excluded from SARS) and 101 non-infected medical staff who might have been exposed to SARS-CoV. Another control group contained 190 healthy, non-related Taiwanese people. Initially, during the analysis of SARS infected patients and the high-risk medical staff, the researchers found that HLA-B*4601 (OR = 2. 08, *P* = 0. 04, Pc = n. s.) and HLA-B*5401 (OR = 5. 44, *P* = 0. 02, Pc = n. s.) might be the most probable factors assisting SARS-CoV infection. When comparing the "severe patient" group (selected from the SARS patient group) and the high-risk medical staff group, the researchers found that the severity of SARS was significantly correlated with HLA-B*4601 (*P* =0. 0008 or Pc=0. 0279). Until recently, no SARS patient had been found among local Taiwanese whose genes were different from ordinary Taiwanese. They carry no HLA-B*4601 gene but have HLA-B*1301 at a high frequency. However, the increased HLA-B*4601 allele frequency found in the suspected SARS patient group was significantly higher in severe patient group. These results support the hypothesis that the HLA-B*4601 gene in Asian populations is correlated with the severity of SARS infection.

Another study also showed that SARS infection was correlated with Chinese HLA. This study determined a strong correlation between SARS development and HLA-B*0703 (OR, 4. 08; 95% CI, 2. 03-8. 18; *P*=0. 00072 [Bonferroni corrected *P* value, Pc<0. 0022]) and DRB1*0301 (OR, 0. 06; 95%, 0. 01-0. 47; *P* =0. 00008 [Bonferroni corrected, Pc<0. 0042]), through the human leukocyte antigen (HLA) A, B, DR, or DQ allele type analysis of 90 serologically diagnosed Chinese SARS patients. Compared with the expected value (0. 4%) in ordinary people, the joint inheritance rate of B*0703 and B60 (9. 6%; 95% CI, 4. 6% - 19%) showed a significant increase in the SARS patient group ($P = 3\times10^{-9}$).

Evidences of the SARS-HLA correlation has also been found in other Asian populations. In Vietnam 44 out of 62 SARS patients participated in a study. The control groups were 103 individuals who had contact with SARS patients and 50 individuals who had not. Compared with the control groups, HLA-DRB1*12 occurred more often in the SARS patient group (corrected P = 0. 042). HLA-DRB1*1202, the dominate gene in Vietnamese, showed the strongest correlation with SARS in the dominant model (corrected P = 0. 0065 and 0. 0052, depending on the size of the control group).

However, some studies resulted in the opposite conclusions. Xiong P, *et al.* conducted correlation studies of HLA gene polymorphism and SARS in Cantonese after their initial infection by SARS, but did not find a correlation. The study included 95 SARS rehabilitation patients and 403 genetically unrelated healthy people (control group). HLA –A, B, and DRB1 allele analysis was conducted by sequence-specific primer polymerase chain reactions. The severity of disease was evaluated by assisted ventilation and lymphopenia based on their history of pulmonary infiltrates. Although the frequencies of A23, A34, B60, and DRB1*12 alleles were slightly higher in SARS group and the frequency of A33, -B58, and -B61 alleles in SARS group were all lower than those in control group, the Pc values indicated no statistical significance. Similarly, the correlation between HLA alleles and disease severity was not found. Therefore, the main organization of MHC variation appears not to have significant correlation with Cantonese SARS predisposition or severity.

4. The revelations SARS brought to people

Early in Feb. 2005 on an annual meeting of Association for the Advancement of Science (AAAS), an American microbiologist Kathryn Holmes, who had long been engaged in coronavirus researches, pointed out that it was not impossible to have another outbreak of severe acute respiratory syndrome (SARS) in the world like the one 2 years ago. The SARS-CoV used to spread in populations might only exist in laboratory samples. Her words shocked the world. It has been 10 years since the SARS pandemic. Many scholars conducted broad and indepth studies but have not achieved breakthroughs with respect to the origin of SARS CoV. On the contrary, the new influenza A virus (H1N1) that spread worldwide in April 2009 was studied thoroughly during the first 2 months of its spreading. It has 8 types of genes coming from 4 pedigrees and is very similar to the North American popular triple ligand swine H1N1 virus. Different from other viruses, there has been no SARS patient other than lab infections after the widespread infections in January 2004. SARS-CoV does not exist in nature or people now. Hence the natural SARS epidemic history has some extraordinary abnormalities. What are the reasons? The most important reason could be that there is no direct ancestor of SARS-CoV in nature. It had an "unusual evolution". It is very likely that it was "unnaturally" introduced to populations, so it did not follow the normal epidemic transmission rules.

SARS-CoV has an unordinary phylogeny. It has a fast and obvious "reverse evolution. " "Reverse evolution" is defined as "regaining the ancestor's state" and is an evolution component that commonly exists in the biosphere, including microbial communities. In the long course of natural evolution, "reverse evolution" might be largely supplemental and it might coordinate "forward evolution" , acting as the twists and turns of mainstream evolution. However, the "reverse evolution" of SARS-CoV appears earlier and more powerfully, and it has more presence and lasts longer. In the early state of its epidemic, it had already lost the genes related to host adaptability (characteristic 29-ntORF8 gene) and presented "reverse evolution" of key amino acids on the virulence and transmission-related receptor's binding site. The SARS-CoV outbreak in 2003-2004 in Guangzhou was phylogenetically closer to earlier viruses in the 2002-2003 epidemics than the later viruses. Under natural conditions, it is not possible that the adaptive evolution of Bt-SLCoV could have developed to the human level through carnivores in such a short time. Therefore, the only possible explanation is that SARS-CoV was produced through "unusual evolution (UE)," via processes such as like GM technology.

There have already been some debates about the technical maturity of transforming animal virus to human virus (for example, GM technology). However, it would be indisputable now, as in May and June 2012, a top international journal published 2 papers, which shocked the international natural science field in 2011 and clarified this problem by facts. However, according to some international information sources, in 2000 or earlier some scientists were studying or had already mastered these technologies at those early dates.

Therefore, Xu D *et al.* reasoned that there was no storage host of SARS-CoV in nature and it was made by "unnatural ways (GM technology)"from Bt-SLCoV, which means we had already entered a new era where a "novel artificial virus" could cause a global epidemic. We can further explain the unnatural origin of SARS from its apparently abnormally epidemiological and clinical characteristics: 1) in the early and middle stages of the epidemic, all Cantonese patients were from the west and the south of Guangzhou while there was not even 1 patient from the north or the east; 2) During December 2003 to January 2004, 4 cases in Guangzhou had only mild symptoms and no sustainability due to the reverse evolution of SARS-CoV in the population. However, during March and April 2004, the outbreak from a laboratory (9 cases and 1 death) was super transmissible, which was the same as in the 2002-2003 epidemic, without reverse evolution; and 3) As a specific infection source, infected civets were found only in 2 animal markets in Guangzhou and Shenzhen and could have been used for unnatural introduction. Therefore, we are facing unprecedented threats today, and we must deal with them together.

5. Conclusions

The investigation of the SARS in-out flow epidemic transmission network in mainland China shows that Beijing and Guangdong were the places where the exported cases and self-transmission cases were the most severe. Guangzhou was the origin of the transmission of

SARS and the main import source of the early-stage regional cases of infection in most areas, but it did not cause significant radiation of transmission to its neighboring regions. Nevertheless, the in-out flow between Beijing and its neighboring regions did not start until the middle to late stages of the epidemic transmission. The transmission, however, was able to radiate significantly across regions. There have been no other cases reported among people and among animals except for laboratory infections and 4 mild infections reported in Guangzhou in December 2003 and January 2004. This is different from the trend of typical epidemic transmissions, and it is different from the correlation between the HLA gene polymorphism and SARS, as demonstrated by many studies. The HLA alleles that are closely related to the infection of SARS, such as B*4601, B*5401, Cw0801, and DRB1*0301, as found among populations from Taiwan, Hong Kong, and mainland China, are types of HLA alleles that are relatively common in the Chinese population. Why were only people in limited regions infected? Further, why did the transmission disappear rapidly?

The study of Xu D *et al.* appeared to provide a good explanation to the paradox between the HLA gene polymorphism and the genetic predisposition to SARS. Because of the unusual virus phylogeny of SARS-CoV, with rapid and evident "reverse evolution," it is likely that SARS CoV was produced through an unnatural mechanism (such as gene modification techniques). The SARS CoV from the outbreak in Guangzhou during 2003-2004 was phylogenetically closer to earlier viruses in the 2002-2003 epidemics than the later viruses, which led to its rapid decrease in virulence. Therefore, the correlation would be expected to disappear because of the reverse genetics of SARS-CoV, regardless of whether the susceptible gene existed in the Chinese population. Of course, these conclusions can be supported and the nature of this mysterious disease can be explained only with the support of a large number of valid and convincing investigational results.

Acknowledgements

Supported by grants from the State Key Development Program for Basic Research of China (No.2003CB515509 and 2009CB522401) and from National Natural Scientific Foundation of China(No.81070450 and 30470751) to Dr. X.-Y.Z.

Author details

Yuying Sun and Yongzhi Xi*

*Address all correspondence to: xiyz@yahoo. com

Department of Immunology and National Center for Biomedicine Analysis, Beijing Hospital Affiliated to Academy of Medical Sciences, Beijing, PRC

References

[1] Wang SF, Chen KH, Chen M, et al. Human-leukocyte antigen class I Cw 1502 and class II DR 0301 genotypes are associated with resistance to severe acute respiratory syndrome (SARS) infection. Viral Immunol. 2011, 24(5):421-6.

[2] Oh HL, Chia A, Chang CX, et al. Engineering T cells specific for a dominant severe acute respiratory syndrome coronavirus CD8 T cell epitope. J Virol. 2011, 85(20): 10464-71.

[3] Liu J, Wu P, Gao F, et al. Novel immunodominant peptide presentation strategy: a featured HLA-A*2402-restricted cytotoxic T-lymphocyte epitope stabilized by intra-chain hydrogen bonds from severe acute respiratory syndrome coronavirus nucleo-capsid protein. J Virol. 2010, 84(22):11849-57.

[4] Liu J, Sun Y, Qi J, et al. The membrane protein of severe acute respiratory syndrome coronavirus acts as a dominant immunogen revealed by a clustering region of novel functionally and structurally defined cytotoxic T-lymphocyte epitopes. J Infect Dis. 2010, 202(8):1171-80.

[5] Zhao K, Yang B, Xu Y, et al. CD8+ T cell response in HLA-A*0201 transgenic mice is elicited by epitopes from SARS-CoV S protein. Vaccine. 2010, 28(41):6666-74.

[6] Chen YZ, Liu G, Senju S, et al. Identification of SARS-COV spike protein-derived and HLA-A2-restricted human CTL epitopes by using a new muramyl dipeptidederivative adjuvant. Int J Immunopathol Pharmacol. 2010, 23(1):165-77.

[7] Lv Y, Ruan Z, Wang L, et al. Identification of a novel conserved HLA-A*0201-restricted epitope from the spike protein of SARS-CoV. BMC Immunol. 2009, 10:61.

[8] Sin FW, Cheng SC, Chan KT, et al. Mouse studies of SARS coronavirus-specific immune responses to recombinant replication-defective adenovirus expressing SARS coronavirus N protein. Hong Kong Med J. 2009, Suppl 2:33-6.

[9] Kohyama S, Ohno S, Suda T, et al. Efficient induction of cytotoxic T lymphocytes specific for severe acute respiratory syndrome (SARS)-associated coronavirus by immunization with surface-linked liposomal peptides derived from a non-structural polyprotein 1a. Antiviral Res. 2009, 84(2):168-77.

[10] Kong SL, Chui P, Lim B, et al. Elucidating the molecular physiopathology of acute respiratory distress syndrome in severe acute respiratory syndrome patients. Virus Res. 2009, 145(2):260-9.

[11] Ohno S, Kohyama S, Taneichi M, et al. Synthetic peptides coupled to the surface of liposomes effectively induce SARS coronavirus-specific cytotoxic T lymphocytes and viral clearance in HLA-A*0201 transgenic mice. Vaccine. 2009, 27(29):3912-20.

[12] Keicho N, Itoyama S, Kashiwase K, et al. Association of human leukocyte antigen class II alleles with severe acute respiratory syndrome in the Vietnamese population. Hum Immunol. 2009, 70(7):527-31.

[13] Cheung YK, Cheng SC, Sin FW, et al. Investigation of immunogenic T-cell epitopes in SARS virus nucleocapsid protein and their role in the prevention and treatment of SARS infection. Hong Kong Med J. 2008, Suppl 4:27-30.

[14] Yang J, James E, Roti M, et al. Searching immunodominant epitopes prior to epidemic: HLA class II-restricted SARS-CoV spike protein epitopes in unexposed individuals. Int Immunol. 2009, 21(1):63-71.

[15] Røder G, Kristensen O, Kastrup JS, et al. Structure of a SARS coronavirus-derived peptide bound to the human major histocompatibility complex class I molecule HLA-B*1501. Acta Crystallogr Sect F Struct Biol Cryst Commun. 2008, 64(Pt 6): 459-62.

[16] Lundegaard C, Lamberth K, Harndahl M, et al. NetMHC-3. 0: accurate web accessible predictions of human, mouse and monkey MHC class I affinities for peptides of length 8-11. Nucleic Acids Res. 2008, 36(Web Server issue):W509-12.

[17] Xiong P, Zeng X, Song MS, et al. Lack of association between HLA-A, -B and -DRB1 alleles and the development of SARS: a cohort of 95 SARS-recovered individuals in a population of Guangdong, southern China. Int J Immunogenet. 2008, 35(1):69-74.

[18] Libraty DH, O'Neil KM, Baker LM, et al. Human CD4(+) memory T-lymphocyte responses to SARS coronavirus infection. Virology. 2007, 368(2):317-21.

[19] Cheung YK, Cheng SC, Sin FW, et al. Induction of T-cell response by a DNA vaccine encoding a novel HLA-A*0201 severe acute respiratory syndrome coronavirus epitope. Vaccine. 2007, 25(32):6070-7.

[20] Gu J, Korteweg C. Pathology and pathogenesis of severe acute respiratory syndrome. Am J Pathol. 2007, 170(4):1136-47.

[21] Zhan J, Deng R, Tang J, et al. The spleen as a target in severe acute respiratory syndrome. FASEB J. 2006, 20(13):2321-8.

[22] Oscarsson J, Kanth A, Tegmark-Wisell K, et al. SarA is a repressor of hla (alpha-hemolysin) transcription in Staphylococcus aureus: its apparent role as an activator of hla in the prototype strain NCTC 8325 depends on reduced expression of sarS. J Bacteriol. 2006, 188(24):8526-33.

[23] Zhou M, Xu D, Li X, et al. Screening and identification of severe acute respiratory syndrome-associated coronavirus-specific CTL epitopes. J Immunol. 2006, 177(4): 2138-45.

[24] Tsao YP, Lin JY, Jan JT, et al. HLA-A*0201 T-cell epitopes in severe acute respiratory syndrome (SARS) coronavirus nucleocapsid and spike proteins. Biochem Biophys Res Commun. 2006, 344(1):63-71.

[25] Chen YM, Liang SY, Shih YP, et al. Epidemiological and genetic correlates of severe acute respiratory syndrome coronavirus infection in the hospital with the highest nosocomial infection rate in Taiwan in 2003. J Clin Microbiol. 2006, 44(2):359-65.

[26] Zhang GL, Khan AM, Srinivasan KN, et al. Neural models for predicting viral vaccine targets. J Bioinform Comput Biol. 2005, 3(5):1207-25.

[27] Senn MM, Bischoff M, von Eiff C, et al. sigmaB activity in a Staphylococcus aureus hemB mutant. J Bacteriol. 2005, 187(21):7397-406.

[28] Xu X, Gao X. Immunological responses against SARS-coronavirus infection in humans. Cell Mol Immunol. 2004, 1(2):119-22.

[29] Blicher T, Kastrup JS, Buus S, et al. High-resolution structure of HLA-A*1101 in complex with SARS nucleocapsid peptide. Acta Crystallogr D Biol Crystallogr. 2005, 61(Pt 8):1031-40.

[30] Chen H, Hou J, Jiang X, et al. Response of memory CD8+ T cells to severe acute respiratory syndrome (SARS) coronavirus in recovered SARS patients and healthy individuals. J Immunol. 2005, 175(1):591-8.

[31] Ingavale S, van Wamel W, Luong TT, et al. Rat/MgrA, a regulator of autolysis, is a regulator of virulence genes in Staphylococcus aureus. Infect Immun. 2005, 73(3): 1423-31.

[32] Wang YD, Chen WF. Detecting specific cytotoxic T lymphocytes against SARS-coronavirus with DimerX HLA-A2: Ig fusion protein. Clin Immunol. 2004, 113(2):151-4.

[33] Srinivasan KN, Zhang GL, Khan AM, August JT, Brusic V. Prediction of class I T-cell epitopes: evidence of presence of immunological hot spots inside antigens. Bioinformatics. 2004, Suppl 1:i297-302.

[34] Ng MH, Lau KM, Li L, et al. Association of human-leukocyte-antigen class I (B*0703) and class II (DRB1*0301) genotypes with susceptibility and resistance to the development of severe acute respiratory syndrome. J Infect Dis. 2004, 190(3):515-8.

[35] Wang YD, Sin WY, Xu GB, et al. T-cell epitopes in severe acute respiratory syndrome (SARS) coronavirus spike protein elicit a specific T-cell immune response in patients who recover from SARS. J Virol. 2004, 78(11):5612-8.

[36] Wang C, Xia CQ. Changes in monocyte counts and expression of mCD (14) and HLA-DR in the peripheral blood of patients with severe acute respiratory syndrome. Chin Med J (Engl). 2004, 117(4):624-6.

[37] Lin M, Tseng HK, Trejaut JA, et al. Association of HLA class I with severe acute respiratory syndrome coronavirus infection. BMC Med Genet. 2003, 4:9.

[38] Xu D, Zhang Lei, Sun H, et al. Unnatural origin of SARS CoV. Negative. 2013, 4(4): 6-9.

[39] Xu D, Sun H, Tan Y. SARS CoV no longer exists in nature and population. Negative. 2013, 4(1): 22-26.

Chapter 13

Influence of Human Leukocyte Antigen on Susceptibility of Tropical Pulmonary Infectious Diseases and Clinical Implications

Attapon Cheepsattayakorn

Additional information is available at the end of the chapter

http://dx.doi.org/10.5772/58288

1. Introduction

Human leukocyte antigen (HLA) is the most polymorphic genetic system in humans, with numerous alleles, and subsequently, various possible combinations [1]. These genes, the products of histocompatibility complex (MHC) [2] are located in the short arm of chromosome 6 at band p 21.3 [2] and are divided into three classes, I, II and III [1]. HLA class I is responsible for coding the molecules HLA-A, -B and -C, present in almost all somatic cells with killing of viral infected targets by class I antigens restrict cytotoxic T-cell (CD8+) function [2] while HLA class II genes code the molecules HLA-DR, -DQ and -DP [1] by presentation of exogenous antigens to T-helper cells (CD4+) or antigen presenting cells (APC) [2]. This polymorphism contributes to the differences in susceptibility to diseases among genetically distinct groups [1]. The molecules coded for by the HLA system are responsible for the antigen presentation [1]. The T lymphocytes that are linked to HLA molecules only recognize antigens by the antigen-specific cell surface receptor-antigens interaction [2], thus the HLA antigens [1] and MCH molecules [2] apparently participate in controlling susceptibility and resistance to various diseases. Some infectious diseases were considered as familial before the finding of the causative microorganism and early twin studies indicated that there was a substantial host genetic influence on susceptibility to diseases such as polio and tuberculosis (TB) [3]. At present, it has been confirmed that human genetic variation demonstrates a major influence on the course of diseases caused by several infectious microorganisms [3].

2. Severe Acute Respiratory Syndrome and HLA

Recently, Itoyama *et al* reported that the deletion of the 287 bp *Alu* repeat (D allele) in intron 16 of the angiotensin converting enzyme 2 (*ACE 2*) gene is associated with hypoxemia and diffuse alveolar damage in patients with severe acute respiratory syndrome (SARS) [4] and may protect acute lung injury and respiratory failure [5]. Nevertheless, there may be potential confounders to a genetic association study as the following: 1) the dead patients were excluded from this study, 2) hypoxemia was defined as requiring oxygen supplementation, and 3) only 44 patients were studied [6]. Some HLA subtypes, particularly *HLA-B*0703* and *HLA-DRB1*0301* alleles have been demonstrated to be more prevalent in patients with SARS [7] and those with poorer outcomes [8]. On the other hand, the polymorphism in *ACE II* gene, coding for a functional receptor of the SARS-coronavirus, was not associated with the susceptibility or outcome of SARS [9]. A previous study revealed that *CXCL10(-938AA)* gene is always protective from SARS infection whenever it appears only jointly with either *Fg12(+158T/*)* or *HO-1 (-497A/*)*, whereas *Fg12(+158T/*)* is associated with higher SARS-infection susceptibility unless combined with *CXCL10/IP-10(-938AA)* which is associated with lower susceptibility [10]. Chan *et al* concluded that the *ACE I/D* polymorphism was not directly associated with increasing susceptibility to SARS-coronavirus infection and was not associated with poor outcome after SARS-coronavirus infection [6]. A recent study in Taiwan demonstrated that *HLA-Cw*1502* [11], *-DR*0301* [11], and *-A*2402* [12] alleles conferred resistance against SARS infection. CD209L homozygote individuals [13] and low-mannose-binding-lectin-producing genotypes [14] have been demonstrated to have a significantly lower risk and increased risk of SARS infection, respectively. A previous study among Vietnamese population with SARS revealed that polymorphisms of two interferon-inducible genes, *2′, 5′-oligoadenylate synthetase 1* (*OAS-1* (G-allele in exon 3 and the one in exon 6)) and *myxovirus resistance-A* (*MxA*) were associated with SARS infection [15]. The single nucleotide polymorphisms (SNPs) in *MxA* was associated with the progression of SARS [15]. The SNPs in *OAS-1* were associated with SARS-coronavirus infection or SARS development [15]. The GG genotype and G-allele of G/T-SNP at position -88 in the *MxA* gene promoter were demonstrated more frequent in hypoxemic group of patients with SARS than non-hypoxemic group [15]. They may be related to the response of SARS patients to interferons (IFNs), particularly those with AA genotype of the A/G-SNP in exon 3 of *OAS-1* may respond to IFN treatment more effectively than those with AG or GG genotype [15]. If SARS re-emerges, IFN could be a promising candidate to treat patients with SARS [16-23]. These findings may contribute to the perception of IFN-induced antiviral response to SARS infection. SARS-coronavirus infection elicited both CD^{4+} and CD^{8+} T-cell responses to the M protein in recovered SARS patients that persisted for a long period of time [24]. This may have significant implications in developing SARS vaccines [24]. A previous study indicated that a *HLA-A*0201*-restricted decameric epitope P15 (S411-420, KLPDDFMGCV) derived from the S protein that was found to localized within the angiotensin-converting enzyme 2 receptor-binding region of the S1 domain could significantly enhance the expression of *HLA-A*0201* molecules on the T2 cell surface [25]. P15 then stimulated IFN-γ-producing cytotoxic-T lymphocytes (CTLs) from the peripheral blood mononuclear cells of former SARS patients and induced specific CTLs from P15-immunized *HLA-A*2.1*-transgenic mice *in vivo* [25]. Significant P15-specific CTLs then were induced by *HLA-A*2.1*-trangenic mice that was immunized by a deoxyribonucleic-acid (DNA) vaccine encoding the S protein [25]. This suggested that P15 was a naturally processed epitope [25]. Thus, P15 could be a novel SARS-associated coronavirus-specific epitope and a potential target for evaluation of candidate SARS vaccines and characterization of virus control mechanisms [25].

3. Tuberculosis and HLA

HLA studies conducted in India revealed that there was association of *HLA-DQ 1* and *-DR 2* antigens with susceptibility of pulmonary TB [26]. A study in North Indian patients demonstrated that the allele *DRB 1*1501* of *HLA-DR 2* was higher compared with *DRB 1*1502* [26] whereas *HLA-DQB 1*0601* (a subtype of *HLA-DQ 1*), *-DRB 1*1501* and *DPB 1*02* were demonstrated to be positively associated with pulmonary susceptibility among South Indian patients [26]. Antigen processing gene 2 and mannose-binding protein (MBP) genes along with *HLA-DR2* have been associated with pulmonary TB [26]. Mannose-binding lectin-54 heterozygotes may be associated with protection against TB meningitis [26]. *HLA-DQB 1*0601* and *HLA-DRB 1*0803* were associated with TB disease progression in Korean populations [27]. The frequencies of *HLA-DQB 1*0402* and antigens DR4 and DR8 were significantly decreased in patients with pulmonary TB but the frequencies of *HLA-DQA1*0101, -DQB1*0501,* and *-DRB1*1501* were significantly increased in immunocompetent patients with pulmonary TB [28]. An increased frequency of *HLA-B*27* in the Greeks, *HLA-A*2* and *-B*5* in the Egyptians, *HLA-B*5, -B*15* and *-DR*5* in the North American blacks, *HLA-B*8* in the Canadians was observed [26] whereas *HLA-DQB1*0502* and *-DQB1*0503* alleles were demonstrated among the Thai and Vietnamese TB patients, respectively [26, 29]. *HLA-B*17-tumor-necrosis-factor-*α*-238/A, -tumor-necrosis-factor-*α*-308/2* and *-tumor-necrosis-factor-*β*-2* have been shown to be associated with TB bacteriological relapse among Indian population [30]. Recently, a novel *HLA-DR*-restricted peptide E7 from the ESAT-6 protein of *Mycobacterium tuberculosis* before and during TB treatment was used to prepare modified *HLA-DR*08032/E7* and *HLA-DR*0818/E7* tetramers to monitor tetramer-positive CD4+ T-cells in direct staining of single specimen and flow cytometric analyses and resulted in 0.1 to 8.8% in the initial pulmonary TB patients' blood, 0.1 to 10.7% in pleural fluid of the initial tuberculous pleuritis patients, 0.02 to 2.2% in non-TB patients' blood, 0.02 to 0.48% in healthy donors' blood and mostly resulted in 0 to 0.2% in umbilical cord blood [31]. After 90-120 days of initial TB symptoms, levels of tetramer-positive $CD4^+$-T cells in tetramer-positive $CD4^+$-T cells reached and kept at low even normal at 0.03 to 0.3% [31]. Tetramer-positive, interferon-γ-producing and/or tumor-necrosis-factor-α-producing $CD4^+$-T cells in pulmonary granuloma, lymph node and cavernous tissues of TB patients could be detected by *in situ* staining [31]. Sensitivity and specificity of tetramer molecules should be confirmed in the future in order to develop possible diagnostic reagents and research [31].

4. Human Immunodeficiency Virus Infection (HIV)/Acquired Immunodeficiency Syndrome (AIDS) — Related tropical pulmonary infectious diseases and HLA

The World Health Organization (WHO) estimates that 8-10 million new cases of TB globally occur each year [32]. Although AIDS is the same disease as HIV disease in all part of the world, this microorganism is mostly in many tropical countries [32]. In tropical countries, TB and bacterial pneumonia represent the major pulmonary infections among the patients with HIV-infection/AIDS [32]. Although the spectrum of HIV disease/AIDS is quite broad, the majority of the pulmonary infections in HIV-1 infected patients are similar to those observed in non-HIV infected persons [32]. The geographical differences are primarily due to varying frequencies rather than the kinds of infections [32]. Of all the pulmonary infections encountered in the tropics obviously *Mycobacterium tuberculosis* is one of the most significant pathogenic micro-organisms [32]. A recent study on HLA and AIDS in children with AIDS revealed that the presence of homozygous *HLA-B* or *-C* alleles was associated with more rapid disease progression, in contrast, the presence of *HLA-B*27* or *-B*57* alleles was associated with slower disease progression which remained significant after adjustment for age, gender, race, and baseline HIV-1 log ribonucleic acid (RNA), $CD4^{+}$-T cell count and percent and weight for age Z score or other genetic variants including *CCR5-wt/Δ32* (CCR5 = chemokine (C-C motif) receptor 5), *-59029-G/A, CCR2-wt/64I* (CCR2 = chemokine (C-C motif) receptor 2), CX_3CR1*-249-V/I* (CX_3CR1 = chemokine (C-C motif) ligand 3-like 1), *-280-T/M, SDF-1-180-G/A* (SDF-1 = stromal cell-derived factor-1), *MCP-1-G/A* (MCP-1 = monocyte chemotactic protein-1), *MBL2-A/O* (MBL = mannose-binding lectin), *MBL2-X/Y* (MBL = mannose-binding lectin), *MBL2-P/Q* (MBL = mannose-binding lectin), and *MBL2-H/L* (MBL = mannose-binding lectin) [33]. Additionally, the *HLA-A*24* allele was associated with more rapid central nervous system (CNS) impairment and the *HLA-Cw2* allele protected against disease progression [33]. For HLA class II, the presence of the *HLA-DQB1*2* allele protected against both HIV-1 disease progression and CNS impairment [33]. HLA concordance between a mother and her infant is associated with increased risk of HIV transmission whereas HLA discordance decreases the risk of mother-to-child HIV transmission [34, 35]. HLA class I homozygosity [36, 37] and children who have the same HLA class I alleles at both sites with their mothers at one of more HLA locus [38] are at increased risk for more rapid disease progression.

4.1. HIV-infection/AIDS-TB Co-infection and HLA

Studies from Haiti and sub-Saharan Africa have demonstrated that 17% to 66% of TB cases are HIV-1 seropositive while 50% of HIV-seropositive patients with pulmonary symptoms are sick with TB [32]. A previous study in Brazilians by Figueiredo *et al* revealed that *HLA-A*31, HLA-B*41, HLA-DQB1*5,* and *HLA-DRB1*10* alleles, were over- represented in acquired-immuno-deficiency-syndrome (AIDS) patients with TB, indicated that these HLA molecules are associated with susceptibility to TB in Brazilian patients with AIDS [39].

4.2. HIV-infection/AIDS-related community acquired pneumonia

A previous study in Kenya in 1976 demonstrated that 20% of patients presenting with pneumonia to Kenyatta National Hospital had pneumococcal bacteremia which was very common among HIV-infected patients (26% of the HIV-1 seropositive group versus 6% of the seronegative group) [40] whereas *Streptococcus pneumoniae* pneumonia has been the most common cause of bacterial pneumonia same as in the pre-AIDS era [32]. Approximately, 17% of medically hospital admissions to the one of East Africa's largest hospital are community acquired pneumonia (CAP) [32]. Gilks *et al* reported that invasive pneumococcal disease among the female prostitutes in Nairobi, Kenya was the most frequently encountered serious HIV-associated infection and was more common than TB [40]. Pneumococcal pneumonia occurred at a significantly higher rate among HIV- seropositive patients, particularly HIV-1 serotype [40]. The clinical presentation of pyogenic pneumonia in HIV-1 seropositive patients was similar to that observed in HIV-seronegative ones [40]. The acute onset of fever and cough was the most common presentation [40]. Although, approximately, 10% of patients with lobar pneumonia in the tropics fail to improve with penicillin treatment, there is no significant difference in penicillin treatment response in both HIV-seropositive and HIV-seronegative patients [40]. In tropical and developing countries, penicillin, because of it antimicrobial tolerance and cheapness, is still the drug of choice for CAP regardless of HIV status [40]. The mortality rate was higher among HIV-1 seropositive patients with CAP than HIV-1 seronegative persons with CAP (17% versus 8%) [40]. Recurrence of pneumococcal disease occurred 22% among the prostitutes in Nairobi, Kenya which rate of recurrence increased both in Kenya and the United States of America [40].

4.3. HIV-infection/AIDS-related pulmonary *Nocardia asteroides* infectionasteroides infection

Nocardiaasteroides is a branching filamentous, beaded Gram-positive-rod microorganism which is usually found worldwide in soil and decaying organic matter and usually produces disease in immunocompromised persons, particularly HIV-1 infected individuals although few cases have been reported from the tropical regions [32]. The earliest report of AIDS patients from Rwanda demonstrated one of 26 cases diagnosing *Nocardia asteroides* pleuropneumonia whereas one of 50 AIDS patients with pulmonary interstitial infiltrates in Zimbabwe was diagnosed pneumonia [32]. In previous studies in Uganda, Cote d' Ivoire, and Zaire, three of the 57, one of 52, and occasional AIDS patients who underwent post-mortem examination revealed histopathologically pulmonary military nocardiosis, respectively [32]. Clinical manifestations of pulmonary nocardiosis in HIV-1 infected patients are usually non-specific [32]. The majority of cases present with fever, cough, night sweats, malaise, and body weight loss [32]. Although nocardiosis is frequently disseminated at the presentation, the lungs are the most common site of involvement, particularly upper lobes [32]. Thus, pulmonary nocardiosis is roentgenographically indistinguishable from pulmonary TB [32]. Because of rarely positive-blood culture, culture of the respiratory specimens is the definitely diagnostic method [32]. Due to 47% of patients was indicated of nocardiosis so the diagnosis should be suspected if the characteristic morphology is detected on Gram staining [41]. This microorganism is also weakly stains the acid fast [32]. According to ability to stain the acid fast coupled with the roentgenographic presentation of this microbial pulmonary infection, it may contribute to be misdiagnosed as pulmonary TB [32]. It is likely that sulphonamides (trimethoprim-sulphamethoxazole) will be effective in HIV-1 infected patients with nocardiosis whereas sulphonamides have been the treatment of choice for nocardiosis in non-HIV-1 infected patients [32]. Other antimicrobial agents with *in vitro* bactericidal activity to *Nocardia ÿsteroids* include amoxicillin-clavulanic acid, minocycline, amikacin, and third-generation cephalosporin [32]. Treatment duration is at least 6 to 12 months and, perhaps, indefinitely since recurrences have been reported [32].

4.4. HIV-infection/AIDS-related pulmonary melioidosis

Melioidosis is caused by the Gram-negative motile bacillus, *Burkholderia (Pseudomonas) pseudomallei* [32]. A previous study in Bangkok, Thailand, 49 cases were observed between 1975 and 1987 [32]. Of these patients, 20 had localized disease while 29 had disseminated disease [32]. Almost all of these patients had an underlying immunocompromised condition like hematological malignancy, collagen vascular disease, and diabetes mellitus [32]. One case had AIDS and presented with left lung infiltrates and recurrent bacteremic melioidosis [32]. More than 750 cases of melioidosis have occurred during the last two decades, and over 75% of the patients were farmers [32]. The disease is endemic in southeast Asia, west Africa, and northern Australia [32]. The clinical manifestations of melioidosis are non- specific but in immunocompromised patients, they usually present with fever and pulmonary infiltrates [32]. The roentgenographic presentation is also non-specific and may demonstrate diffuse infiltrates, hilar adenopathy, lung abscess, or extensive pneumonia, thus the diagnosis requires isolation of this microorganism, particularly by culture of blood and/or respiratory samples in cases with disseminated disease [32]. A previous study by Cheepsattayakorn *et al* at the 10th Zonal Tuberculosis and Chest Disease Center, Chiang Mai, Thailand in 2001 among a number of patients with clinical and roentgenographic presentations mimicked *Burkholderia (Pseudomonas) pseudomallei* pneumonia revealed no detection of the laboratory-confirmed cases but having dramatic response to 6-12 months of tetracycline treatment [42]. A previous study in Thailand reported that 14 immunocompromised melioidosis patients with disease dissemination had a treatment delay or were appropriately treated, all but one were dead [32]. Thus, rapid and early diagnosis and treatment with combined antimicrobials is crucial [32]. It should be emphasized that most HIV- infected/AIDS patients in Thailand are urban dwellers and that most melioidosis cases occur in farmers [32]. Thus, the incidence of melioidosis is expected to increase as the HIV epidemic spread into rural area [32]. *Burkholderia (Pseudomonas) pseudomallei* is usually susceptible to tetracycline, chloramphenicol, trimethoprim-sulphamethoxazole, and third-generation cephalosporin [32]. If the patient is seriously clinical toxic, two antimicrobials are usually recommended during the initial 30 days and followed by 60-150 days of trimethoprim-sulphamethoxazole alone [32]. In septicemic melioidosis, trimethoprim-sulphamethoxazole plus a third-generation cephalosporin are recommended [32]. For patients who are intolerant to trimethoprim-sulphamethoxazole, another antimicrobial listed above should be replaced [32].

4.5. HIV-infection/AIDS-related fungal pneumonia

4.5.1. Pulmonary histoplasmosis

Histoplasma capsulatum is a dimorphic soil dwelling fungus which is rare in Africa before the AIDS epidemic [43]. This microorganism is endemic in the Americas [43]. Histoplasmosis was reported in 1984 in a Zairean AIDS patients and subsequently was identified in a few post-mortem-examined lungs in Zaire [43]. African histoplasmosis is also caused by *Histoplasma duboisii,* a fungal disease which is not increased in Congo but occurs mainly in Central and West Africa [44]. Carme *et al* reported a 26-year-old Congolese male with disseminated *Histoplasma duboisii* infection [45]. In 1987, a white heterosexual European patient was reported with African histoplasmosis [46, 47]. Three Belgian AIDS patients who had lived in Africa disseminated *Histoplasma duboisii* infection whereas one of these patients developed pulmonary disease [48]. An African HIV-2 infected child from Guinea Bissau was reported with disseminated disease [46]. Amphotericin B remains the drug of choice for the treatment of histoplasmosis with AIDS [49]. Ketoconazole, with or without a prior course of amphotericin B, has been used, but sometimes with unacceptable results [50]. After induction therapy, patients should be maintained on lifelong maintenance therapy with either weekly intravenous amphotericin B, oral itraconazole, or oral fluconazole [50].

4.5.2. Pulmonary cryptococcosis

Cryptococcus neoformans, a budding encapsulated yeast is distributed worldwide [50]. In Haiti, the prevalence of cryptococcosis among AIDS patients was approximately 13% whereas as many as 30% of AIDS patients in some areas of subsahara Africa had cryptococcosis [51]. Most of the patients present with disseminated disease or meningitis although the lungs is the usual portal of entry, thus, isolated pulmonary involvement is unusual [32]. A previous study in Bujumbura, Burundi demonstrated that only one patients of 222 cases was diagnosed cryptococcal pneumonia [52] while two of 40 Ugandan patients in a previous study were diagnosed cryptococcal pneumonia [53] but no cases with pulmonary cryptococcosis in Cote d' Ivoire was reported in a post-mortem study [54]. Previous data from Rwanda indicated that cryptococcal pneumonia was common in this country [55, 56]. Between January 1990 and March 1992, 28 Rwandese HIV-1 infected patients were diagnosed cryptococcal pneumonia by isolation from sputum, pleural fluid, and bronchoalveolar lavage (BAL) [55]. The serum cryptococcal antigen testing was negative in all patients without extrapulmonary site of infection [55]. Generally, there are two varieties of *Cryptococcus neoformans,* and gattii [57]. Most HIV-1 infected cases were reported of neoformans variety [57]. Variety gattii is mainly restricted to tropical and subtropical areas [57]. Since 1987, six cases of variety gattii have been reported from Rwanda, Brazil, and Zaire [57]. One Rwandese patient with negative serum and cerebrospinal fluid cryptococcal antigen demonstrated right hilar adenopathy accompanying a right lower lung infiltrate [57]. *Cryptococcus neoformans* variety gattii was isolated from the BAL fluid when the patient did not respond to penicillin and trimethoprim-sulphamethoxazole [57]. Taelman *et al* demonstrated that itraconazole(200 mg/

day) was effective in preventing future disease dissemination for Rwandese patients with isolated pulmonary cryptococcosis [56]. Fluconazole (400-800 mg/day) has been shown to be effective as primary treatment as well as long-term therapy (200- 400 mg/day) [50]. In the USA, the drug of choice for treatment of cryptococcosis is amphotericin B, with or without flucytosine [50]. Nevertheless, these antimicrobials are frequently not available in tropical countries [50].

4.5.3. Pulmonary paracoccidioidomycosis

Paracoccidioidomycosis is caused by the dimorphic fungus *Paracoccidioides brasiliensis* [58]. The patients with paracoccidioidomycosis may present with cutaneous form, isolated pulmonary involvement, or disseminated form [58]. Most patients present with disseminated involvement [58]. Only few cases involving HIV-1 infection have been reported despite its endemicity [58]. The chest roentgenographic findings demonstrate notable diffuse reticulonodular infiltrates, and sometimes with hilar adenopathy [59]. Patients have been successfully treated with various regimens including amphotericin B, imidazole compounds, and sulphadiazine [60]. Itraconazole (100 mg/day) appears to be more effective than ketoconazole (200-400 mg/day) which has been successfully used to treat paracoccidioidomycosis in immunocompetent patients with unknown treatment duration [60]. Nevertheless, the recommended treatment duration is 6 to 18 months [60]. At least two patients have been placed on suppressive therapy with sulphadiazine (1-6 g/day) for lifelong prophylaxis with good early results [60].

4.5.4. Pulmonary penicillosis

This disease caused by the usual dimorphic fungus, *Penicillium marneffei,* both in normal and immunocompromised hosts [61]. This fungus is endemic to southeast Asia and southern China [61]. Most cases have been reported as a systemic mycoses [61]. A previous study from Thailand demonstrated that 11 of the 21 patients had a cough as their presentation [61]. Of the 6 cases with abnormal chest roentgenographic findings, 3 showed diffuse reticulonodular infiltrates, 2 had localized interstitial infiltrates, and 1 had a focal alveolar infiltrate [61]. Definite diagnosis is usually made from cultures of blood, bone marrow, or skin biopsy [61]. The current treatment of choice is 6-8 weeks of Amphotericin B (40 mg/kg) [32]. In in above study in Thailand by Supparapinyo *et al*, 6 of 8 patients who were treated with Amphotericn B responded well [61]. Nevertheless, 6 of 9 patients who were treated with 400 mg itraconazole for eight weeks also well responded [61]. Unfortunately, 4 patients died before treatment started [61]. *Penicillium marneffei* infection may become more common as HIV-infection/AIDS move into rural areas as with melioidosis [32].

4.5.5. Pneumocystis jeroveci (carinii) pneumonia (Pulmonary pneumocystosis)

Currently, the taxonomy of *Pneumocystis jeroveci (carinii)* is in question, but recent data demonstrated it is closely related to fungus [62]. Generally, *Pneumocystis jeroveci (carinii)* is a ubiquitous microorganism found every region of the world [63]. During the course of HIV disease/AIDS, 75% of the patients may develop *Pneumocystis jeroveci (carinii)* pneumonia (PCP) [64]. A previous study by Cheepsattayakorn *et al* at the 10th Zonal Tuberculosis and Chest Disease center, Chiang Mai, Thailand between 1999 and 2000 among 49 HIV-infected/AIDS patients who had clinical manifestations and chest roentgenographic findings compatible with PCP revealed that only one patient demonstrated induced sputum-reverse transcriptase polymerase chain reaction (RT-PCR)- confirmed PCP whereas two patients were confirmed by blood RT-PCR [65]. Nevertheless, the frequency of PCP is quite different in tropical countries [66]. Blaser *et al* reported that 20% of PCP occurred among HIV-infected/AIDS individuals native to the tropics (35%) was significantly lower than for HIV-infected/AIDS individuals in more developed countries (73%) [66]. PCP has been detected in 37% of AIDS patients of African origin in the USA and in 14-24% of African patients with AIDS treated in Europe [67]. The question is whether the exposure to *Pneumocystis jeroveci (carinii)* occurred in Africa or after leaving is not known. A previous study from Zimbabwe reported that of 50 HIV-infected/AIDS patients with acute interstitial pneumonia, 17 and 16 were diagnosed PCP and TB, respectively [68]. By using sputum induction with hypertonic saline, researchers in Tanzania reported that 3 of 83 specimens (3-6%) were positive for *Pneumocystis jeroveci (carinii)* [69]. A number of previous studies in 229 AIDS cases from Haiti indicated that PCP was detected in only 7% of 131 cases compared with 71% of the first 80 AIDS patients noted at the New York Hospital in New York City, USA [70]. Chequer *et al* reported their study in Brazil of 2,135 adult AIDS patients and demonstrated that 425 cases (20%) were diagnosed PCP whereas PCP plus another infection was detected in 265 cases (12%) [71] whereas 45% of homosexual urban AIDS patients in southern Brazil were diagnosed PCP [72]. The clinical and roentgenographic presentations of PCP are likely to be similar among the different regions [68]. Nevertheless, the frequent occurrence of TB in developing countries makes differentiation of the two diseases difficult [68], but in one study, the clinical picture most consistent with PCP was a respiratory rate of over 40/minute [68]. In contrast, the coarse reticulonodular infiltrates on the chest roentgenogram is most likely to be TB [68]. Currently, the treatment of choice for PCP is trimethoprim-sulphamethoxazole [32]. Other alternative antipneumocystis drugs are often not available in the tropical countries [32]. It has been postulated that HIV-infected/AIDS patients in the tropics die before they become immunocompromised enough to develop PCP [54, 73, 74].

4.6. HIV-infection/AIDS-related parasitic pneumonia

4.6.1. Pulmonary strongyloidiasis

Very few parasitic diseases have been reported to cause pneumonia in HIV- infected/AIDS patients [32]. A helminth, *Strongyloides stercoralis* which is commonly found in many tropical and subtropical areas, has occasionally been reported as the cause of pulmonary disease [32]. The prevalence of this helminth in stool specimen varies from region to region as the following : 26-48% in subsahara Africa, 15-82% in Brazil, 1-16% in Ecuador, and 4-40% in the USA [75]. Although the prevalence of strongyloides infection in southeast Asia is high, but no cases have been reported in the English language literature [32]. There have been relatively few cases reported of helminth infection in AIDS patients in the tropics despite its high prevalence [32]. In a previous study in Brazil, 10% of 100 AIDS patients were infected with *Strongyloides stercoralis* [76] whereas in a study in Zambia, 6% of 63 HIV-infected patients with chronic diarrhea were infected with *Strongyloides stercoralis* [77]. The parasitic females live in the mucous membrane (wall) of small intestine of humans, particularly in the lamina propria of the duodenum and proximal jejunum whereas the parasitic males remain in the lumen of the bowel and they have no capability to penetrate the mucous membrane [78]. The rhabditiform larvae that emanating from the eggs pierce the mucous membrane and reach the lumen of the bowel [78]. These larvae are then passed with feces and can penetrate the intestinal epithelium or perianal skin without leaving the host by metamorphosing into filariform larvae in the lumen of small intestine [78]. This contributes to autoinfection and persistence of infection for 20 to 30 years in individuals who have left the endemic regions [79]. Most patients with hyperinfection present with cough, fever, and breath shortness and usually diffuse pulmonary infiltrates [80]. The definite diagnosis is identifying the helminth in the respiratory specimens or stool [80]. Previous reports demonstrated that at least two cases with strongyloides hyperinfection had concomitant PCP [81, 82]. In a previous review of the literature revealed that only surviving patients were treated with thiabendazole, 25 mg/kg twice a day for five days with three courses 10 days apart followed by monthly course of thiabendazole whereas the duration of treatment in HIV-1 infected individual is unknown [82]. Generally, most patients have died directly or indirectly from their strongyloides hyperinfection [82]. It seem cautious to treat any patient who is infected with *Strongyloides stercoralis* detected in the stool despite the rarity of clinically significant strongyloides infection in HIV-infected/AIDS patients [82].

4.6.2. Pulmonary ascariasis

Ascaris lumbricoides is the most common intestinal helminthic infection [83]. Both fertilized and unfertilized eggs are passed in the feces and released in the soil [84]. Infection occurs through soil contamination of hand or food with eggs and then swallowed [84]. The eggs hatch into larvae in the small bowel, call " first stage ", then moult into second-stage larvae in the lumen of the small bowel. The second-stage larvae penetrate the wall of the intestine and migrate via lymphatics and capillaries to the hepatic circulation and to the right side of the heart and then reach the lungs [84]. The second-stage larvae larvae moult twice more in the alveoli to produce third- and fourth-stage larvae. The fourth-stage larvae which are formed 14 days after ingestion migrate upward to the trachea and then are swallowed to reach back the small bowel [84]. The fourth-stage larvae take approximately 10 days for migration from the lungs to the small intestine [84]. It takes 10-25 days to produce eggs after initial ingestion [84]. The migrating larvae can induce tissue- and lung- granuloma formation with macrophages, neutrophils, and eosinophils [85]. This may produce a hypersensitivity in the lungs and result in peribronchial inflammation, increased bronchial mucus production and finally, bronchospasm [85]. *Ascaris lumbricoides* can produces both specific and polyclonal IgE [85]. Elevation of IgG4 levels in patients with ascariasis have also been reported [86]. Symptomatic pulmonary involvement may range from mild cough to a Loffler's syndrome which is a self-limiting lung inflammation and is associated with blood and pulmonary eosinophilia, particularly childhood ascariasis [87, 88]. This syndrome can occur as a result of exposure to various drugs. Clinical Presentation may vary from malaise, fever, loss of appetite, myalgia, and headache [87, 88] to respiratory symptoms which include sputum-productive cough, chest pain, hemoptysis, shortness of breath, and wheezing [89]. Chest roentgenographic findings usually demonstrate peripherally basal opacities, but occasionally show unilateral, bilateral, transient, migratory, non-segmental opacities of various sizes [90].

4.6.3. Pulmonary ancylostomiasis

4.6.3.1. Ancylostoma duodenale

Ancylostoma duodenale can live only one year [91, 92]. Female *Ancylostoma duodenale* produces 10,000 to 30,000 eggs per day [91, 92]. Man is the only definite host [91, 92]. *Ancylostoma duodenale* larvae can enter the human host via the oral route in addition to the entry through the skin and reach pulmonary circulation through the lymphatics and venules [91]. *Ancylostoma duodenale* larvae can developmentally get arrested in the intestine or muscle and restart development when environmental conditions become favorable [93]. Bronchitis and bronchopneumonia can occur when the larvae break through the pulmonary capillaries to enter the alveolar spaces [32, 91, 92]. Pulmonary larval migration can develop peripheral blood eosinophilia [32, 91, 92]. Hookworm larvae can release a family of protein called " ancylostoma-secreted proteins (ASP) " [32, 91, 92] and can secrete low-molecular weight polypeptides which inhibit clotting factor Xa and tissue factor VIIa [94]. During pulmonary larval migration, the patients may present with cough, fever, wheezing, and transient pulmonary infiltrates that is associated with blood and pulmonary eosinophilia [32]. Both albendazole (single dose of 400 mg) and mebendazole (100 mg twice daily for three days) are drug of choice for treatment of hookworm [32]. Pyrantel pamoate (single dose of 11 mg/kg with maximum dose of 1 g, orally) is an alternative drug of choice [32]. A previous study revealed that ivermectin can effectively treat hookworm infections [32].

4.6.3.2. Necator americanus

Necator americanus larvae can infect human only through the skin [91]. The larvae reach the lungs same mechanisms as the *Ancylostoma duodenale* [32]. The interval between the time of skin penetration and laying of eggs by adult worms is about six weeks [32]. Bronchitis and bronchopneumonia can occur when the larvae break through the pulmonary capillaries to enter the alveoli [32]. Drugs of choice for treatment of *Necator americanus* are the same as the drugs of choice for treatment of *Ancylostoma duodenale* [32].

4.6.4. Pulmonary paragonimiasis

In Asia, nearly 20 million people are infected with *Paragonimus* species such as *Paragonimus westernmani* which is the main species in humans, *Paragonimus mexicanus*, *Paragonimus africa-*

nus, Paragonimus miyazakii, Paragonimus phillipinensis, Paragonimus kellicotti, Paragonimus skrjabini, Paragonimus heterotremus, and *Paragonimus uterobilateralis* [95-97]. Paragonimiasis is a food-borne zoonoses [32]. Humans get *Paragonimus* species when ingest raw crayfishes or crabs infected with infective metacercariae [95]. The parasite from the human gut passes through several organs and tissues to reach the lungs [95]. Adult worm live in the lungs and the eggs are voided in the sputum or feces [95]. Pulmonary paragonimiasis manifests as chronic cough, hemoptysis, chest pain, and fever [98]. Pneumothorax or pleural effusion is an important manifestation in paragonimiasis [99]. Chest roentgenographs may demonstrate infiltrates, nodules, and cavities [100]. The parasitic eggs can be shown in sputum specimens, bronchoalveolar lavage fluid or lung biopsy specimens [32].Peripheral blood eosinophilia and elevated serum IgE levels are demonstrated in more than 80% of cases with paragonimiasis [95, 99]. *Paragonimus westernmani* adult excretory-secretory products are composed of cysteine proteases which are involved in immunological reactions during parasitic infection [101, 102]. Immunoglobulin G4 antibodies to an excretory-secretory product of *Paragonimus heterotremus* had accuracy, sensitivity, specificity, and positive and negative predictive values of 97.6%, 100%, 96.9%, 90%, and 100%, respectively [103]. Paragonimiasis can be treated with praziquantel 75 mg/kg/day for three days), triclabendazole (20 mg/kg in two equal doses), niclofolan (2 mg/kg as a single dose), or bithionol (30 to 40 mg/kg in 10 days on alternative days) [95, 104, 105].

4.6.5. Pulmonary schistosomiasis

Schistosoma species that cause human disease are *Schistosoma hematobium, Schistosoma japonicum,* and *Schistosoma mansoni* [106]. The schistosome eggs are passed in feces (*Schistosoma japonicum* and *Schistosoma mansoni*) or in urine (*Schistosoma hematobium*) [32]. The infective cercariae in water are ingested to penetrate the human gut or penetrate human skin and finally reside at the mesenteric beds (*Schistosoma japonicum* and *Schistosoma mansoni*) and the urinary bladder vesicle beds (*Schistosoma hematobium*) [32]. Pulmonary schistosomiasis can clinically present as acute or chronic form [32]. Acute manifestations, called " Katayama syndrome " can develop three to eight weeks after skin penetration [107, 108]. The acute form presents with dry cough, wheezing, shortness of breath, chill, fever, weight loss, abdominal pain, diarrhea, urticarial, myalgia [108, 109], and small pulmonary nodules in chest roentgenographs or computed tomography in immunocompromised patients [110]. Patients with chronic form present with pulmonary hypertension and cor-pulmonale [111, 112] whereas massive hemoptysis and lobar consolidation and collapse have been reported [113]. Hepatosplenomegaly due to portal hypertension has been reported in patients infected with *Schistosoma japonicum* and *Schistosoma mansoni* [106]. In chronic form, peripheral blood eosinophilia with mild leukocytosis, IgE levels, and abnormal liver function test are reported [106]. Acute and chronic schistosomiasis can be treated with corticosteroids alone followed by praziquantel (20-30 mg/kg orally in two doses within 12 hours) and then praziquantel is repeated several weeks later to eradicate the adult flukes [106]. Acute form can be treated with artemether, an artemisinin derivative [106].

4.6.6. Pulmonary hydatid disease

Human hydatid disease is caused by *Echinococcus multilocularis* and *Echinococcus granulosus* [32]. Hydatid cysts are mainly formed in the lungs and liver [32]. Pulmonary alveolar echinococcosis (AE) is caused by hematogenous spreading from hepatic lesions [114]. The adult *Echinococcus granulosus* resides mainly in the small gut of the dogs [32]. Humans are infected by ingestion of parasitic eggs excreted in the feces of the dogs [32]. Clinical pulmonary manifestations include cough, dyspnea, chest pain, and fever [32]. Rupture of hydatid cysts into a bronchus may result in expectoration of cystic fluid containing parasite membrane, hemoptysis, asthma-liked symptoms, respiratory distress, persistent pneumonia, anaphylactic shock, and sepsis [115, 116] and elevation of IgG and eosinophilia [117]. Immunodiagnostic tests using purified *Echinococcus granulosus* antigens have preferable sensitivity and specificity for the diagnosis of AE [118]. Chest roentgenographs demonstrate solitary or multiple round opacificaties mimicking lung tumors [119]. It has been experimentally revealed that magnetic resonance imaging can detect early pulmonary AE [120]. Many year-treatment with mebendazole, praziquantel or albendazole is useful, particularly in inoperably recurrent and multiple cysts, but treatment of hydatid cyst is primary surgical [121]. The treatment of AE is radical surgical resection of entire parasitic lesion [121] but should avoid segmentectomy, lobectomy, and pneumonectomy [122-124].

4.6.7. Pulmonary trichinellosis

The most important species that infect humans is *Trichinella spiralis* [125]. Humans get parasitic infection from ingestion of raw and infected pig's muscle containing larval trichinellae [126]. The larvae develop into adults in the duodenum and jejunum [126]. The larvae undergo encystment in the muscle and a host capsule develops around the larvae and later on may get calcified [126]. Clinical pulmonary features include cough, dyspnea, and pulmonary infiltrates on the chest roentgenographs [127]. The important laboratory findings are elevation of serum aminotransferase, serum adolase, serum lactate dehydrogenase, and serum creatine phosphokinase, leukocytosis, and eosinophilia [127]. An enzyme-linked immunosorbent assay (ELISA) for identification of anti-*Trichinella* antibodies using excretory-secretory antigens may be useful in the diagnosis of *Trichinella spiralis* infection [128], a definite diagnosis can be performed by muscle biopsy (preferably deltoid muscle) [127]. Treatment of choice is with mebendazole, 200 to 400 mg, three times a day for three days followed by 400 to 500 mg, three times a day for 10 days [32]. The alternative drug of choice is albendazole, 400 mg per day for three days followed by 800 mg per day for 15 days [32]. Symptomatic treatment of trichinosis is analgesics and corticosteroids [32].

5. Filarial parasites — Related tropical pulmonary eosinophilia and HLA

This syndrome results from immunological hyperresponsiveness to human filarial parasites, *Wuchereria bancrofti* and *Brugia malayi* [129]. Tropical pulmonary eosinophilia (TPE) is one of the main causes of pulmonary eosinophilia in the tropical countries and is prevalent in filarial endemic regions of the world particularly Southeast Asia [129, 130]. Clinical findings are cough, fever, chest pain, and body weight loss in association with massive blood eosinophilia [131]. Chest roentgenographs demonstrate military infiltrates of both lungs mimic military TB [132]. Additionally, there may be prominent hila with heavy vascular markings [133-136], but 20% of cases present with normal chest roentgenographs [137]. Some previous studies of computed tomographic scan of the chest demonstrated air trapping, mediastinal lymphadenopathy, calcification, and bronchiectasis [138]. At least 120 million people are globally infected with mosquito-borne lymphatic filariasis [137], but only less than 1% of filarial infection causes TPE [139] whereas various studies have demonstrated that filarial infection is the cause of TPE [129, 140]. A positive immediate reaction to intradermal skin tests with *Dirofilaria immitis* antigens have been demonstrated in patients with TPE [141]. Microfilariae, anatomical features of *Wuchereria bancrofti* had demonstrated in the lungs, liver, and lymph nodes of the patients with TPE [142-144], but are rarely identified in the blood [142]. A recent study revealed that the CD45RA$^+$ and CD45RA$^-$ effector cells in patients with chronic lymphatic filarial infection demonstrated a reduced activation state based on their lower expression of *HLA-DR*, contrasting with findings identified in patients with HIV-1 infection [145]. An inverse correlation between the percentage of CD8$^+$ HLA-DR$^+$ lymphocytes pokeweed mitogen-induced proliferation was observed [146]. These findings indicated that activated CD8$^+$- T lymphocytes may be involved in the pathogenesis of chronically obstructive lymphatic form of filariasis [146]. A previous study conducted by Sasisekhar *et al* demonstrated that monocytes from microfilaremic (MF) patients revealed an inability to respond to lipopolysaccharide compared to monocytes from endemic normal individuals of from patients with lymphedema [147]. Serum from MF patients demonstrated reduction of adherence and spreading of normal monocytes which was a finding not observed with serum from other clinical individuals [147]. Surprisingly, there was a significant correlation between the adherence of normal lymphocytes and the production of interleukin (IL)-1β with spontaneous secretion of IL-10 [147]. The effects noted were not a result of diminished viability or alteration in the expression of the cell surface markers *HLA-DR* and CD14 [147]. This study indicates that monocyte function is dampened in MF patients [147]. A previous study in Sri Lanka and India demonstrated that 30% of Sri Lankan patients with elephantiasis and 28% of Southern Indian patients with elephantiasis were significantly associated with *HLA-B*15* compared to 4% of Sri Lankan controls and 10% of Southern Indian controls [148]. Filarial specific IgG and IgE concentration elevation have been observed in TPE [149]. Peripheral basophils from patients with TPE was released more greater amounts of histamine when they were challenged with *Wuchereria* or *Brugia* antigens than with *Dirofilaria* antigen [149]. This indicated that TPE resulted from immunological hyperresponsiveness to human filarial parasites [149]. Leukocyte adhesion phenomenon in sera from patients with TPE using *Wuchereria bancrofti* revealed maximal positive results compared with *Dirofilaria immitis* and *Dirofilaria repens* [150]. Demonstration of living adult *Wuchereria bancrofti* in the lymphatic vessels of the spermatic cord of the patients with TPE is evidenced by ultrasound examination [151] and biopsy of a lump in the spermatic cord shows degenerating adult female filarial worm with uteri full of microfilariae [152]. There is a marked reduction of filarial-specific IgG and IgE levels in the lung epithelial lining fluid [153] and roentgenological improvement [154, 155] after 6-14 days of therapy with dethylcarbamazine citrate (DEC). The standard treatment recommended by the World Health Organization is oral DEC (6 mg/kg/day) for three weeks [156]. The usefulness of DEC in the treatment of TPE further focuses attention on its filarial etiology [157, 158].

6. Pulmonary malaria and HLA

Four types of malarial parasites (*Plasmodium falciparum, Plasmodium malariae, Plasmodium vivax,* and *Plasmodium ovale*), the protozoa of the genus *Plasmodium* causes malaria and is primarily transmitted by the bite of an infected female *Anopheles* mosquito to infect humans [159]. A previous study in a Thai population demonstrated that the allele frequencies of *HLA-B*46, -B*56,* and *-DRB1*1001* were statistically different between non- cerebral severe malaria and cerebral malaria, between mild malaria and non-cerebral malaria, and mild malaria and cerebral malaria, respectively [160]. A recent study revealed that the NK cell repertoire shaped by the *KIR2DL3-HLA-C1* interaction demonstrates certain functional responses that facilitates the development of cerebral malaria [161]. The frequency of the *KIR2DL3-HLA-C1* combination was found to be significantly lower in malaria high-endemic populations [161]. This indicates that natural selection has reduced the frequency of the *KIR2DL3-HLA-C1* combination in in malaria high-endemic populations because of the propensity of interaction between *KIR2DL3* and *C1* to favor development of cerebral malaria [161]. Young *et al* conducted a study in Mali and Gambia and reported that either malaria parasite types cp26 or cp29 were found to be less, not more common in Mali population with *HLA-B*35* (37%) compared to non-*HLA-B*35*-bearing hosts (55%) whereas 51% of *HLA-B*35*-bearing Gambian population were infected with either cp26 or cp29 compared to 42% of non-*HLA-B*35*-bearing hosts [162]. A previous study in West African children demonstrates that *HLA-Bw*53, -DRB1*1302,* and *-DQB1*0501* which are common in West Africans are independently associated with protection from severe malaria [163]. *HLA-DR*04* alleles were observed more frequently among patients with severe malaria [164]. Additionally, carriers of the amino acid methionine at position 11 of the *DPA1* allele were more often infected with merozoite surface antigen (MSA)-1 K1 malaria parasites and less frequently with MSA-1 RO33 malaria parasite infection [164]. The main finding of patients with falciparum malaria which is the most deadly type of malaria infection is sequestration of erythrocytes containing mature forms of *Plasmodium falciparum* in the microvasculature of the organs and is quantified by measurement of *Plasmodium falciparum* specific histidine-rich protein 2 (PfHRP2) using a quantitative antigen-capture enzyme-linked immunosorbent assay [159]. Gas exchange is significantly impaired in patients with severe malaria [165]. The gold standards for the diagnosis of malaria are light microscopic examination of thin and thick stained blood smears [78, 166]. Human urine and saliva PCR detection of *Plasmodium falciparum* has been introduced [166]. In severe falciparum malaria, the roentgenographic presentations include diffuse interstitial edema, pulmonary edema, pleural effusion, and lobar consolidation [166]. Intravenous chloroquine is the drug of choice for chloroqiune-susceptible *Plasmodium falciparum* infections and those rare cases of life-threatening malaria caused by *Plasmodium* *vivax, Plasmodium malariae*, and *Plasmodium ovale* [78, 166]. A point mutation in the *Plasmodium falciparum* chloroqiune-resistance transporter (PfCRT) gene is responsible for chloroqiune-resistant falciparum malaria [167] whereas diaappearance of the K76T mutation in PfCRT is associated with chloroquine susceptibility [168]. Oral artemisinin -based combination therapies (artesunate + mefloquine, artesunate + sulfadoxine-pyrimethamine, artesunate + amodioquine, or artemether + lumefantrine) are the best antimalarial drugs [169, 170]. Additionally, the World Health Organization (WHO) recommends oral treatment of dihydroartemisinin plus piperaquine as soon as the patients is able to take oral medication but not before a minimum of 24 hours of parenteral treatment [171]. The WHO recommended that intravenous artesunate can be used preferentially over quinine for the treatment of severe malaria caused by any *Plasmodium* species in both children and adults [172]. Oral artemisinin-based combination therapies have also demonstrated equivalent (if not better) efficacy in the treatment of uncomplicated malaria caused by all *Plasmodium* species and chloroquine-resistant *Plasmodium vivax* in both children and adults [172]. Hence, conventional therapeutic regimens continue to be efficacious [172]. Insecticide-treated bed-nets in which insecticide is incorporated into the net fibers is evidenced to be the best way to prevent malaria [173]. It is demonstrated that RTS, S/ASO2, a vaccine has demonstrated promising results in endemic areas [173].

7. Pulmonary amoebiasis and HLA

Pulmonary amoebiasis that caused by the protozoan parasite, *Entamoeba histolytica* occurs mainly by the extension from the amoebic liver abscess [174, 175]. In a nine-year prospective study in a cohort of preschool children in Dhaka, Bangladesh demonstrated that a single amino acid polymorphism (Q223R) in the leptin receptor was associated with increased susceptibility to *Entamoeba histolytica* infection [176]. Children with two arginine alleles (223R) were nearly four times more likely to infect with *Entamoeba histolytica* as compared to those homozygous for glutamine (223Q) [176]. An *in vitro* study demonstrated that leptin signaling protected human epithelial cells from amoebic killing via a STAT3- dependent pathway [177]. It was identified that children who were heterozygous for the HLA class II *DQB1*0601/DRB1*1501* haplotype were more likely to *Entamoeba histolytica* negative [178]. The immune mechanism that explains why only a subset of *Entamoeba histolytica*-exposed persons develops clinical disease is not fully understood [179]. The effect of microbiota on immune response to *Entamoeba histolytica* and its virulence is not yet known [179]. The presence of cysts or trophozoites of amoeba in the stool does not imply that the disease is caused by *Entamoeba histolytica* as other two non-pathogenic species found in humans (*Entamoeba dispar* and *Entamoeba moshkovskii*) are morphologically indistinguishable, but can be rapidly, accurately, and effectively diagnosed by a single-round PCR [78, 180, 181]. Other diagnostic methods include culture of *Entamoeba histolytica*, ELISA, indirect fluorescent antibody test (IFAT), and indirect hemagglutination test (IHA) [78, 180, 181]. A combination of serological tests with identification of the parasite by PCR or antigen detection is the best diagnostic approach [182]. Active trophozoites of *Entamoeba histolytica* can be identified in sputum or pleural specimen [78]. Physical examination reveals fever, chest pain, tender hepatomegaly, and cough are indicated pleuropulmonary amoebiasis [78]. Some patients may present with hemoptysis, expectoration of anchovy source-liked pus, respiratory distress, and shock [78]. Chest roentgenographic findings include pleural effusion, basal pulmonary involvement, and elevation of hemidiaphragm [78]. Metronidazole is the treatment of choice [183]. Diloxanide furoate, a luminal amoebiacidal drug can eliminate intestinal *Entamoeba* cysts [184]. Lactoferrin and lactoferricins, amoebicidal drugs, can be co-administered with a low dose of metronidazole to reduce metronidazole toxicity [184]. Identification of possible vaccine candidates against amoebiasis are in progressive studies [185].

8. Pulmonary leishmaniasis and HLA

Pulmonary or visceral leishmaniasis, also called " Kala azar " is caused by *Leishmania donovani* and and *Leishmania chagasi* or *infantum* [186] is transmitted by various species of *Phebotomus*, a type of sand fly [187]. *Leishmania amastigotes* can be identified in pulmonary septa, alveoli, and the BAL fluid [188, 189]. Pleural effusion, mediastinal lymphadenopathy, and pneumonitis have been reported in HIV-infected patients with visceral leishmaniasis and lung transplant patients [188, 189]. The expansion of the HIV- infection/AIDS epidemic over leishmaniasis, particularly visceral leishmaniasis endemic regions has increased the number of co-infected patients [190] indicating that visceral leishmaniasis is an opportunistic disease in HIV-infected/AIDS patients although not yet considered an AIDS-defining disease [191]. According to sharing of immune-compromising mechanisms of both infections with *Leishmania infantum* and HIV-1 that may affect the parasite control in visceral leishmaniasis co-infected patients [191]. In comparison to patients with visceral leishmaniasis alone, co-infected patients present a more severe disease with increased parasite burden, frequent relapses, and anti-leishmanial drug resistance [190, 192]. On the other hand, Leishmania infection can impair both the chronic immune activation and the lymphocyte depletion and can accelerate progression to AIDS, particularly in HIV-1-infected individuals [193, 194]. Hence, serological testings for latent infection due to *Leishmania* species are indicated in the pre-transplantation screening from endemic areas [195]. A recent study in two populations from Brazil (cases) and India (controls) demonstrated that the *HLA-DRB1-HLA-DQA1 HLA* class II region strongly contributed to visceral leishmaniasis susceptibility, indicating shared risk factors for visceral leishmaniasis that cross the epidemiological divides of geography and parasite species [196]. Several previous studies of *Leishmania donovani* in mice model demonstrated dramatic differences in visceral disease in spleens and livers in congenic mice with different H-2 haplotypes [197]. There was evidenced that noncuring and curing responses mapped to the HLA-class II molecules by using recombinant congenic mice [198] and functional analysis blocking IA or IE (corresponding to DQ and DR, respectively) molecules *in vivo* with monoclonal antibodies [199]. A significant role for $CD8^+$ T-cells has also been shown in *Leishmania donovani* [200, 201]. A previous case-control study in Tunisia demonstrated that visceral leishmaniasis was associated with *DR/DQ* class II genes but not with *TNF/LTA* or *HSP70* class III loci [202]. Associations between delayed-type hypersensitivity-positive asymptomatic persons and *TNF* alleles were identified [203]. Positive associations between polymorphisms and various clinical phenotypes for cutaneous leishmaniasis have been demonstrated in a number of small case-control studies [204]. A recent study demonstrated a trend towards susceptibility to cutaneous leishmaniasis for alleles *HLA-DRB1*13, HLA- B*35,* and *HLA-B*44* [205]. *HLA-B*49* allele tended towards susceptibility to recurrent American cutaneous leishmaniasis (ACL), and *HLA-B*52* to re-infection whereas presence of *HLA-B*45* tended towards protection of against the cutaneous form of ACL [205]. *A*02B*44 DRB1*07* and *A*24B*35 DRB1*01* alleles, the most frequent haplotypes may be associated with susceptibility to ACL [205]. Immune activation can profoundly impact the visceral lieshmaniasis clinical course and prognosis, leading to increase the risk of death even under treatment of leishmaniasis [206]. Pentavalent antimonials, pentamidine, and amphotericin B, particularly the liposome formulations, and miltefosine are the drugs for the treatment of lieshmaniasis [207]. A previous study demonstrated that Poly/hsp/pcDNA vaccine can significantly decrease parasite load in spleen and liver indicating a feasible, effective, and practical approach for visceral leishmaniasis [208].

9. Pulmonary trypanosomiasis and HLA

Human African trypanosomiasis (HAT) or sleeping sickness is caused by an extracellularly protozoan parasite, called " *Trypanosoma brucei gambiense* " [209], "*Trypanosoma brucei rhodesiense* " [210] and " *Trypanosoma cruzi* " which was discovered by Carlos Chagas in 1909 [211] and endemic to West Africa and Central Africa, mostly in Democratic Republic of Congo, Angola, Chad, Central African Republic, Uganda, and Sudan [209]. HAT continues to threat more than 60 million people in 36 sub-Saharan countries [209, 212]. In mice model, hypercellularity and edema of alveolar walls, approximately 10 times thicker than normal alveolar wall are identified and results in wall thickening although parasites are not demonstrated in alveoli [211]. Thickening and edema of bronchial walls of small and medium size bronchi due to parasite infiltration and significant inflammatory reaction (except large bronchi) in mice model were observed [211]. These bronchial inflammatory changes result in bronchial lumen reduction [211]. Most infected mice demonstrated infiltration of the walls of large blood vessels with extensive clusters of parasites in the myocytes of the muscular stratum and accompanying by an inflammatory reaction, interstitial edema, and rupture of muscle fibers [211]. These pathologically lung changes can contribute to pulmonary alveolar hemorrhage, bronchiolitis, and pneumonitis [211]. Pulmonary emphysema was also observed in the lungs of infected rats [213]. By the statistical analysis, the difference between experimental groups in lung-parasitic distribution and the degree of inflammatory reaction demonstrated no statistical difference [211]. Most Mexican strains demonstrated cardiomyotropism [211] and could cause pulmonary hypertension that could result in a dilatation of the right ventricle which is a typical characteristic of Chagas' disease caused by *Trypanosoma cruzi* without affecting the left ventricle [211]. However, many cases of Chagas' disease with pulmonary hypertension associated with right ventricular dilatation could attribute to left ventricular failure [214]. Several HLA alleles and haplotype associated with Chagas' disease have studied [215]. The highly polymorphic HLA class I (A, B, and C) and II (DR, DQ, and DP) molecules determine the efficiency of presentation of *Trypanosoma cruzi* epitopes to $CD8^+$ and $CD4^+$ T-cells, respectively [215]. A previous study in Mexican population demonstrated that *HLA –B*39* and *HLA-DR4* alleles were associated with *Trypanosoma cruzi* infection while *HLA-A*68* and *HLA-DR16* allele were markers of protection of development of chronic Chagas' cardiomyopathy (CCC) and heart damage susceptibility, respectively [216]. Another study in Mexico revealed that *HLA-B*39* and *HLA-DR*4* alleles were also more frequently identified in patients with Chagas' disease [1]. A previous study in south-eastern Brazil demonstrated that *HLA-A*30* and *HLA-DQB1*06* alleles were associated with susceptibility to Chagas' disease and protection of Chagas' disease, respectively in regardless of the clinical form of the disease, respectively [217] while *HLA-DR2* allele was associated with susceptibility to chronic Chagas' disease [218]. Nevertheless, in another previous study revealed that polymorphism of *HLA-DR* and *HLA-DQ* alleles did not influence on the susceptibility to different clinical forms of Chagas' disease or the progression to severe Chagas' cardiomyopathy [219]. A study in Chile, it was found that *HLA-B*40* antigen in the presence of Cw3 was significantly lower in patients with CCC [220] and was higher expressed in subjects without cardiac disease in the city of Santiago [221]. A previous study in Venezuela in comparison of HLA class II allele frequencies between patients with Chagas' disease and controls demonstrated a higher frequency of *DQB1*0501*, *DRB1*01*, and *DRB1*08* alleles, and a decreased frequency of *DQB1*0303* and *DRB1*14* alleles whereas patients with congestive heart failure and arrhythmia revealed decreased frequency of *DRB1*1501* allele [222]. A higher frequency of the *HLA-DPB1*0401* allele and *DPB1*0401-HLA-DPB1*2301* or *DPB1*0401-DPB1*3901* haplotype was identified in patients with cardiac manifestations in an endemic area of central Venezuela [223] whereas susceptibility between *HLA-C*03* allele and CCC was confirmed [224]. In several Latin American mestizos from different countries and patients with CCC, there was an increase frequency of *HLA-A*31*, -*B*39*, and -*DR8* alleles and a decrease of frequency of *HLA-DQ1*, -*DQ3*, -*DR4*, and -*DR5* alleles [225]. A study in Bolivia revealed that *HLA-DRB1*0102*, - *DRB*1402*, and *MICA*011* alleles were in strong linkage disequilibrium and there was association between the *HLA-DRB1*01-B*14-MICA*011* haplotype and the resistance against chronic Chagas' disease whereas the frequencies of *HLA-DRB1*01* and *HLA- B*1402* alleles were significant lower in patients with electrocardiogram alteration and/or megacolon compared with a group of patients with indeterminate clinical form [226]. In a study in Argentine population, the class II alleles *HLA-DRB1*0409* and *HLA-DRB1*1503* were significantly more prevalent in Chagas' disease and *HLA-DRB1*1103* allele was associated with Chagas' disease resistance whereas increased frequency of *DRB1*1503* allele was identified in patients with CCC [227, 228]. A previous study on treatment of relapsing trypanosomiasis in Gambian population demonstrated that a 7-day course of intravenous eflornithine was satisfactory and would result in substantial savings compared with the standard 14-day regimen although the prior regimen was inferior to the standard regimen and could be used by the national control programmes in endemic areas, provided that its efficacy was closely monitored whereas melarsoprol remains the only effectively therapeutic option for new cases [229]. In animal experimental studies, eflornithine and melasoprol synergistically act against trypanosomes since the former drug decreases the trypanothione production, the target of the latter drug [230, 231]. A recent study demonstrated that oxidative stress could contribute to parasite persistence in host tissue and the development of anti-*Trypanosoma cruzi* drugs [232].

10. Pulmonary larval migrans

Toxocara larval migrans caused by *Toxocara canis*, a parasite in dogs' intestine and *Toxocara catis*, a parasite in cats' intestine infected intermediate host, humans by ingestion these embryonated *Toxocara* eggs which hatch into infective larvae in the human intestine [78]. The infective larvae then penetrate the intestinal wall and are carried by blood circulation to many organs including lungs, liver, central nervous system, eyes, and muscles [78]. Granulomata then occur in these organs and later develop fibrosis and calcification [78]. A previous study indicated that *Toxocara* species infections were associated with a polarized CD4 Th2-dominat immunity and eosinophilia, mediated mainly be HLA class II molecules, and Foxp3^{+} CD4^{+}CD25^{+}-expressing T regulatory (Treg) cells play a role in regulation of the immunopathology of *Toxocara* granulomas in experimental animals and in enhancing the expression of TGF-β1, which is an important function of Treg demonstrated during *Toxocara canis* invasion in the mouse' s brain [233]. The potential susceptibility loci HLA class II molecules are considered to be involved in regulation of a Th2-dominant immunity which is highly controlled by stimulation through TGF-β1 [233]. Exploration of TGF-β1 polymorphism, Fox3^{+} CD4^{+}CD25^{+} Treg cells permit insight into the contribution produced by environmental and genetic factors in influencing disease syndrome type and severity in human toxocariasis [233]. Pulmonary manifestations are found in 80% and present with severe asthma [78]. Clinical manifestations may demonstrate scattered rales and rhonchi on auscultation including fever, cough, hepatosplenomegaly, generalized lymph node enlargement, eye pain, strabismus, white pupil, unilaterally visual loss, abdominal pain, and neurological manifestations [78]. Some cases may present with severe eosinophilic pneumonia and may contribute to respiratory distress syndrome [234-236]. Chest roentgenogram may demonstrate localized patchy infiltrates [78]. This syndrome is usually associated with eosinophilia, elevated antibody titers to *Toxocara canis*, and increased total serum IgE level [237, 238]. About 25% of childhood patients have no eosinophilia [239]. Identification of serum IgE antibodies by ELISA [240] and *Toxocara* excretory-secretory antigens by Western-blotting method have been reported for diagnosis [241]. Nevertheless, serodiagnostic methods cannot distinguish between past and current infections [240, 241]. *Toxocara* eggs or larvae cannot be identified in the feces since human is not the definitive host [78]. Histopathological examination of lung or liver biopsy specimens may reveal granulomas with multinucleated giant cells, eosinophils, and fibrosis [78]. *Toxocara* larval migrans may be spontaneous resolution, therefore, mild to moderate symptomatic patients need not any treatment [78]. However, patients with severe *Toxocara* larval migrans can be treated with diethylcarbamazine 6 mg/kg/day, 21 days) [242], mebendazole (20-25 mg/kg/day, 21 days) [243] or albendazole (10 mg/kg/day, 5 days) [244]. Exacerbation of the inflammatory reactions in the tissues due to killing of the larvae may occur, therefore, antihelminthics plus corticosteroids is recommended [78].

11. Pulmonary toxoplasmosis and HLA

A celled protozoan parasite, called " *Toxoplasma gondii* " which are primarily carried by cats is causal microorganism [245]. Humans are infected by ingestion of parasitic cyst- contaminated uncooked milk product, vegetables or meat [78]. The clinical manifestations are influenza-liked illness, myalgia or enlarged lymph nodes [78] which is the most common recognized clinical manifestation [246]. Pulmonary involvement has been increasingly reported in HIV-infected/AIDS patients [78]. Pulmonary manifestations may be interstitial pneumonia, diffuse alveolar damage or necrotizing pneumonia [247]. Nevertheless, obstructive or lobar pneumonia has been reported in a 49-year-old Spanish heterosexual man [246]. Early pregnancy with toxoplasmosis can cause fetal death, and chorioretinitis and neurological symptoms in the newborn whereas chronic disease can cause chorioretinitis, jaundice, convulsion, and encephalitis [78]. Association between the *HLA-DQ*3* allele and the susceptibility to toxoplasmic encephalitis in HIV-infected/AIDS patients has been reported [248]. A previous study among Caucasians demonstrated that the *DQ3* gene frequency was significantly higher in infected infants with hydrocephalus than subjects without hydrocephalus [249]. In infected- mice model, human major histocompatibility MHC-class II transgenes reduced parasite burden and brain necrosis that was consistent with the observed association between *HLA-DQ*3* allele and hydrocephalus in human infants [249]. In the murine model, the *DQ3* (*DQ8*, *DQB1*0302*) gene protected less than *DQ1* (*DQ6*, *DQB1*0601*) [249]. These significant findings can provide characterization of the human immune responses that are pathogenic or protective in *Toxoplasma gondii* infections. Diagnosis of toxoplasmosis is based on detection of the protozoan parasites in the body tissues [78]. Sputum examination was used in diagnosis of pulmonary or disseminated toxoplasmosis in a 14-year-old allogeneic bone marrow recipient with graft- versus-host disease by identification of *Toxoplasma gondii* tachyzoites in sputum smears [250]. Serodiagnosis is unable to discriminate between active and chronic *Toxoplasma gondii* infection due to ability to increase the antibody levels without active disease [78]. A real-time-PCR-based assay in BAL fluid has been performed in HIV-infected/AIDS patients [251]. Toxoplasmosis can be treated with a combination regimen of pyrimethamine and sulfadiazine [78].

12. Pulmonary dengue viral infection and HLA

This disease is caused by dengue virus (DENV) that belong to the family *Flaviviridae,* genus *Flavivirus,* and is transmitted to humans by *Aedes* mosquitoes, mainly *Aedes aegypti* [252]. Four serotypes of virus have been identified ; DENV-1, DENV-2, DENV-3, and DENV-4 [252]. An estimated 50 million-infected people occur each year and more than 2.5 billion people are being at risk of infection [253]. Epidemic with high incidences of dengue hemorrhagic fever have been linked to primary infection with DENV-1 followed by infection with DENV-2 or DENV-3 whereas it indicated that the longer the interval between primary and secondary infections, the higher the risk of developing severe disease [254-256]. In adults, primary infections with each of four DENV serotypes, especially with DENV-1 and DENV-3, frequently results in dengue fever whereas some outbreak of primary infections with DENV-2 have been predominantly subclinical [257]. However, adult- dengue infections are frequently accompanied by a tendency for severe hemorrhage [258] and can be life-threatening when infections occur in patients with chronic diseases such as asthma and diabetes [259-261]. Several HLA class I alleles, female sex, AB blood group, a single-nucleotide polymorphism in the tumor necrosis factor gene, and a promoter variant of the DC-SIGN receptor gene are the host factors that increase the risk of severe dengue disease [262-267]. Notably, the first outbreak in the Americas occurred in 1981, which coincided with the introduction of the possibly more virulent DENV-2 Southeast Asian genotype whereas the less virulent indigenous DENV-2 genotype was already circulating in the region [259, 268-270]. Age has been demonstrated to influence the disease outcome following a secondary infection with heterologous DENV [271]. In Asia, the risk of severe disease is greater in children than in adults, in contrast to the Americas [272, 273]. Nevertheless, the finding that dengue hemorrhagic fever or dengue shock syndrome is noted primarily in a relative small percentage of secondary DENV infections and to a much lesser extent in primary infections although with virulent strains indicates that host factors must be critical determinants of severe DENV disease development [252]. There is evidence that DENV antigen is present in the pulmonary vascular endothelium [274] whereas liver is the organ commonly involved in human DENV infections including mouse model [275, 276]. Glucose-6-phosphate dehydrogenase deficiency which is highly prevalence identified among African population [277] can cause abnormal cellular redox, therefore affecting production of hydrogen peroxide, superoxide, and nitric oxide indicating oxidative stress [278]. Viral proliferation and virulence by increasing viral receptors on target cells or increasing of viral particles is known to be affected by oxidative stress [278], therefore, glucose-6-phosphate dehydrogenase deficiency may contribute to increased replication of DENV in monocytes [277]. Several human HLA class I alleles *(-A*01, -A*0207, -A*24, - B*07, -B*46, -B*51)* [262, 264, 279] and HLA class II alleles *(-DQ*1, -DR*1, -DR*4)* [263, 280] are associated with development of dengue hemorrhagic fever. Additionally, a recent study demonstrated that significantly higher frequency of *HLA-A*33* allele in dengue fever patients, *HLA-A*0211* allele in dengue hemorrhagic fever cases compared to controls and dengue fever cases, respectively [281]. The frequency of *HLA-B*18* and *HLA-Cw*07* alleles were significantly higher in DENV-infected cases compared to controls [281]. The combined frequency of *HLA-Cw*07* with *HLA-DRB1*07/*15* genotype was significantly higher in dengue hemorrhagic fever cases as compared to dengue fever cases and controls but the frequency of combination of *HLA-Cw*07* allele without *HLA-DRB1*07* allele was significantly higher in dengue fever cases compared to controls [281]. This study results indicate that *HLA-A*33* allele may be associated with development of dengue fever whereas *HLA-B*18* and *HLA-Cw*07* alleles may be associated with symptomatic dengue infection requiring hospitalization [281]. A previous study demonstrated that *HLA-A*0207* and *HLA-B*51* alleles was associated with dengue hemorrhagic fever in patients having secondary DENV-1 or DENV-2 infection only and children with *HLA-A*24* allele were more likely to develop dengue hemorrhagic fever [282]. After secondary dengue infections, *HLA-B*44, -B*62, -B*76,* and *-B*77* alleles revealed to protect against development of clinical disease [282]. Clinical findings in early febrile stage include fever, headache, malaise, rash, body pain, and later develops pleural effusion [258, 283], both lower lobes infiltration [283], bilateral perihilar edema [284], ascites, bleeding, thrombocytopenia (platelet < 100,000 per mm^3), hematocrit > 20%, and clinical warning signs such as restlessness, severe and continuous abdominal pain, persistent vomiting and a sudden reduction in body temperature associated with profuse perspiration, adynamia (vigor or loss of strength) and sometimes fainting which can be indicative of shock due to plasma extravasation [258]. Dengue disease must be excluded from two syndromes related to hantavirus, hemorrhagic fever with renal syndrome (HFRS) in Eurasia and hantavirus pulmonary syndrome (HPS) in Americas [285-287]. HPS is typically characterized by acute noncardiogenic pulmonary edema and circulatory shock whereas fever, hemorrhagia, and acute renal failure are hallmark findings in HFRS [288]. Laboratory diagnosis of DENV infection include virus isolation, serodiagnostic tests (MAC-ELISA, IgG ELISA, IgG : IgM ratio, neutralization assay), nucleic acid-amplification tests (real-time PCR, reverse-transcriptase PCR, nucleic acid- sequence based amplification assay (NASBA)), and antigen detection (NS1 antigen and antibody detection) [258]. DENV complications include massive hemorrhage, disseminated intravascular coagulation, non-cardiogenic pulmonary edema, respiratory failure, and finally develops multiple organ failure [258]. In uncomplicated dengue cases, treatment is only supportive, but in cases with prolonged or recurrent dengue shock, intravenous fluids should be administered carefully according to dosage and age to prevent pulmonary edema [258]. DENV control and prevention strategies include vector control and vaccine development [258]. Current approaches to vaccine development involve using deoxyribonucleic acid vaccine, chimeric viruses using yellow fever vaccine, subunit vaccine, inactivated viruses, attenuated viruses, and attenuated dengue viruses as backbones [289-294]. An Acambis/Sanofi Pasteur yellow fever-dengue chimeric vaccine is in advanced Phase II testing in children in Thailand [258]. A possible licensed vaccine will be available in less than 10 years [258].

13. Pulmonary leptospirosis and HLA

Leptospirosis is a zoonotic disease caused by genus *Leptospira* which belongs to the phylum of spirochaetes [295]. The 8 pathogenic species of this genus are *Leptospira interrogans, Leptospira borgpetersenii, Leptospira noguchii, Leptospira santarosai, Leptospira kirschneri, Leptospira alstonii, Leptospira alexanderi,* and *Leptospira weilii* [295]. Transmission of leptospirosis requires continuous enzoonotic circulation of the pathogen among animal reservoir or as commonly referred-maintenance host [295]. *Leptospira* serovars reveal specific host preferences with regard to their ability to produce high-grade carriage [295]. Rats (genus *Rattus*) serve as reservoirs for the Icterohaemorrhagiae serogroup while house mice (*Mus musculus*) are the reservoir for the Ballum serogroup [295]. Additionally, serovars often do not cause significant disease in highly adapted-reservoir hosts [295]. A previous study demonstrated that *HLA-DQ*6* allele increased risk of laboratory-confirmed leptospirosis [296]. Pathogenic species produce a systemic infection after an environmental exposure, establish persistent renal and urinary shedding in reservoir animals and cause tissue damage in multiple organs of susceptible hosts [295]. Humans are incidental hosts in which leptospirosis produces acute disease manifestations and does not induce a disease carrier state [295]. The incubation period varies from 2 to 30 days [295]. Clinical presentation in human leptospirosis includes acute febrile illness that often cannot be differentiate from other causes of acute fever illness [295]. The clinical manifestations include fever, headache, myalgia (especially calf muscle), and prostration associated with any of the following symptoms or signs: cough, hemoptysis, breathlessness, conjunctival suffusion, jaundice, oliguria or anuria, internal organ hemorrhages, skin rash, cardiac arrhythmia or failure, and meningeal irritation [297]. Leptospirosis-associated pulmonary hemorrhage syndrome was first described in China and Korea and then was brought to global attention by a large outbreak of severe-from disease in Nicaragua in 1995 [295]. The risks of developing severe leptospirosis include a critical threshold of qPCR- determined leptospiremia, identification of the infective strain, and early laboratory results [298]. The illness usually resolves after the first week of symptoms [295]. The presumptive diagnosis was made from a positive result of a rapid screening test such as latex agglutination test, IgM ELISA, dipstick, lateral flow, etc [297]. The confirmatory diagnosis includes isolation of the organism from blood or other clinical specimens, a positive PCR result, and fourfold or greater rise in titer or seroconversion in microscopic agglutination test (MAT) on paired samples obtained at least 2 weeks apart [297]. Severe case usually treated with intravenous benzylpenicillin (30 mg/kg up to 1.2 g intravenously and 6-hourly for 5-7 days) [297]. Oral administration of doxycycline (2 mg/kg up to 100 mg, 12-hourly for 5-7 days), amoxicillin, ampicillin, or tetracycline is the treatment of choice in less severe cases [297]. The third-generation cephalosporins, such as ceftriazone and cefotaxime, quinolone antimicrobials may also be effective, but Jarrisch-Herxheimer reactions can occur after the start of antimicrobial treatment [297]. The patients should be appropriate monitored and care supported, such as mechanical ventilation, dialysis, etc [297]. A recent study in Thailand demonstrated that only the latex test could be considered cost-effective when compared to the no-antimicrobial option, and that latex test, microcapsule agglutination test, and lateral flow were still inferior to empirical treatment (7-day course of doxycycline, 100 mg bid treatment) [299]. A recent study on vaccine candidates for protection of leptospirosis successfully demonstrated LBJ_2271 as a protein candidate for further study of antigenic immune stimulation for vaccine development [300] whereas another recent study revealed that czcA and its four subunit vaccine peptides could be ideal T-cell driven efficacious vaccine against this disease [301]. Until epidemiologically-validated immune correlates are determined and discovery of vaccine candidates will likely continue to rely on the search for new virulence factors and outer membrane proteins of the organism.

14. Conclusions

Most of several studies have inconclusively demonstrated statistical association between HLA class I and II molecules and susceptibility to a range of complex tropical pulmonary infectious diseases, particularly parasitic pulmonary diseases. The globalization of neglected tropical pulmonary infectious diseases can alert the healthcare providers in diagnosis in recent immigrants or travelers from endemic areas who present with respiratory manifestations and peripheral blood or tissue eosinophilia. A complete re-evaluation of the true impact of HLA/MHC genes on susceptibility to tropical pulmonary infectious diseases. Summary of association between known HLA alleles and susceptibility of some tropical pulmonary infectious diseases are shown in Table 1.

Disease	Known HLA	Influence	Reference
SARS	*HLA-B*0703, HLADRB1*0301*	More prevalent and more poorer outcome	7, 8
	CXCL10(-938AA)/Fg12(+158T/)* or *CXCL10(-938AA)/ HO-1(-497A/*)*	Protective	10
	Fg12(+158T/)*	Susceptible	10
Tuberculosis	*HLA-DQB1*0601, HLA-DRB1*1501HLA-DPB1*02, HLA-DRB1*0803, HLA-DQA1*0101, HLA-DQB1*0501HLA-DRB1*1501, HLA-DQB1*0502, HLA-DQB1*0503*	Susceptible	26, 27, 28, 29
	*HLA-DQB1*0402*	Decreased frequency	28
	*HLA-B*17-tumor-necrosis-factor-α-238/A, HLA-tumor-necrosis-factor-α-308/2, HLA-tumor-necrosis-factor-β-2*	Relapse	30
HIV-Infection/AIDS	*HLA-B*27, HLA-B*57*	Slow progression	33
	*HLA-A*24*	More rapid central nervous system impairment	33
	*HLA-Cw*2*	Protective against disease progression	33
	*HLA-DQB1*2*	Protective against both disease progression and central nervous system impairment	33
	*HLA-A*31, HLA-B*41, HLA-DQB1*5, HLA-DRB1*10*	Susceptible to TB disease	39
Filariasis	*CD8⁺ HLA-DR⁺*	Susceptible to chronically obstructive lymphatic form	146
	*HLA-B*15*	Susceptible	148
Malaria	*HLA-B*46, HLA-B*56, HLA-DRB1*1001, HLA-B**	Susceptible	160, 162
	*KIR2DL3-HLA-C1, HLA-Bw*53, HLA-DRB1*1302, HLA-DQB1*0501*	Protective	161, 163
Amoebiasis	*HLA-DQB1*0601/DRB1*1501*	Protective	178
Leishmaniasis	*HLA-DRB1, HLA-DQA1*	Susceptible to visceral or pulmonary leishmaniasis	196
	*HLA-DRB1*13, HLA-B*35, HLA-B*44, HLA-A*02, HLA-B*44, HLA-DRB1*07, HLA-A*24, HLA-DRB1*01*	Susceptible to cutaneous leishmaniasis	205

Disease	Known HLA	Influence	Reference
	*HLA-B*49*	Susceptible to recurrent cutaneous leishmaniasis (American type)	205
	*HLA-B*52*	Susceptible to re-infected cutaneous leishmaniasis American type)	205
	*HLA-B*45*	Protecive against cutaneous leishmaniasis (American type)	205
Trypanosomiasis	*HLA-B*39, HLA-DR4, HLA-A*30, HLA-DQB1*0501, HLA-DRB1*01, HLA-DRB1*08, HLA-DPB1*0401, HLA—DPB1*2301, HLA-DPB1*3901, HLA-C*03, HLA-A*31, HLA-B*39, HLA-DR8, HLA-DRB1*0409, HLA-DRB1*1503*	Susceptible to infection and development of Chagas' disease	1, 216, 217, 222, 223, 224, 225, 227, 228
	*HLA-A*68, HLA-DR*16, HLA-DQB1*06, HLA-B*40, HLA-DQB1*0303, HLA-DRB1*14, HLA-DRB1*1501, HLA-DQ1, HLA-DQ3, HLA-DR4, HLA-DR5, HLA-DRB1*0102, HLA-DRB*1402, HLA-MICA*011, HLA-DRB1*1103*	Protective against development of chronic Chagas' cardiomyopathy and cardiac damage	216, 217, 220, 225, 226, 227, 228
Toxoplasmosis	*HLA-DQ*3*	Human hydrocephalus	249
	*HLA-DQ*6, HLA-DQB1*0601*	Protective in murine model	249
Dengue	*HLA-A*01, HLA-A*0207, HLA-A*24, HLA-B*07, HLA-B*46, HLA-B*51, HLA-DQ*1, HLA-DR*1, HLA-DR*4, HLA-A*0211, HLA-Cw*07* (in combination with *HLA-DRB1*07/*15* genotype)	Susceptible to development of dengue hemorrhagic fever	263, 280, 281
	*HLA-A*33, HLA-HLA-Cw*07*	Susceptible to development of dengue fever	281
	*HLA-B*18, HLA-Cw*07*	Susceptible to symptomatic dengue infection	281
Leptospirosis	*HLA-DQ*6*	Increased risk of laboratory confirmation	296

Table 1. Association between some Tropical Pulmonary Infectious Diseases and known Human Leukocyte Antigens

http://dx.doi.org/10.5772/58288

Author details

Attapon Cheepsattayakorn[1,2]

Address all correspondence to: attaponche@yahoo.com

1 10th Zonal Tuberculosis and Chest Disease Centre, Chiang Mai, Thailand

2 10th Office of Disease Prevention and Control, Department of Disease Control, Ministry of Public Health, Thailand

References

[1] Alves C, Souza T, Meyer I. Immunogenetics and infectious diseases : special reference to the major histocompatibility complex. Bra J Infect Dis 2006 ; 10 (2) : 122-131.

[2] Singh N, Agrawal S, Rastogi AK. Infectious diseases and immunity : special reference response to major histocompatibility complex. Emerg Infect Dis 1997 ; 3 (1) : 42-49.

[3] Hill AVS. Genetics and genomics of infectious disease susceptibility. Br Med Bull 1999 ; 55 (2) : 401-413 C.

[4] Itoyama S, Keicho N, Quy T, Phi NC, Long HT, Ha le D, *et al.* ACE1 polymorphism and progression of SARS. Biochem Biophys Res Commun 2004 ; 323 (3) : 1124-1129.

[5] Kuba K, Imai Y, Rao S, Huan Y, Guo F, Guan B, *et al.* A crucial role of angiotensin converting enzyme 2 (ACE2) in SARS coronavirus-induced lung injury. Nat Med 2005 ; 11 (8) : 875-879.

[6] Chan KCA, Tang NLS, Hui DSC, Chung GTY, Wu AKL, Chim SSC, *et al.* Absence of association between angiotensin converting enzyme polymorphism and development of adult respiratory distress syndrome in patients with severe acute respiratory syndrome : a case control study. BMC Infect Dis 2005 ; 5(NA) : 26. DOI : 10.1186/1471-5-26

[7] Ng MH, Lau KM, Li L, Cheng SH, Chan WY, Hui PK, *et al.* Association of human-leukocyte-antigen class I (B*0703) and class II (DRB1*0301) genotypes with susceptibility and resistance to the development of severe acute respiratory syndrome. J Infect Dis 2004 ; 190 (3) : 515-518. Epub 2004 Jul 07.

[8] Lin M, Tseng HK, Trejaut JA, Lee HL, Loo JH, Chu CC, *et al.* Association of HLA class I with severe acute respiratory syndrome coronavirus infection. BMC Med Genet 2003 Sep 12 ; 4(NA) : 9.

[9] Chiu RWK, Tang NL, Hui DS, Chung GT, Chim SSC, Chan KCA, *et al.* ACE2 gene polymorphisms do not affect outcome of severe acute respiratory syndrome. Clin Chem 2004 ; 50 (9) : 1683-1686.

[10] Hsieh Y-H, Chen CWS, Schmitz S-F H, King C-C, Chen W-J, Wu Y-C, *et al.* Candidate genes associated with susceptibility for SARS-coronavirus. Bull Math Biol 2009 ; 72 (1) : 122- 132. DOI : 10.1007/s11538-009-9440-8

[11] Wang SF, Chen KH, Chen M, Li WY, Chen YJ, Tsao CH, *et al.* Human-leukocyte antigen class I Cw 1502 and class II DR 0301 genotypes are associated with resistance to severe acute respiratory syndrome (SARS) infection. Viral Immunol 2011 ; 24 (5) : 421-426.

[12] Liu J, Wu P, Gao F, Qi J, Kawana-Tachikawa A, Xie J, *et al.* Novel immunodominant peptide presentation strategy : a featured HLA-A*2402-restricted cytotoxic T-lymphocyte epitope stabilized by intrachain hydrogen bonds from severe acute respiratory syndrome coronavirus nucleocapsid protein. J Virol 2012 ; 84 (22) : 11849-11857.

[13] Chan VS, Chan KY, Chen Y, Poon LL, Cheung AN, Zheng B, *et al.* Homozygous LSIGN (CLEC4M) plays a protective role in SARS coronavirus infection. Nat Genet 2006 ; 38 (1) : 38-46.

[14] Ip WK, Chan KH, Law HK, Tso GH, Kong EK, Wong WH, *et al.* Mannose-binding lectin in severe acute respiratory syndrome coronavirus infection. J Infect Dis 2005 ; 191 (10) : 1697-1704.

[15] Hamano E, Hijikata M, Itoyama S, Quy T, Phi NC, Long HT, *et al.* Polymorphisms of interferon-inducible genes OAS-1 and MxA associated with SARS in the Vietnamese population. Biochem Biophys Res Commun 2005 ; 329 (4) : 1234-1239.

[16] Haagmans BL, Kuiken T, Martina BE, Fouchier RA, Rimmelzwaan GF, Amerongen van, *et al.* Pegylated interferon-alpha protects type 1 pneumocytes against SARS coronavirus infection in macaques. Nat Med 2004 ; 10 (3) : 290-293.

[17] Cinatl J, Morgenstern B, Bauer G, Chandra P, Rabenau H, Doerr HW. Treatment of SARS with human interferons. Lancet 2003 ; 362 (9380) : 293-294.

[18] Hensley LE, Frizt LE, Jahrling PB, Karp CL, Huggins JW, Geisbert TW. Interferon-beta 1a and SARS coronavirus replication. Emmerg Infect Dis 2004 ; 10 (2) : 317-319.

[19] Spiegel M, Pichlmair A, Muhlberger E, Haller O, Weber F. The antiviral effect of interferon-beta against SARS-coronavirus is not mediated by MxA protein. J Clin Virol 2004 ; 30 (3) : 211-213.

[20] Stroher U, DiCaro A, Li Y, Strong JE, Aoki F, Plummer F, *et al.* Severe acute respoiratory syndrome-related coronavirus is inherited by interferon-alpha. J Infect Dis 2004 ; 189 (7) : 1164-1167.

[21] Tan EL, Ooi EE, Lin CY, Tan HC, Ling AE, Lim B, *et al.* Inhibition of SARS coronavirus infection *in vitro* with clinically approved antiviral drugs. Emerg Infect Dis 2004 ; 10 (4) : 581-586.

[22] Zheng B, He ML, Wong KL, Lum CT, Poon LL, Peng Y, *et al.* Potent inhibition of SARS-associated coronavirus (SCOV) infection and replication by type I interferons (IFN-alpha/beta) but not by type II interferon (IFN-gamma). J Interferon Cytokine Res 2004 ; 24 (7) : 388-390.

[23] Sainz JrB, Mossel EC, Peters CJ, Garry RF. Interferon-beta and interferon-gamma synergistically inhibit the replication of severe acute respiratory syndrome-associated coronavirus (SARS-Cov). Virology 2004 ; 329 (1) : 11-17.

[24] Yang L, Peng H, Zhu Z, Gang L, Huang Z, Zhao Z, *et al.* Persistent memory $CD4^{+}$ and $CD8^{+}$ T-cell responses in recovered severe acute respiratory syndrome (SARS) patients to SARS coronavirus M antigen. J Gen Virol 2007 ; 88 (Pt 10) : 2740-2748.

[25] Zhou M, Xu D, Li X, Li H, Shan M, Tang J, *et al.* Screening and identification of severe acute respiratory syndrome-associated coronavirus-specific CTL epitopes. J Immunol 2006 ; 177 (4) : 2138-2145.

[26] Selvaraj P. Host genetics and tuberculosis susceptibility. Curr Sci 2004 ; 86 (1) : 115-121.

[27] Kim HS, Park MH, Song EY, Park H, Kwon SY, Han SK, et al. Association of HLA-DR and HLA-DQ genes with susceptibility to pulmonary tuberculosis in Koreans : preliminary evidence of association with drug resistance, disease severity, and disease recurrence. Hum Immunol 2005 ; 66 (10) : 1074-1081.

[28] Teran-Escandon D, Teran-Ortiz L, Camarena-Olvera A, Gonzalez-Avila G, Vaca-Marin MA, ranados J, et al. Human leukocyte antigen-associated susceptibility to pulmonary tuberculosis : molecular analysis of class II alleles by DNA amplification and oligonucleotide hybridization in Mexican patients. Chest 1999 ; 115 (2) : 428-433.

[29] Vejbaesya S, Chierakul N, Luangtrakool K, Srinak D, Stephens HA. Associations of HLA class II alleles with pulmonary tuberculosis in Thais. Eur J Immunol 2002 ; 29 (5) : 431-434.

[30] Selvaraj P, Sriram U, Mathan KS, Reetha AM, Narayanan PR. Tumor necrosis factor alpha (-238 and -308) and beta gene polymorphisms in pulmonary tuberculosis : haplotype analysis with HLA-A, B and DR genes. Tuberculosis (Edinb) 2001 ; 81 (5-6) : 335-341.

[31] Li Y, Zhu Y, Zhou L, Fang Y, Huang L, Ren L, *et al.* Use of HLA-DR*08032/E7 and HLA-DR*0818/E7 tetramers in tracking of epitope-specific CD4+ T cells in active and convalescent tuberculosis patients compared with control donors. Immunobiology 2011 ; 216 (8) : 947-960.

[32] Daley CL. Pulmonary infections in the tropics : impact of HIV infection. Thorax 1994 ; 49 (4) : 370-378.

[33] Singh KK, Spector SA. Host genetic determinants of human immunodeficiency virus infection and disease progression in children. Pediatr Res 2009 ; 65 (5 Pt 2) : 55R-63R.

[34] Mackelprang RD, John-Stewart G, Carrington M, Richardson B, Rowland-Jones S, Gao X, *et al.* Maternal HLA homozygosity and mother-child HLA concordance increase the risk of vertical transmission of HIV-1. J Infect Dis 2008 ; 197 (8) ; 1156-1161.

[35] Polycarpou A, Ntais C, Korber BT, Elrich HA, Winchester R, Krogstad P, *et al.* Association between maternal and infant class I and II HLA alleles and of their concordance with the risk of perinatal HIV type 1 transmission. AIDS Res Hum Retroviruses 2002 ; 18 (11) : 741-746.

[36] O' Brien SJ, Gao X, Carrington M. HLA and AIDS : a cautionary tale. Trends Mol Med 2001; 7 (9) : 379-381.

[37] Carrington M, O' Brien SJ. The influence of HLA genotype on AIDS. Annu Rev Med 2003 ; 54 (NA) : 535-551.

[38] Kuhn L, Abrams EJ, Palumbo P, Bulterys M, Aga R, Louie L, *et al.* Maternal versus paternal inheritance of HLA class I alleles among HIV-infected children : consequences for clinical disease progression. AIDS 2004 ; 18 (9) : 1281-1289.

[39] Figueiredo JF, Rodrigues Mde L, Deghaide NH, Donadi EA. HLA profile in patients with AIDS and tuberculosis. Bra J Infect Dis 2008 ; 12 (4) : 278-280.

[40] Gilks CF, Otieno LS, Brindle RJ, Newnham RS, Lule GN, Were JB, *et al.* The presentation and outcome of HIV-related disease in Nairobi. Q J Med 1992 ; 82 (297) : 25-32.

[41] Javaly K, Horowitz HW, Wormser GP. Nocardiosis in patients with human immunodeficiency virus infection ; report of 2 cases and review of the literature. Medicine (Bultimore) 1992 ; 71(3) : 128-138.

[42] Cheepsattayakorn A, Sutachai V. Identification of Burkholderia (Pseudomonas) pseudomallei at 10th Zonal Tuberculosis and Chest Disease Center, Chiang Mai, Thailand. Thai J Tuberc Chest Dis 2001 ; 22 (2) : 105-111.

[43] Carme B, Itoua-Ngaporo A, Bourgarel J, Poste B. Histoplasma capsulatum histoplasmosis. Apropos of a disseminated form with skin lesions in a woman from Zaire. Bull Soc Pathol Exot Filiales 1984 ; 77 (5) : 653-657.

[44] Carme B, Ngolet A, Ebikili B, Itoua N. Is African histoplasmosis an opportunistic fungal infection in AIDS? Trans R Soc Trop Med Hyg 1990 ; 84 (2) : 293.

[45] Carme B, Ngaporo A, Ngolet A, Ibara J, Ebikili B. Disseminated African histoplasmosis in a Congolese patient with AIDS. J Med Vet Myco 1992 ; 30 (3) : 245-248.

[46] Peeters P, Depre' G, Rickaert F, Coremans-Pelseneer J, Serruys E. Disseminated African histolasmosis in a white heterosexual male patient with AIDS. Mykosen 1987 ; 30 (10) : 449-453.

[47] Depre' G, Coremans-Pelseneer J, Peeters P, Rickaert F, Struelens M, Serruys E. Histoplasmose africaine dissemenee associee a un syndrome d' immunodeficience acquise. Bull Soc Franc Mycol Med 1987 ; 16 (NA) : 75-80.

[48] Arendt V, Gerard M, Pelseneer J, Gottlob R, Clumeck N. African histoplasmosis in three HIV patients. In : VI International AIDS Conference. San Francisco : 1990, 396.

[49] Stansell J. Pulmonary fungal infections in HIV-infected persons. Sem Resp Infect dis 1993 ; 8 (2) : 116-123.

[50] Diamond R. The growing problem of mycoses in patients infected with the human immunodeficiency virus. Rev Infect Dis 1991 ; 13 (3) : 480-486.

[51] Homberg K, Meyer R. Fungal infections in patients with AIDS and AIDS-related complex. Scand J Infect Dis 1986 ; 18 (NA) : 179-192.

[52] Kamanfu G, Mlika-Cabanne N, Girard P-M, Nimubona S, Mpfizi B, Cishako A, *et al.* Pulmonary complications of human immunodeficiency virus infection in Bujumbura, Burundi. Am Rev Respir Dis 1993 ; 147 (3) : 658-663.

[53] Serwadda D, Goodgame R, Lucas S, Kocjan G. Absence of pneumocystosis in Ugandan AIDS patients. AIDS 1989 ; 3 (1) : 47-48.

[54] Abouya YL, Beaumel A, Lucas S, Dago-Akribi A, Coulibaly G, N'Dhatz M, *et al.* Pneumocystis carinii pneumonia : an uncommon cause of death in African patients. Am Rev Respir Dis 1992 ; 145 (3) : 617-620.

[55] Taelman H, Bogaerts J, Batungwanayo J, Van de Perre P, Lucas S, Allen S. Value of the cryptococcal serum antigen test in diagnosing pulmonary cryptococcosis in HIV-infected Rwandese patients. In : IX International Conference on AIDS. Berlin ; 1993, 364.

[56] Taelman H, Batungwanayo J, Bogaerts J, Clerinx J, Kagame A, Van de Perre P. Maintenance therapy with itraconazole prevents disseminated cryptococcal disease in HIV-infected patients with isolated pulmonary cryptococcosis. In : IX International Conference on AIDS. Berlin ; 1993, 364.

[57] Bogaerts J, Taelman H, Batungwanayo J, Van de Perre P, Swinne D. Two cases of HIV-associated crptococcosis due to the variety of gattii in Rwanda. Trans R Soc Trop Med Hyg 1993 ; 87 (1) : 63-64.

[58] Goldani L, Coelho I, Machado A, Martinez R. Paracoccidioidomycosis and AIDS. Scand J Infect Dis 1991 ; 23 (3) : 393.

[59] Bakos L, Kronfeld M, Hampe S, Castro I, Zampese M. Disseminated paracoccidioidomycosis with skin lesions in a patient with acquired immunodeficiency syndrome. J Am Acad Dermatol 1989 ; 20 (5 Pt 1) : 854-855.

[60] Restrepo A. Paracoccidioides brasiliensis. In : Mandell G, Douglas R, Bennett J. (eds.) Principles and practice of infectious diseases. New York : Churchill Livingstone; 1990 : p2018-2031.

[61] Supparapinyo K, Chiewchanvit S, Hirunsri P. Uthammachai C, Nelson K, Sirisanthana T. Penicillium marneffei infection in patients infected with human immunodeficiency virus. Clin Infect Dis 1992 ; 14 (4) : 871-874.

[62] Edman J, Kovacs J, Masur H, Santi D, Elwood H, Sogin M. Ribosomal RNA sequence shows Pneumocystis carinii to be a member of the fungi. Nature 1988 ; 334 (6182) : 519-522.

[63] Smulian A, Sullivan D, Linke M, Halsey N, Quinn T, MacPhail A, *et al*. Geographic variation in the humoral response to Pneumocystis carinii. J Infect Dis 1993 ; 167 (5) : 1243-1247.

[64] Meduri G, Stein D. Pulmonary manifestations of AIDS. Clin Infect Dis 1993 ; 14 (NA) : 98-113.

[65] Cheepsattayakorn A, Punjaisri S, Chanwong S. Pneumocystis carinii pneumonia detection by sputum and blood polymerase chain reaction. Thai J Tuberc Chest Dis Crit Care 2003 ; 24 (2) : 125-135.

[66] Blaser M, Cohn D. Opportunistic infections in patients with AIDS : clues to the epidemiology of AIDS and the relative virulence of pathogens. Rev Infect Dis 1986 ; 8 (1) : 21-30.

[67] Kreiss J, Castro K. Special consideration for managing suspected human immunodeficiency virus infection and AIDS in patients from developing countries. J Infect Dis 1990 ; 162 (4) : 955-960.

[68] Malin A, Gwanzura L, Klein S, Musvaire P, Robertson V, Mason P. A bronchoscopic study of acute interstitial pneumonia in Zimbabwe ; difficulties in distinguishing Pneumocystis carinii pneumonia from disseminated pulmonary tuberculosis. In : IX International Conference on AIDS. Berlin ; 1993, 431.

[69] Atzori C, Bruno A, Chichino G, Gatti S, Scaglia M. Pneumocystis carinii pneumonia and tuberculosis in Tanzanian patients infected with HIV. Trans R Soc Trop Med Hyg 1993 ; 87(1) : 55-56.

[70] Pape JW, Liautaud B, Thomas F, Mathurin JR, St Amand MM, Boncy M, *et al*. The acquired immunodeficiency syndrome in Haiti. Ann Intern Med 1985 ; 103 (5) : 674-678.

[71] Chequer P, Hearst N, Hudes E. Determinants of survival in adult Brazilian AIDS patients, 1982-1989. AIDS 1992 ; 6 (5) : 483-487.

[72] Kronfeld M, LeHugeur D, Rotbland A, de Quadros A, Dias D, dos Santos L, *et al*. Acquired immunodeficiency syndrome in the State of Rio Grand do Sul : a report of 40 cases. Rev Hosp Clin Porto Allegre 1988 ; 8 (NA) : 9-19.

[73] Elvin K, Lumbwe C, Luo N, Bjorkman A, Kallenius G, Linder E. Pneumocystis carinii is not a major cause of pneumonia in HIV-infected patients in Lusaka, Zambia. Trans R Soc Trop Med Hyg 1989 ; 83 (4) : 553-555.

[74] Lucas S. Missing infections in AIDS. Trans R Soc Trop Med Hyg 1990 ; 84 (Suppl 1) : 34-38.

[75] Genta R. Global prevalence of strongyloidiasis : critical review with epidemiologic insights into the prevention of disseminated disease. Rev Infect Dis 1989 ; 11(5) : 755-767.

[76] Neto V, Pasternak J, Moreira A, Duarte M, Campos R, Braz L. Strongyloides stercoralis hyperinfection in the acquired immunodeficiency syndrome. Am J Med 1989 ; 87 (5) : 602-603.

[77] Conlon C, Pinching A, Perera C, Moody A, Luo N, Lucas S. HIV-related enteropathy in Zambia : a clinical, microbiological, and histopathological study. Am Trop Med Hyg 1990 ; 42 (1) : 83-88.

[78] Vijayan VK. Tropical parasitic lung diseases. Indian J Chest Dis Allied Sci 2008 ; 50 (1) : 49-66.

[79] Scowden EB, Schaffner W, Stone WJ. Overwhelming strongyloidiasis : an unappreciated opportunistic infection. Medicine (Baltimore) 1978 ; 57 (6) : 527-544.

[80] Gompels MM, Todd J, Peters BS, Main J, Pinching AJ. Disseminated strongyloides in AIDS : uncommon but important. AIDS 1991 ; 5 (3) : 329-332.

[81] Armignacco O, Capecchi A, De Mori P. Strongyloides stercoralis hyperinfection and the acquired immunodeficiency syndrome. Am J Med 1989 ; 86 (2) : 258.

[82] Maayan S, Wormser G, Widerhorn J, Sy E, Kim Y, Ernst J. Strongyloides stercoralis hyperinfection in a patient with the acquired immune deficiency syndrome. Am J Med 1987 ; 83 (5) : 945-948.

[83] Crompton DWT. How much human helminthiasis is there in the world ? J Parasitol 1999 ; 85 (3) : 379-403.

[84] Peng W, Zhou X, Gasser RB. Ascaris egg profile in human feces : biological and epidemiological implications. Parasitology 2003 ; 127 (Pt 3) : 283-290.

[85] Yaziciogølu M, Ones U, Yalcin I. Peripheral and nasal eosinophilia and serum total immunoglobulin E levels in children with ascariasis. Turk J Pediatric 1996 ; 38 (4) : 477-484.

[86] Santra A, Bhattacharya T, Chowdhury A, Ghosh A, Ghosh N, Chatterjee BP, et al. Serodiagnosis of ascariasis with specific IgG4 antibody and its use in epidemiological study. Trans R Soc Trop Med Hyg 2001 ; 95 (3) : 289-292.

[87] Loffler W. Zur differential-diagnose der lungeninfiltrieurgen : 11 Uber fluchtige succedan-infiltrate (mit eosinophile). Bietr Klin Tuberk 1932 ; 19 (NA) : 368-392.

[88] Ford RM. Transient pulmonary eosinophilia and asthma : a review of 20 cases occurring in 5,702 asthma sufferers. Am Rev Respir Dis 1996 ; 93 (5) : 797-803.

[89] Liu LX, Weller PF. Strongyloidiasis and other intestinal nematode infections. Infect Dis Clin North Am 1993 ; 7 (3) : 655-682.

[90] Citro LA, Gordon ME, Miller WT. Eosinophilic lung disease (or how to slice PIE). Am J Roentgenol Rad Ther Nuc Med 1973 ; 117 (NA) : 787-797.

[91] Hoagland KE, Schad GA. Necator americanus and Ancylostoma duodenale : life history parameters and epidemiological implications of two sympatric hookworms on humans. Exp Parasitol 1978 ; 44 (1) : 36-49.

[92] Hotez P. Human hookworm infection. In : Farthing MJG, Keusch GT, Wakelin D. (eds.) Intestinal Helminths. London : Chapman and Hall ; 1995. p129-150.

[93] Nawalinski TA, Schad GA. Arrested development in Ancylostoma duodenale : cause of self-induced infections in man. Am J Trop Med Hyg 1974 ; 23 (5) : 895-898.

[94] Cappello M, Clyne LP, MacPhedram P, Hotez PJ. Ancylostoma factor Xa inhibitor : partial purification and its identification as a major hookworm-derived anticoagulant in vitro. J Infect Dis 1993 ; 167 (6) : 1474-1477.

[95] Nakamura-Uchiyama F, Mukae H, Nawa Y. Paragonimiasis : a Japanese perspective. Clin Chest Med 2002 ; 23 (2) : 409-420.

[96] Blair D, Xu ZB, Agatsuma T. Paragonimiasis and the genus paragonimus. Adv Parasitol 1999 ; 42 (NA) : 113-222.

[97] King CH. Pulmonary flukes. In : Mahamoud AAF. (ed.) Lung Biology in Health and Disease : Parasitic Lung Disease. New York : Marcel Dekker ; 1997. p157-169.

[98] Xu ZB. Studies on clinical manifestations, diagnosis and control of paragonimiasis in China. Southeast Asian J Trop Med Pub Health 1991 ; 22 (Suppl. 1) : 345-348.

[99] Mukae H, Taniguchi H, Matsumoto N, Liboshi H, Ashitani J, Matsukura S, *et al*. Clinicoradiological features of pleuropulmonary Paragonimiasis (westernmani) on Kyushu Island, Japan. Chest 2001 ; 120 (NA) : 514-520.

[100] Suwanik R, Harinasuta C. Pulmonary paragonimiasis : an evaluation of roentgen findings in 38 positive sputum patients in an endemic area in Thailand. Am J Roentgenol 1959 ; 81 (2) : 236-244.

[101] Lee EG, Na BK, Bae YA, Kim SH, Je EY, Ju JW, *et al.* Identification of immunodominant excretory-secretory cysteine proteases of adult Paragonimus westernmani by proteome analysis. Proteomics 2006 ; 6 (4) : 1290-1300.

[102] Na BK, Kim SH, Lee EG, Kim TS, Bae YA, Kang I, *et al.* Critical roles for excretory-secretory cysteine proteases during tissue invasion of Paragonimus westernmani newly excysted metacercariae. Cell Microbiol 2006 ; 8 (6) : 1034-1046.

[103] Wongkham C, Intapan PM, Maleewong W, Miwa M. Evaluation of human IgG subclass antibodies in the serodiagnosis of *Paragonimus heterotremus*. Asian Pac J Allergy Immunol 2005 ; 23 (4) : 205-211.

[104] Vele'z ID, Ortega JE, Vela'squez LE. Paragonimiasis : a review from Columbia. Clin Chest Med 2002 ; 23 (2) : 421-431.

[105] Keiser J, Engels D, Buscher G, Utzinger J. Triclabendazole for treatment of fascioliasis and paragonimiasis. Expert Opin Investig Drugs 2005 ; 14 (12) : 1513-1526.

[106] Schwartz E. Pulmonary schistosomiasis. Clin Chest Med 2002 ; 23 (2) : 433-443.

[107] Schwatz E, Rozenman J, Perelman N. Pulmonary manifestations of early Schistosoma infection in nonimmune travelers. Am J Med 2000 ; 109 (9) : 718-722.

[108] Walt F. The Katayama syndrome. A Afr Med J 1954 ; 28 (5) : 89-93.

[109] Doherty JF, Moody AH, Wright SG. Katayama fever ; an acute manifestation of schistosomiasis. Br Med J 1996 ; 313 (7064) : 1071-1072.

[110] Nguyen LQ, Estrella J, Jett EA, Grunvald EL, Nocholson L, Levin DL. Acute schistosomiasis in nonimmune travelers : chest CT findings in 10 patients. Am J Roentgenol 2006 ; 186 (5) : 1300-1303.

[111] Lapa MS, Ferreira EV, Jardim C, Martins BC, Arakaki JS, Souza R. Clinical characteristics of pulmonary hypertension patients in two reference centers in the city of Sao Paulo. Rev Assoc Med Bras 2006 ; 52 (3) : 139-143.

[112] Morris W, Knauer M. Cardiopulmonary manifestations of schistosomiasis. Semin Respir Infect 1997 ; 12 (2) : 159-170.

[113] Sersar SI, Abulmaaty RA, Elnahas HA, Moussa SA, Shisa UA, Ghafar WA, *et al.* A diagnostic dilemma of right lower lobe collapse caused by pulmonary bilharsiasis. Heart Lung Circ 2006 ; 15 (1) : 50-52.

[114] Gottstein B, Reichen J. Hydatid lung disease (echinococcosis/hydatidosis). Clin Chest Med 2002 ; 23 (2) : 397-408.

[115] Kuzucu A. Parasitic diseases of the respiratory tract. Curr Opin Pulm Med 2006 ; 12 (3) : 212-221.

[116] Fanne RA, Khamaisi M, Mevorach D, Leitersdorf E, Berkman N, Laxer U, *et al*. Spontaneous rupture of lung echinococcal cyst causing anaphylactic shock and respiratory distress syndrome. Thorax 2006 ; 61 (6) : 550.

[117] Savani DM, Sharma OP. Eosinophilic lung disease in the tropics. Clin Chest Med 2002 ; 23 (2) : 377-396.

[118] Ito A, Sako Y, Yamasaki H, Mamuti W, Nakaya K, Nakao M, *et al*. Development of Em 18- immunoblot and Em 18-ELISA for specific diagnosis of alveolar echinococcosis. Acta Trop 2003 ; 85 (2) : 173-182.

[119] Gencer M, Ceylan E. Pulmonary echinococcosis with multiple nodules mimicking metastatic lung tumor in chest radiography. Respiration. http://www.ncbi.nlm.nih.gov/sites/entrez/ (accessed 30 August 2013). DOI : 10.1159/000091141.

[120] Asanuma T, Kawahara T, Inanami O, Nakao M, Nakaya K, Ito A, *et al*. Magnetic resonance imaging of alveolar echinococcosis experimentally induced in the rat lung. J Vet Med Sci 2006 ; 68 (1) : 15-20.

[121] Gottstein B, Reichen J. Hydatid lung disease. In : Sharma OP (ed.) Lung Biology in Health and Disease : Tropical Lung Disease ; 2nd ed. New York : Taylor and Francis Group ; 2006. p327-350.

[122] Kavukcu S, Kilic D, Tokat AO, Kutlay H, Cangir AK, Enon S, *et al*. Parenchyma-preserving surgery in the management of pulmonary hydatid cysts. J Invest Surg 2006 ; 19 (1) : 61-68.

[123] Hasdiraz L, Og@uzkaya F, Bilgin M. Is lobectomy necessary in the treatment of pulmonary hydatid cysts? ANZ J Surg 2006 ; 76 (6) : 488-490.

[124] Dincer SI, Demir A, Sayar A, Gunluoglu MZ, Kara HV, Gurses A. Surgical treatment of pulmonary hydatid disease : a comparison of children and adults. J Pediatr Surg 2006 ; 41 (7) : 1230-1236.

[125] Pozio E, La Rosa G, Murrell KD, Lichtenfels JR. Taxonomic revision of genus Trichinella. J Parasitol 1992 ; 78 (4) : 654-659.

[126] Despommier DD. How does Trichinella spiralis make itself at home? Parasitol Today 1998 ; 14 (8) : 318-323.

[127] Bruschi F, Murrell K. Trichinellosis. In : Guerrant RL, Walker DH, Weller PF. (eds.) Tropical Infectious Diseases : Principles, Pathogens and Practice ; Vol. II. Philadelphia : Churchill Livingstone (Elsevier Science Health Science Divn) ; 1999. p917-925.

[128] Engvall E, Ljungstrom I. Detection of human antibodies to Trichinella spiralis by enzyme- linked immunosorbent assay (ELISA). Acta Pathol Microbiol Scand 1975 ; 83 (NA) : 231-237.

[129] Vijayan VK. Tropical pulmonary eosinophilia : pathogenesis, diagnosis and management. Curr Opin Pulm Med 2007 ; 13 (5) : 428-433.

[130] Ottesen EA. Immunological aspects of lymphatic filariasis and onchocerciasis. Trans R Soc Trop Med Hyg 1984 ; 73 (suppl) : 9-18.

[131] Frimodt-Mo@ller C, Barton RM. A pseudo-tuberculosis condition associated with eosinophilia. Indian Med Gaz 1940 ; 75 (10) : 607-613.

[132] Weingarten RJ. Tropical eosinophilia. Lancet 1943 ; 1 (NA) : 103-105.

[133] Kamat SR, Pimparkar SD, Store SD, Warrier NVU, Fakey YC. Study of clinical, radiological and pulmonary function patterns and response to treatment in pulmonary eosinophilia. Indian J Chest Dis 1970 ; 12 (3) : 91-100.

[134] Basu SP. X-ray appearance in lung fields in tropical eosinophilia. Indian Med Gaz 1954 ; 89 (NA) : 212-217.

[135] Islam N, Huque KS. Radiological features of tropical eosinophilia. J Trop Med Hyg 1965 ; 68 (NA) : 117-180.

[136] Khoo FY, Danaraj TJ. The roentgenographic appearance of eosinophilic lung (tropical eosinophilia). Am J Roentgenol Radium Ther Nucl Med 1960 ; 86 (NA) : 251-259.

[137] World Health Organization, Division of Control of Tropical Diseases. Lymphatic filariasis infection and disease : control strategies, 1994 (TDR/CTD/FIL/Penang) ; p1-30.

[138] Sandhu M, Mukhopadhyay S, Sharma SK. Tropical pulmonary eosinophilia : a comparative evaluation of plain chest radiography and computed tomography. Australas Radiol 1996 ; 40 (1) : 32-37.

[139] Johnson S, Wilkinson R, Davidson RN. Tropical respiratory medicine. IV : Acute tropical infection and the lung. Thorax 1994 ; 49 (NA) : 714-718.

[140] Ottensen EA, Nutman TB. Tropical pulmonary eosinophilia. Ann Rev Med 1992 ; 43 (NA) : 417-424.

[141] Danaraj TJ, Schacher JF. I/D test with Dirofilaria immitis extract in eosinophilic lung (tropical eosinophilia). Am J Trop Med Hyg 1959 ; 8 (6) : 640-643.

[142] Webb JKB, Job OK, Gault EW. Tropical eosinophilia : demonstration of microfilariae in lung, liver and lymph nodes. Lancet 1960 ; 275 (7129) : 835-842.

[143] Joshi VV, Udwadia FE, Gadgil RK. Etiology of tropical eosinophilia : a study of lung biopsies and review of published reports. Am J Trop Med Hyg 1969 ; 18 (2) : 231-240.

[144] Danaraj TJ, Pachecco G, Shanmugaratnam K, Beaver PC. The etiology and pathology of eosinophilic lung (tropical eosinophilia). Am J Trop Med Hyg 1966 ; 15 (2) : 183-189.

[145] Steel C, Nutman TB. Altered T-cell Memory and effector cell development in chronic lymphatic filarial infection that is independent of persistent parasite antigen. PLoS ONE 2011 ; 6 (4) : e19197. DOI : 10.1371/journal.pone.0019197

[146] Lal RB, Kumaraswami V, Krishnan N, Nutman TB, Ottesen EA. Lymphocyte subpopulations in Bancroftian filariasis : activated (DR^+) $CD8^+$-T cells in patients with chronic lymphatic obstruction. Clin Exp Immunol 1989 ; 77 (1) : 77-82.

[147] Sasisekhar B, Aparna M, Augustin DJ, Kaliraj P, Kar SK, Nutman TB, *et al*. Diminished momnocyte function in microfilaremic patients with lymphatic filariasis and its relationship to altered lymphoproliferative responses. Imfect Immun 2005 ; 73 (6) : 3385-3393.

[148] Chan SH, Dissanayake S, Mak JW, Ismail MM, Wee GB, Srinivasan N, *et al*. HLA and filariasis in Sri Lankans and Indians. The Southeast Asian J Trop Med Public Health 1984 ; 15 (3) : 281-286.

[149] Ottesen EA, Neva FA, Paranjape RS, Tripathy SP, Thiruvengadam KV, Beaver MA. Specific allergic sensitization to filarial antigens in tropical pulmonary eosinophilia. Lancet 1979 ; 314 (8153) : 1158-1161.

[150] Viswanathan R, Bagai RC, Raran R. Leukocyte adhesion phenomenon in pulmonary eosinophilia (tropical eosinophilia). Am Rev Respir Dis 1973 ; 107 (NA) : 298-300.

[151] Dreyer G, Noroes J, Rocha A, Addiss D. Detection of living adult *Wuchereria bancrofti* in a patient with tropical eosinophilia. Braz J Med Biol Res 1996 ; 29 (NA) : 1005-1008.

[152] Perera CS, Perera LM, de Silva C, Abeywickreme W, Dissanaike AS, Ismail MM. An eosinophilic granuloma containing an adult female *Wuchereria bancrofti* in a patient with tropical eosinophilia. Trans R Soc Trop Med Hyg 1992 ; 86 (5) : 542.

[153] Nutman TB, Vijayan VK, Pinkston P, Steel R, Crystal RG, Ottesen EA. Tropical pulmonary eosinophilia : analysis of antifilarial antibody localized to the lung. J Infect Dis 1989 ; 160 (6) : 1042-1050.

[154] Vijayan VK. Tropical eosinophilia : bronchoalveolar lavage and pulmonary pathophysiology in relation to treatment. PhD thesis. University of Madras, Madras, India; 1988.

[155] Vijayan VK, Kuppurao KV, Sankaran K, Venkatesan P, Prabhakar R. Tropical eosinophilia : clinical and physiological response to diethylcarbamazine. Respir Med 1991 ; 85 (1) : 17-20.

[156] World Health Organization. Final report : Joint WPRO/SEARO Working Group on Brugian Filariasis. Manila : WHO ; 1979. p1-47.

[157] Ganatra RD, Sheth UK, Lewis RA. Diethylcarbamazine (Hetrazan) in tropical eosinophilia. India J Med Resi 1958 ; 46 (2) : 205-222.

[158] Baker SJ, Rajan KT, Davadutta S. Treatment of tropical eosinophilia : a controlled trial. Lancet 1959 ; 274 (7095) : 144-147.

[159] Dondorp AM, Desakorn V, Pongtavornpinyo W, Sahassananda D, Silamut K, Chotivanich K, Newton PN, *et al.* Estimation of the total parasite biomass in acute falciparum malaria from plasma PfHRP2. PLoS Med 2005 ; 2 (8) : e204. DOI : 10.1371/journal.pmed.0020204

[160] Hananantachai H, Patarapotikul J, Ohashi J, Naka I, Looareesuwan S, Tokunaga K. Polymorphisms of the HLA-B and HLA-DRB1 genes in Thai malaria patients. Jpn J Infect Dis 2005 ; 58 (1) : 25-28.

[161] Hirayasu K, Ohashi J, Kashiwase K, Hananantachai H, Naka I, Okawa A, *et al.* Significant association of KIR2DL3-HLA-C1 combination with cerebral malaria and implications for co-evolution of KIR and HLA. PLoS Pathog 2012 ; 8(3) : e1002565. DOI : 10.1371/journal.ppat.1002565

[162] Young K, Frodsham A, Doumbo OK, Gupta S, Dolo A, Hu JT, *et al.* Inverse associations of human leukocyte antigen and malaria parasite types in two West African populations. Infect. Immun. 2005 ; 73 (2) : 953-955.

[163] Hill AVS, Allsopp CEM, Kwiatkowski D, Anstey NM, Twumasi P, Rowe PA, *et al.* Common West African HLA antigens are associated with protection from severe malaria. Nature 1991 ; 352 (6336) : 595-600.

[164] May J, Meyer CG, Kun JFJ, Lell B, Luckner D, Dippmann AK, *et al.* HLA class II factors associated with Plasmodium falciparum merozoite surface antigen allele families. J Infect Dis 1999 ; 179 (4) : 1042-1045.

[165] Maquire GP, Handojo T, Pain MC, Kenangalem E, Price RN, Tjitra E, *et al.* Lung injury in uncomplicated and severe falciparum malaria : a longitudinal study in Papua, Indonesia. J Infect Dis 2005 ; 192 (11) : 1966-1974.

[166] Mharakurwa S, Simoloka C, Thuma PE, Shiff CJ, Sullivan DJ. PCR detection of Plasmodium falciparum in human urine and saliva samples. Malar J 2006 Nov 8 ; 5 (NA) : 103. DOI :10.1186/1475-2875-5-103

[167] Djimde' A, Doumbo OK, Cortese JF, Kayentao K, Doumbo S, Diourte Y, *et al.* A molecular marker for chloroquine-resistant falciparum malaria. N Engl J Med 2001 ; 344 (4) : 257-263.

[168] Laufer MK, Thesing PC, Eddington ND, Masonga R, Dzinjalamala FK, Takala SL, *et al.* Return of chloroqiune antimalarial efficacy in Malawi. N Engl J Med 2006 ; 355 (19) : 1959-1966.

[169] Mutabingwa TK. Artemisinin-based combination therapies (ACTs) : best hope for malaria treatment but inaccessible to the needy! Acta Trop 2005; 95 (3) : 305-315.

[170] World Health Organization. Guidelines for the treatment of malaria. Geneva : World Health Organization ; 2006. p1-266.

[171] World Health Organization. Management of severe malaria : a practical handbook, 3rd ed. WHO ; 2012. http://www.who.int/malaria (accessed 16 December 2013).

[172] Kiang KM, Bryant PA, Shingadia D, Ladhani S, Steer AC, Burgner D. The treatment of imported malaria in children : an update. Arch Dis Child Educ Prac Ed 2013 ; 98 (1) : 7-15.

[173] Greenwood BM, Bojang K, Whitty CJ, Targett GA. Malaria. Lancet 2005 ; 365 (9469) : 1487-1498.

[174] Ackers JP, Mirelman D. Progress in research on Entamoeba histolytica pathogenesis. Curr Opin Microbiol 2006 ; 9 (4) : 367-373.

[175] Shamsuzzaman SM, Hashiguchi Y. Thoracic amoebiasis. Clin Chest Med 2002 ; 23 (2) : 479-492.

[176] Duggal P, Guo X, Haque R, Peterson KM, Rickklefs S, Mondal D, et al. A mutation in the Leptin receptor is associated with Entamoeba histolytica infection in children. J Clin Invest 2011 ; 121 (3) : 1191-1198. DOI : 10.1172/JC145294

[177] Marie CS, Verkerke HP, Paul SN, Mackey AJ, Petri WA Jr. Leptin protects host cells from Entamoeba histolytica cytotoxicity by a STAT3-dependent mechanism. Infect Immun 2012 ; 80 (5) : 1934-1943.

[178] Duggal P, Haque R, Roy S, Mondal D, Sack RB, Farr BM, et al. Influence of human leukocyte antigen class II alleles on susceptibility to Entamoeba histolytica infection in Bangladeshi children. J Infect Dis 2004; 189 (3) : 520-526. DOI : 10.1128/IAI. 06140-11

[179] Moonah SN, Jiang NM, Petri WA Jr. Host immune response to intestinal amoebiasis. PLoS Pathog 2013 ; 9 (8) : e1003489. DOI : 10.1371/journal.ppat.1003489

[180] Hamzah Z, Petmitr S, Mungthin M, Leelayoova S, Chavalitshewinkoon-Petmitr P. Differential detection of Entamoeba histolytica, Entamoeba dispar and Entamoeba moshkovskii by a single-round PCR assay. J Clin Microbiol 2006 ; 44 (9) : 3196-3200.

[181] Haque R, Petri WA Jr. Diagnosis of amoebiasis in Bangladesh. Arch Med Res 2006 ; 37 (2) : 273-276.

[182] Tanyuksel M, Petri WA Jr. Laboratory diagnosis of amoebiasis. Clin Microbiol Rev 2003 ; 16 (4) : 713-729.

[183] Garcia-Rubio I, Martinez-Cocera C, Santos Magadan S, Rodriguez-Jimenez B, Vasquez-cortes S. Hypersentivity reactions to metronidazole. Allergol Immunopathol (Madr) 2006 ; 34 (2) : 70-72.

[184] Leo'n-Sicairos N, Reyes-Lo'pez M, Ordaz-Pichardo C, de la Garza M. Microbicidal action of lactoferrin and lactoferricin and their synergic effect with metronidazole in Entamoeba histolytica. Biochem Cell Biol 2006 ; 84 (3) : 327-336.

[185] Lotter H, Tannich E. The current status of an amoebiasis vaccine. Arch Med Res 2006 ; 37 (2) : 292-296.

[186] Basu R, Roy S, Walden P. HLA class I-restricted T-cell epitopes of the kinetoplastid membrane protein-11 presented by Leishmania donovani-infected human macrophages. J Infect Dis 2007 ; 195 (9) : 1378-1380.

[187] Piscopo TV, Mallia AC. Leishmaniasis. Postgrad Med J 2006 ; 82 (972) : 649-657.

[188] Russo R, Laguna F, Lopez-Velez R, Medrano FJ, Roenthal E, Cacopardo B, *et al.* Visceral leishmaniasis in those infected with HIV : clinical aspects and other opportunistic infections. Ann Trop Med Parasitol 2003 ; 97 (Suppl.1) : S99-S105.

[189] Benzie AA, Goldin RD, Walsh J. A case report of seronegative pulmonary leishmaniasis in an HIV-hepatitis C co-infected patient. HIV Med 2006 ; 7 (Suppl. 1) : 36 (abstract no. P100).

[190] Alvar J, Aparicio P, Aseffa A, Boer MD, Cañavate C, Dedet JP, et al. The relationship between leishmaniasis and AIDS : the second 10 years. Clin Microbiol Rev 2008 ; 21 (2) : 334-359.

[191] Barreto-de-Souza V, Pacheo GJ, Silva AR, Castro-Faria-Neto HC, Bozza PT, Saraiva EM, *et al.* Increased leishmania replication in HIV-1-infected macrophages is mediated by tat protein through cyclooxygenase-2 expression and prostaglandin E 2 synthesis. J Infect Dis 2006 ; 194 (6) : 846-854.

[192] Cota GF, de Sousa MR, Rabello A. Predictors of visceral leishmaniasis relapse in HIV-infected patients : a systematic review. PLoS Negl Trop Dis 2011 ; 5 (6) : Article ID e1153.

[193] Santos-Oliveira JR, Giacoia-Gripp CBW, de Oliveira PA, Amato VS, Lindoso JA, Goto H, *etal.* High levels of T-lymphocyte activation in Leishmania-HIV-1 co-infected individuals despite low HIV viral load. BMC Infect Dis 2010 ; 10 (NA) : 358-363.

[194] Alexandro-de-Oliveira P, Santos-Oliveira JR, Dorval MEC, Da-Costa Fd, Pereira GR, da Cunha RV, *et al.* HIV/AIDS-associated visceral leishmaniasis in patients from an endemic area in Central-west Brazil. Mem Inst Oswaldo Cruz 2010 ; 105 (5) : 692-697.

[195] Morales P, Torres JJ, Salavert M, Pema'n J, Lacruz J, Sole' A, *et al.* Visceral leishmaniasis in lung transplantation. Transplantation Proc 2003 ; 35 (5) : 2001-2003.

[196] LeishGEN Consortium ; Wellcome Trust Case Control Consortium, Fakiola M, Strange A, Cordell HJ, Miller EN, Pirinen M, Su Z, *et al.* Common variants in the

HLADRB1-HLA-DQA1 HLA class II region are associated with susceptibility to visceral leishmaniasis. Nat Genet 2013 ; 45 (2) : 208-213.

[197] Blackwel JM, Freeman J, Bradley D. Influence of H-2 complex on acquired resistance to Leishmania donovani infection in mice. Nature 1980 ; 283 (5742) : 72-74.

[198] Blackwel JM. Leishmania donovani infection in heterozygous and recombinant H-2 haplotype mice. Immunogenetics 1983 ; 18 (2) : 101-109.

[199] Blackwel JM, Roberts MB. Immunomodulation of murine visceral leishmaniasis by administration of monoclonal anti-Ia antibodies : differential effects of anti-I-A vs anti-I-E antibodies. Eur J Immonol 1987 ; 17 (11) : 1669-1672.

[200] Polley R, Stager S, Prickett S, Maroof A, Zubairi S, Smith DF, *et al.* Adoptive immunotherapy against experimental visceral leishmaniasis with $CD8^+$ T-cells requires the presence of cognate antigen. Infect Immun 2006 ; 74 (1) : 773-776.

[201] Stern JJ, Oca MJ, Rubin BY, Anderson SL, Murray HW. Role of L3T4+ and LyT-2+ cells in experimental visceral leishmaniasis. J Immunol 1988 ; 140 (11) : 3971-3977.

[202] Medddeb-Garnaoui A, Gritli S, Garbouj S, Ben Fadhel M, El kares R, Mansour L, *et al.* Association analysis of HLA class II and class III gene polymorphisms in the susceptibility to Mediterranean visceral leishmaniasis. Hum Immunol 2001 ; 62 (5) : 509-517.

[203] Karplus TM, Jeronimo SM, Chang H, Helms BK, Burns TL, Murray C, *et al.* Association between the tumor necrosis factor locus and the clinical outcome of Leishmania/chagasi infection. Infect Immun 2002 ; 70 (12) : 6919-6925.

[204] Blackwell JM, Jamieson SE, Burgner D. HLA and infectious diseases. Clin Microbiol Rev 2009 ; 22 (2) : 370-385.

[205] Ribas-Silva RC, Ribas AD, dos Santos MCG, da Silva Jr WV, Lonardoni MVC, Borelli SD, *et al.* Association between HLA genes and American cutaneous leishmaniasis in endemic regions of southern Brazil. BMC Infect Dis 2013 ; 13 (NA) : 198. DOI : 10.1186/1471-2334-13-198

[206] Santos-Oliveira JR, Da-Cruz AM. Lipopolysaccharide-induced cellular activation may participate in the immunopathogenesis of visceral leishmaniasis alone or in HIV co-infection. Int J Microbiol 2012, Article ID 364534, 4 pages. DOI : 10.1155/2012/364534

[207] Croft SL, Engel J. Miltefosine : discovery of the antileishmanial activity of phospholipid derivatives. Trans R Soc Trop Med Hyg 2006 ; 100 (Suppl. 1) : 54-58.

[208] Sachdeva R, Banerjea AC, Malla N, Dubey ML. Immunogenicity and efficacy of single antigen Gp63, polytope and polytopeHSP70 DNA vaccines against visceral leishmaniasis in experimental mouse model. PLoS ONE 2009 ; 4 (12) : e7880. DOI : 10.1371/journal.pone.0007880

[209] Bouteille B, Buguet A. The detection and treatment of human African trypanosomiasis. Res. Rep. Trop. Med. 2012 ; 3 (NA) : 35-45.

[210] Ayub M, Shah SA, Irfan M, Khan JA, Hashmi SN. A case of human African trypanosomiasis during United Nation Mission in Liberia. Pak. Armed. Forces. Med. J. 2011 ; 8 (1) : NA. http://www.pafmj.org/showdetails.php?id=187&t=c (accessed 26 December 2013).

[211] Melnikov VG, Velasco FF, Go'mez FE, Rodriguez FG, Dobrovinskaya OR. Pathologic changes in lungs caused by Mexican isolates of Trypanosoma cruzi in the acute phase of infection in mice. Am J Trop Med Hyg 2005 ; 73 (2) : 301-306.

[212] Ši'ma M, Havelkova' H, Quan L, Svobodova' M, Jaros◉i'kova' T, Vojti's◉kova' J, *et al*. Genetic control of resistance to Trypanosoma brucei infection in mice. PLoS Negl Trop Dis 2011 ; 5 (6) : e1173.

[213] Biswas D, Choudhury A, Misra KK. Histopathology of Trypanosoma (Trypanosoon) evani infection in bandicoot rat I visceral organs. Exp Parasitol 2001 ; 99 (3) : 148-159.

[214] Nuñes Mdo C, Barbosa Mde M, Brum VA, Rocha MO. Morphofunctional characteristics of the right ventricle in Chagas' dilated cardiomyopathy. Int J Cardiol 2004 ; 94 (1) : 79-85.

[215] Ayo CM, Dalalio MMdeO, Visentainer JEL, Reis PG, Sippert EA, Jarduli LR, *et al*. Genetic susceptibility to Chagas' disease : an overview about the infection and about the association between disease and the immune response genes. Biomed Res Int 2013 ; Article ID 284729, 13 pages. http://dx.doi.org/10.1155/2013/284729

[216] Cruz-Robles D, Reyes PA, Monteo'n-Padilla VM, Ortiz-Muñiz AR, Vargas-Alarco'n G. MHC class I and class II genes in Mexican patients with Chagas' disease. Hum Immunol 2004 ; 65(1) : 60-65.

[217] Deghaide NH, Dantas RO, Donadi EA. HLA class I and II profiles of patients presenting with Chagas' disease. Dig Dis Sci 1998 ; 43 (2) : 246-252.

[218] de Oliveira Dala'lio MM, Vissentainer JEL, Moliterno RA, Sell AM, Petzel-Erler ML. Association of HLA-DR2 with chronic chagasic cardiopathy in a population at Parana' Northeast region, Brazil. Acta Scientiarum 2002 ; 24 (3) : 727-730.

[219] Fae' KC, Drigo SA, Cunha-Neto E, Ianni B, Mady C, Kalil J, *et al*. HLA and β-myosin heavy chain do not influence susceptibility to Chagas' disease cardiomyopathy. Microbes Infect 2000 ; 2 (7) : 745-751.

[220] Llop E, Rothhammer F, Acuña M, Apt W. HLA antigens in cardiomyopathic Chilean chagasics. Am J Hum Genet 1988 ; 43 (5) : 770-773.

[221] Llop E, Rothhammer F, Acuña M, Apt W, Arribada A. HLA antigens in Chagas cardiomyopathy : new evidence-based on a case-control study. Rev Med Chil 1991 ; 119 (6) :633-636.

[222] Fernandez-Mestre MT, Layrisse Z, Montagnani S, Acquatella H, Catalioti F, Mastos M, *et al*. Influence of HLA class II polymorphism in chronic Chagas' disease. Parasite Immunol 1998 ; 20 (4) : 197-203.

[223] Colorado IA, Acquatella H, Catalioti F, Fernandez MT, Layrisse Z. HLA class IIDRB1, DQB11, DPB1 polymorphism and cardiomyopathy due to Trypanosoma cruzi chronic infection. Hum Immunol 2000 ; 61 (3) : 320-325.

[224] Layrisse Z, Fernandez MT, Montagnani S, Mastos M, Balbas O, Herrera F, *et al*. HLA-C*03 is a risk factor for cardiomyopathy in Chagas' disease. Hum Immunol 2000 ; 61 (9) : 925-929.

[225] Sierp GM, Albert ED, analysis of the HLA data. In : Gorodezky C, Sierp GM, Alberts E. (eds.) Immunogenetics Laboratory 1992 : Proceedings of the 5th Latin American Histocompatibility Workshop.

[226] del Puerto F, Nisshizawa JE, Kikuchi M, Roca Y, Avilas C, Gianella A, *et al*. Protective human leukocyte antigen haplotype, HLA-DRB1*01-B*14, against chronic Chagas' disease in Bolivia. PLoS Negl Trop Dis 2012 ; 6 (3) : Article e1587.

[227] Borra's SG, Diez C, Cotorruelo C, *et al*. HLA class II DRB1 polymorphism in Argentinians undergoing chronic trypanosome cruzi infection. Ann Clin Biochem 2006 ; 43 (Pt 3) : 214-216.

[228] Borrs SG, Racca L, Cotorruelo C, Biondi C, Beloscar J, Racca A. Distribution of HLA-DRB1 alleles in Artgentinean patients with Chagas' disease cardiomyopathy. Immunol Invest 2009 ; 38 (3-4) : 268-275.

[229] Pe'pin J, Khonde N, Maiso F, Doua F, Jaffar S, Ngampo S, *et al*. Short-course eflornithine in Gambian trypanosomiasis : a multicentre randomized controlled trial. Bull World Health Organ 2000 ; 78 (11) : 1284-1295.

[230] Fairlamb AH. Future prospects for chemotherapy of human trypanosomiasis 1. Novel approaches to the chemotherapy of trypanosomiasis. Trans R Soc Trop Med Hyg 1990 ; 84 (5) : 613-617.

[231] Jennings FW. Future prospects for the chemotherapy of human trypanosomiasis : combination therapy and African trypanosomiasis. Trans R Soc Trop Med Hyg 1990 ; 84 (5) : 618-621.

[232] Paiva CN, Feijo' DF, Dutra FF, Carneiro VC, Freitas GB, Alves LS, *et al*. Oxidative stress fuels Trypanosoma cruzi infection in mice. J Clin Invest 2012 ; 122 (7) : 2531-2542.

[233] Science Alerts Social Network. Factors affecting disease manifestation in humans : genetics and environment. http://sciencealerts.com/stories/2234502/Factors_affecting_disease_manifestation_of_to... (accessed 3 January 2014).

[234] Feldman GJ, Parker HW. Visceral larval migrans associated with the hypereosinophilic syndrome and the onset of severe asthma. Ann Intern Med 1992 ; 116 (10) : 838-840.

[235] Roig J, Romeu J, Riera C, Texido A, Domingo C, Morera J. Acute eosinophilic pneumonia due to toxocariasis with bronchoalveolar lavage findings. Chest 1992 ; 102 (1) : 294-296.

[236] Bartelink AK, Kortbeek LM, Huidekoper HJ, Meulenubelt J, van Knapen F. Acute respiratory failure due to toxocara infections. Lancet 1993 ; 342 (8881) : 1234.

[237] Magnaval JF, Glickman LT, Dorchies P, Morassin B. Highlights of human toxocariasis. Korean J Parasitol 2001 ; 39 (1) : 1-11.

[238] Glickman LT, Magnaval JF, Domanski LM, Shofer FS, Lauria SS, Gottstein B, *et al.* Visceral larval migrans in French adults : a new disease syndrome ? Am J Epidemiol 1987 ; 125 (6) : 1019-1034.

[239] Nathwani D, Laing RB, Currie PF. Covert toxocariasis-a cause of recurrent abdominal pain in childhood. Br J Clin Pract 1992 ; 46 (4) : 271.

[240] Magnaval JF, Fabre R, Maurieres P, Charlet JP, de Larrard B. Evaluation of an immunenzymatic assay detecting specific anti-Toxocara immunoglobulin E for diagnosis and post-treatment follow-up of human toxocariasis. J Clin Microbiol 1992 ; 30 (9) : 2269-2274.

[241] Magnaval JF, Fabre R, Maurieres P, Charlet JP, de Larrard B. Application of the Western-blotting procedure for the immunodiagnosis of human toxocariasis. Parasitol Res 1991 ; 77 (8) : 697-702.

[242] Rasmussen LN, Dirdal M, Birkeback NH. Covert toxocariasis in a child treated with low-dose diethylcarbamazine. Acta Paediatr 1993 ; 82 (1) : 116-118.

[243] Magnaval JF. Comparative efficacy of diethylcarbamazine and mebendazole for the treatment of human toxocariasis. Parasitology 1995 ; 110 (Pt 5) : 529-533.

[244] Sturchler D, Schubarth P, Gualzata M, Gottstein B, Orettli A. Thiabendazole vs albendazole in treatment of toxocariasis : a clinical trial. Ann Trop Med Parasitol 1989 ; 83 (5) : 473-478.

[245] Dodds EM. Toxoplasmosis. Curr Opin Ophthalmol 2006 ; 17 (6) : 557-561.

[246] Monso' E, Vidal R, de Gracia X, Moragas A. Pulmonary toxoplasmoma presenting as obstructive pneumonia. Thorax 1986 ; 41 (6) : 489-490.

[247] Nash G, Kerschmann RL, Herndier B, Dubey JP. The pathological manifestations of pulmonary toxoplasmosis in the acquired immunodeficiency syndrome. Hum Pathol 1994 ; 25 (7) : 652-658.

[248] Elsevier, Inc. Toxoplasmosis causes, diagnosis and treatment-clinical key. https://www.clinicalkey.com/topics/infectious-disease/toxoplasmosis.html (accessed 7 January 2014).

[249] Mack DG, Johnson JJ, Roberts F, Roberts CW, Estes RG, David C, *et al.* HLA-class II genes modify outcome of Toxoplasma gondii infection. Int J Parasitol 1999 ; 29 (9) : 1351-1358.

[250] Laibe S, Ranque S, Curtillet C, Faraut F, Dumon H, Franck J. Timely diagnosis of disseminated toxoplasmosis by sputum examination. J Clin Microbiol 2006 ; 44 (2) : 646-648.

[251] Petersen E, Edvinsson B, Lundgren B, Benfield T, Evengard B. Diagnosis of pulmonary infection with Toxoplasma gondii in immunocompromised HIV-positive patients by real-time PCR. Eur J Clin Microbiol Infect Dis 2006 ; 25 (6) : 401-404.

[252] Martina BEE, Koraka P, Osterhaus ADM. Dengue virus pathogenesis : an integrated view. Clin Microbiol Rev 2009 ; 22 (4) : 564-581.

[253] Guha-Sapir D, Schimmer B. Dengue fever : new paradigms for a changing epidemiology. Emerg Themes Epidemiol 2005 ; 2 (1) : 1.

[254] Guzman MG, Kouri G. Dengue and dengue hemorrhagic fever in the Americas : lessons and challenges. J Clin Virol 2003 ; 27 (1) : 1-13.

[255] Halstead SB. Dengue. Lancet 2007 ; 370 (9599) : 1644-1652.

[256] Ong A, Sandar M, Chen MI, Sin LY. Fatal dengue hemorrhagic fever in adults during a dengue epidemic in Singapore. In J Infect Dis 2007 ; 11 (3) : 263-267.

[257] Guzma'n MG, Kouri G, Valdes L, Bravo L, Alvalez M, Vazques S, *et al.* Epidemiologic studies on dengue in Santiago de Cuba, 1997. Am J Epidemiol 2000 ; 152 (9) : 793-799.

[258] UNICEF, UNDP, World Bank, WHO. Evaluating diagnostics-Dengue : a continuing global threat. http://www.nature.com/reviews/micro (accessed 8 January 2014).

[259] Kouri GP, Guzma'n MG, Bravo JR. Why dengue hemorrhagic fever in Cuba? 2. An integral analysis. Trans R Soc Trop Med Hyg 1987 ; 81 (5) : 821-823.

[260] Halstead SB, Nimanitaya S, Cohen SN. Observations related to pathogenesis of dengue hemorrhagic fever : Relation of disease severity to antibody response and virus recovered. Yale J Biol Med 1970 ; 42 (5) : 311-328.

[261] Lee MS, Hwang KP, Chen TC, Lu PL, Chen TP. Clinical characteristics of dengue and dengue hemorrhagic fever in a medical center of southern Taiwan during the 2002 epidemic. J Microbiol Immunol Infect 2006 ; 39 (2) : 121-129.

[262] Stephens HA, Klaythong R, Sirikong M, Vaughn DW, Green S, Kalayanarooj S, *et al.* HLA-A and HLA-B allele associations with secondary dengue virus infections corre-

late with disease severity and the infecting viral serotype in ethnic Thais. Tissue Antigens 2002 ; 60 (4) : 309-318.

[263] LaFleur C, Granados J, Vargas-Alarcon G, Ruiz-Morales J, Villarreal-Garza C, Hiqueral L, *et al*. HLA-DR antigen frequencies in Mexican patients with dengue virus infection : HLA-DR4 as a possible genetic resistance factor for dengue hemorrhagic fever. Hum Immunol 2002 ; 63 (11) : 1039-1044.

[264] Loke H, Bethell DB, Phuong CX, Dung M, Schneider J, White NJ, *et al*. Strong HLA class I- restricted T-cell responses in dengue hemorrhagic fever : a double-edged sword ? J Infect Dis 2002 ; 184 (11) : 1369-1373.

[265] Sakuntabhai A, Turbpaiboon C, Casade'mont I, Chuansumrit A, Lowhoo T, Kajaste-Rudnitski A, *et al*. A variant in CD209 promoter is associated with severity of dengue disease. Nature Genet 2005 ; 37 (5) : 507-513.

[266] Fernandez-Mastre MT, Gendzekhadze K, Rivas-Vetencourt P, Layrisse Z. TNF-α-308A allele, a possible severity risk factor of hemorrhagic manifestation in dengue fever patients. Tissue Antigens 2004 ; 64 (4) : 469-472.

[267] Kalayanarooj S, Gibbons RV, Vaughn D, Green S, Nisalak A, Jarman RG, *et al*. Blood group AB is associated with increased risk for severe dengue disease in secondary infections. J Infect Dis 2007 ; 195 (7) : 1014-1017.

[268] Rico-Hesse R. Molecular evolution and distribution of dengue viruses type 1 and 2 in nature. Virology 1990 ; 174 (2) : 479-493.

[269] Rico-Hesse R, Harrison LM, Salas RA, Tovar D, Nisalak A, Ramos C, *et al*. Origins of dengue type 2 viruses associated with increased pathogenicity in the Americas. Virology 1997; 230 (2) : 244-251.

[270] Rodriguez-Roche RM, Alvarez M, Gritsun T, Halstead S, Kouri G, Gould EA, *et al*. Virus evolution during a severe dengue epidemic in Cuba, 1997. Virology 2005 ; 334 (2) : 154-159.

[271] Guzma'n MG, Kouri G, Bravo J, Valdes L, Vazquez S, Halstead SB. Effect of age on outcome of secondary dengue 2 infections. Int J Infect Dis 2002 ; 6 (2) : 118-124.

[272] Cologna R, Rico-Hesse R. American genotype structures decrease dengue virus output from human monocytes and dendritic cells. J Virol 2003 ; 77 (7) : 3929-3938.

[273] Leitmeyer KC, Vaughn DW, Watts DM, Salas R, Villalobos I, de Chacon, *et al*. Dengue virus structural differences that correlate with pathogenesis. J Virol 1999 ; 73 (6) : 4738-4747.

[274] Jessie K, Fong MY, Devi S, Lam SK, Wong KT. Localization of dengue virus in naturally infected human tissues, immunohistochemistry and in situ hybridization. J Infect Dis 2004 ; 189 (8) : 1411-1418.

[275] Paes MV, Pinhao AT, Barreto DF, Costa SM, Oliveira MP, Nogueira AC, *et al.* Liver injury and viremia in mice infected with dengue-2 virus. Virology 2005 ; 338 (2) : 236-246.

[276] Seneviratne SL, Malavige GN, de Silva HJ. Pathogenesis of liver involvement during dengue viral infections. Trans R Soc Trop Med Hyg 2006 ; 100 (7) : 608-614.

[277] Nkhoma ET, Poole C, Vannappagari V, Hall SA, Beutler E. The global prevalence of glucose- 6-phosphate dehydrogenase deficiency : a systematic review and meta-analysis. Blood Cells Mol Dis 2009 ; 42 (3) : 267-278.

[278] Wu YH, Tseng CP, Cheng ML, Ho HY, Shih SR, Chiu DT. Glucose-6-phosphate dehydrogenase deficiency enhances human coronavirus 229E infection. J Infect Dis 2008 ; 197 (6) : 812-816.

[279] Zivna I, Green S, Vaughn DW, Kalayanarooj S, Stephens HA, Chandanayingyong D, *et al.* T-cell responses to an HLA-B*07-restricted epitope on the dengue NS3 protein correlate with disease severity. J Immunol 2002 ; 168 (11) : 5959-5965.

[280] Polizel JR, Bueno D, Visentainer JE, Sell AM, Borelli SD, Tsuneto LT, *et al.* Association of human leukocyte antigen DQ1 and dengue fever in a white Southern Brazilian population. Mem Inst Oswaldo Cruz 2004 ; 99 (6) : 559-562.

[281] Alagarasu K, Mulay AP, Sarikhani M, Rashmika D, Shah PS, Celilia D. Profile of human leukocyte antigen class I alleles in patients with dengue infection from Western India. Hum Immunol 2013 ; 74 (12) : 1624-1628.

[282] Malavige GN, Fernando S, Fernando DJ, Seneviratne SL. Dengue viral infection. Postgrad Med J 2004 ; 80 (948) : 588-601.

[283] Likitnukul S, Prappal N, Pongpunlert W, Kingwatanakul P, Poovorawan Y. Dual infections : degue hemorrhagic fever with unusual manifestations and mycoplasma pneumonia in a child. Southeast Asian J Trop Med Public Health 2004 ; 35 (2) : 399-402.

[284] Ali F, Saleem T, Khalid U, Mehwood SF, Jamil B. Crimen-Congo hemorrhagic fever in a dengue-endemic region : lessons for the future. J Infect Dev Ctries 2010 ; 4 (7) : 459-463.

[285] Duchin JS, Koster FT, Peters CJ, Simpson GL, Tempest B, Zaki SR, *et al.* The Hantavirus Study Group. Hantavirus pulmonary syndrome : a clinical description of 17 patients with a newly recognized disease. N Engl J Med 1994 ; 330 (14) : 949-955.

[286] Castillo C, Naranjo J, Sepu'lveda A, Ossa G, Levy H. Hantavirus pulmonary syndrome due to Andes virus in Temuco, Chile : clinical experience with 16 adults. Chest 2001 ; 120 (2) : 548-554.

[287] Vapalahti O, Mustonen J, Lundkvist A, Henttonen H, Plyusnin A, Vaheri A. Hantavirus infections in Europe. Lancet Infect Dis 2003 ; 3 (10) : 653-661.

[288] Rasmuson J, Pourazar J, Linderholm M, Sandstroøm T, Blomberg A, Ahlm C. Presence of activated airway T lymphocytes in human Puumala hantavirus disease. Chest 2011 ; 140 (3) :715-722.

[289] Guirakhoo F, Kitchener S, Morrison D, Forrat R, McCarthy K, Nicholas R, *et al.* Live attenuated chimeric yellow fever dengue type 2 (ChimeriVax-DEN2) vaccine : Phase I clinical trial for safety and immunogenicity : effect of yellow fever pre-immunity in induction of cross neutralizing antibody responses to all 4 dengue serotypes. Hum Vaccine 2006 ; 2 (2) : 60-67.

[290] Durbin AP, Whitehead SS, McArthur J, Perreault JR, Blaney JE Jr, Thumar B, *et al.* rDEN4 Delta 30, a live attenuated dengue virus type 4 vaccine candidate, is safe, immunogenic, and highly infectious in healthy adult volunteers. J Infect Dis 2005 ; 191 (5) : 710-718.

[291] Raviprakash K, Apt D, Brinkman A, Skinner C, Yang S, Dawes G, *et al.* A chimeric tetravalent dengue DNA vaccine elicits neutralizing antibody to all four virus serotypes in rhesus macaques. Virology 2006 ; 353 (1) : 166-173.

[292] Hermida L, Bernardo L, Martin J, Alvarez M, Prado I, Lo′ C, *et al.* A recombinant fusion protein containing the domain III of the dengue-2 envelope protein is immunogenic and protective in nonhuman primates. Vaccine 2006 ; 24 (16) : 3165-3171.

[293] Whitehead SS, Falqout B, Hanley KA, Blaney Jr JE Jr, Markoff L, Murphy BR. A live, attenuated dengue virus type 1 vaccine candidate with a 30-nucleotide deletion in the 3′ untranslated region is highly attenuated and immunogenic in monkeys. J Virol 2003 ; 77 (2) : 1653-1657.

[294] Edelman R, Wasserman SS, Bodison SA, Putnak RJ, Eckels KH, Tang D, *et al.* Phase I trial of 16 formulations of a tetravalent live-attenuated dengue vaccine. Am J Trop Med Hyg 2003 ; 69 (6 Suppl) : 48-60.

[295] Ko AI, Goarant C, Picardeau M. Leptospira : The Dawn of the molecular genetics era for an emerging zoonotic pathogen. Nat Rev Microbiol 2009 ; 7 (10) : 736-747.

[296] Lingappa J, Kuffner T, Tappero J, Whitworth W, Mize A, Kaiser R, *et al.* HLA-DQ*6 and ingestion of contaminated water : possible gene-environment interaction in an outbreak of leptospirosis. Genes and Immun 2004 ; 5 (3) : 197-202.

[297] WHO recommended standards and strategies for surveillance, prevention and control of communicable diseases, 2nd ed. http://www.who.int/emc (accessed 29 January 2014).

[298] Tubiana S, Mikulski M, Becam J, Lacassin F, Lefe`vre P, Gourinat AC. Risk factors and predictors of severe leptospirosis in New Caledonia. PLoS Negl Trop Dis 2013 ; 7 (1) : e1991. DOI : 10.1371/journal.pntd.0001991

[299] Suputtamongkol Y, Pongtavornpinyo W, Lubell Y, Suttinont C, Hoontrakul S, Phimda K, *et al.* Strategies for diagnosis and treatment of suspected leptospirosis : a cost-

benefit analysis. PLoS Negl Trop Dis 2010 ; 4 (2) : e610. DOI : 10.1371/journal.pntd.0000610

[300] Nitipan S, Sritrakul T, Kunjantarachot A, Prapong S. Identification of epitopes in Leptospirosis borgpetersenii leucine-rich repeat proteins. Infect Genet Evol 2013 ; 14 (NA) : 46-57. DOI : 10.1016/j.meegid.2012.10.014.

[301] Umamaheswari A, Pradhan D, Hemanthkumar M. Computered aided subunit vaccine design against pathogenic Leptospira serovars. Interdiscip Sci 2012 ; 4 (1) : 38-45.